F. Vogel

Genetics and the Electroencephalogram

Springer
Berlin
Heidelberg
New York
Barcelona
Hong Kong
London
Milan
Paris
Singapore
Tokyo

F. Vogel

GENETICS and the ELECTRO-ENCEPHALOGRAM

With 76 Figures and 37 Tables

Springer

Professor Dr. Dr. h.c. Friedrich Vogel (em.)
Im Bubenwingert 19
69181 Leimen
Germany

Library of Congress Cataloging-in-Publication Data
Vogel, Friedrich, 1925–
Genetics and the electroencephalogram / F. Vogel.
p. cm.
Includes bibliographical references and index.
ISBN 3-540-65573-5 (softcover : alk. paper)
1. Neurogenetics. 2. Electroencephalography. I. Title
QP356-22-V64 2000
612.8'13--dc21

ISBN 3-540-65573-5 Springer-Verlag Berlin Heidelberg New York

Production: PRO EDIT GmbH, 69126 Heidelberg, Germany
Cover Design: design & production GmbH, 69126 Heidelberg, Germany
Typesetting: STORCH GmbH, 97353 Wiesentheid, Germany
CTF: Saladruck, Berlin, Germany

SPIN: 10684678 27/3136-5 4 3 2 1 0 – Gedruckt auf säurefreiem Papier

This book is dedicated to
Edda Schalt, a companion
of 40 years of research

Preface

This book describes problems and results of research in the gap between two fields: Human genetics, and clinical neurophysiology. Whenever I talked about my research on the genetics of the EEG, the answer of human geneticists was: "Very interesting, but I do not understand anything about the EEG." On the other hand, EEG specialists usually remark: "Very interesting, but I do not understand anything about human genetics." This is why I wrote this book. It tries to summarize results from research - my own and from some others - and to point to problems. In the light of the recent progress especially in human molecular genetics, this field of research promises deep insights into biological mechanisms of brain function, as well as genetic variation involved in mental performance, and personality of humans. However, the logistic problems of such studies are not easy to overcome: It is necessary to study carefully ascertained population samples either of "normal" persons, or of persons selected for phenotypic characteristics that are not easy to diagnose. Moreover, EEG diagnosis and classification must be very specific, and is not trivial at all. All these problems require careful preparations at various levels, long-lasting efforts, and patience. Of this I am sure, however: The results would justify the efforts. I am too old to plan such a program myself; moreover, as an emeritus professor, I do not have the means for such studies. Therefore I can only hope that those of the younger generation will read this book and continue their interest in genetic EEG studies.

I thank many institutions and persons without whose cooperation this work would not have been possible: The late Prof. H. Nachtsheim, my teacher in genetics who gave me freedom for research; Dr. A. Anokhin; Akad. Oberrat J. Krüger; Prof. P. Propping; Doz. Dr. O. Steinlein; and many others, mainly graduate students. The Deutsche Forschungsgemeinschaft financed these studies over almost four decades; and the University of Heidelberg provided for me an independendent position, and the chance to follow my own ways of research. The Flugmedizinisches Institut of the German Air Force permitted studies on Air Force personnel. I also thank all the probands and their fanilies. Above all, I thank Edda Schalt for participating in this research for 40 years as an active partner who did much more than can be expected from a first-class laboratory technician; we discussed all problems and she contributed many ideas of her own. Adelheid Fengler gave indispensible help in preparing this manuscript; and Springer-Verlag, especially Dr. Rolf Lange, did everything possible to produce this book.

FRIEDRICH VOGEL
Heidelberg, Germany, Summer 1999

Contents

CHAPTER 1

1 The Problem

1.1 The Purpose of This Book

This is an old-fashioned book. It deals with phenotypes – phenotypes, however, that are not easy to describe since fairly elaborated techniques are required for their identification and, still more, for their adequate description. The mere fact that the living human brain produces continuous electrical activity has been known for about a century, and the first details, the most important patterns of this activity were described almost exactly 70 years ago not by a physiologist but by a practicing psychiatrist, Hans Berger. Since that time the electroencephalogram (EEG) has been investigated from various points of view. The fact that it proved to be a major tool for diagnosis of many diseases – especially those mainly affecting the brain but also other ones in which the brain was involved – was the main reason for their continuous scientific interest. More recently, this interest has narrowed down somewhat. While the EEG has for a long time been the only method giving a clearcut picture of the present functional state of the brain without intrusion into the integrity of the human body, and without undue molestation of the individual to be examined, other such methods have now been developed. Sometimes they provide even more detailed information. However, the EEG is still an indispensable diagnostic tool; especially for differential diagnosis of diseases in which seizures occur – the epilepsies.

The function of the healthy human brain is guaranteed by an ordered cooperation of neurons and groups of neurons within and between various parts of the central nervous system. The neurons receive information from other neurons by their dendrites which contain thousands of synapses, and pass on information to other neurons by their axon. For passing on informative impulses from one neuron to the next, specific chemical compounds are necessary – the neurotransmitters. They need to be synthesized, excreted by the donor cell following some signals, and taken up by the receiver cell. This cell needs specific receptors on which the neurotransmitters can attach. Within the neuron, the impulse is propagated electrically by changes in the polarity of the cell membrane which is caused by ions. For example, K^+ ions may migrate out of the membrane for a short time while N^+ ions migrate the other way. For these ion migrations, structures of the membrane are necessary that are called ion channels. Hence an ordered function of the entire system requires normal functioning of a number of elements, the most important ones of which are: the single neurons and their normal interconnections. They develop during embryonic and fetal age but their ordered network is completed during childhood and youth – and probably even during adult age – under the influence of function. Even at that anatomical level disturbances are fairly common. These may be caused by external factors such as malnutrition, infectious disease or intoxication (for example, by alcohol.). However, they may also have internal genetic reasons. For example, a number of micromorphological changes have been described in patients suffering from a variety of chromosomal aberrations (see Chap. 8). It even seems as if many types of mental retardation may have in common one micromorphological anomaly; spines on dendrites (i.e., synapses) appear to be thinner, sometimes unusually long, sometimes dilated; however, especially, they are reduced in numbers. In other disturbances of brain function other anomalies of the elements mentioned above might be expected: There may be deviations in chemical composition and synthesis of neurotransmitters; their synthesis, excretion and uptake may be altered, and there may be changes in their action within the cell. Elements within this chain of events that have found much attention in recent years are the neurotransmitter receptors. Other elements that are being considered frequently are the ion channels at the neuronal membrane which are necessary for propagation of impulses; their genetic anomalies may have a strong effect on neuronal function.

1.2 Disturbances Leading to Disease

Disturbances of this system may cause a variety of diseases. For example, disturbances of neurotransmitters, their receptors and their distribution within the CNS could lead to diseases of the motoric system such as parkinsonism or Huntington disease; to mood disorders such as depression, mania, or the mood swings of bipolar disease; and to disturbances of thinking such as those found in schizophrenia. EEG anomalies may be found in such diseases but, as a rule, they are not very characteristic and therefore of moderate diagnostic value only (Chap. 8). As noted, EEG is disturbed in a very specific way, and is therefore of a high diagnostic value, in the epilepsies. Epilepsy is not a disease; it is a symptom or, better, a group of closely related symptoms that may be found in many different diseases. Their common denominator is that neurons or groups of neurons do not discharge, i.e., give impulses to other neurons in an ordered and functionally useful way but many neurons "fire" together leading to a high degree of excitation. The clinical signs of such an "explosion" of neuronal firing may differ, depending on the part of the brain that is mainly involved. For example, if the pathological discharge is widespread, involving, among others, the motoric centers, the grand mal seizure ensues, with involuntary movements and cramps, and loss of conscience. If mainly central brain structures are affected, the petit mal seizure occurs, and a local disturbance may lead to a focal fit- often indicating an anatomical lesion at a specific site of the CNS. Diagnosis of the special type of epilepsy is the task of the epileptologist; the diagnosis must be as specific as ever possible, since the choice of therapy may depend on it. Often, a certain drug or combination of drugs must be selected but in a few instances surgical intervention is the best way of help. It cannot be the task of this book to introduce the reader to the diagnosis of epilepsy nor to speak of treatments. Not even the various EEG patterns seen in different types of epilepsy can be described here; the reader should use the special references that are found, for example, in the classical EEG textbook of Niedermeyer and Lopes da Silva (third edition 1993). Suffice it to say that epileptic fits are one of the clinical signs of many hereditary diseases caused by a disturbing variety of primary genetic and biochemical mechanisms (see Szepetowski and Monaco 1998; Blandfort et al. 1987). In quite a number of genetic diseases, epileptic seizures are even the leading clinical signs; here EEG patterns may be quite characteristic. They often provide guidelines for a correct diagnosis and adequate treatment.

However, even these diseases are not described in this book in any detail. Some of them are mentioned when EEG signs of genetic susceptibility for such diseases are discussed. Recently, however, molecular mechanisms have been elucidated for a few epileptic conditions. These mechanisms are so interesting that they must be discussed in somewhat greater detail; these may indicate in which direction the molecular basis for genetic variation in the "normal" EEG could be found – the main topic of this book.

1.3 Molecular Mechanisms of Some Hereditary Types of Epilepsy

The epilepsies may be classified preliminarily as shown in Table 1.1 (Blandfort et al. 1987). In most instances, they are caused either by genetic factors or by exogenous

Table 1.1. Classification of the epilepsies (Blandfort et al. 1987)

I. Epilepsies with seizures of focal origin
A. Elementary type (Jackson epilepsy) B. Epilepsies with complex partial seizures (psychomotor epilepsy) C. Epilepsies with benign partial seizures a) Epilepsy with centrotemporal sharp waves b) Epilepsy with occipital sharp waves D. Epilepsies with generalized seizures of focal or multifocal origin a) West syndrome b) Lennox-Gastaut syndrome
II. Epilepsies with primary generalized seizures
A. Absences a) Early infantile type b) Childhood absence epilepsy c) Juvenile absence epilepsy B. Centrencephalic myoclonic-astatic petit mal C. Juvenile myoclonic epilepsy *(impulsiv petit mal)* D. Primary generalized grand mal a) Infantile b) Juvenile E. Photogenic epilepsy
III. Epilepsies with unclassified seizures
A. Neonatal convulsions B. Familial neonatal convulsions

effects, or by a combination of the two. The genetic components are heterogeneous; twin studies have shown that MZ twins are more often concordant than DZ twins but there are also discordant MZ twins (Conrad 1936, 1938; Lennox 1951; Inoue 1960). The great majority of all families show a certain accumulation of epileptics but, as a rule, no indication for a monogenic mode of inheritance. In the best preliminary descriptions, multifactorial inheritance - a combination of the actions of an unknown number of different genes in combination with environmental factors - is presumed. Fairly complex threshold models have been constructed to describe adequately the family data (Tsuboi and Christian 1976; Cloninger et al. in Anderson et al. 1982). However, there are quite a few special types of epilepsies for which simple modes of inheritance were described. These types are rare. In 1964 a new syndrome was defined with benign familial neonatal convulsions and a clearcut autosomal dominant mode of inheritance (Rett and Teupel 1964). Seizures in these cases could not be distinguished from neonatal seizures of other origin. They occurred between the second and the 15th day of life, were repeated frequently but stopped spontaneously after a short time. The outcome is usually favorable, but quite a few patients develop epilepsy later in life. As a first step in identification of the responsible gene and its function, this trait was localized by a linkage study to chromosome 20q13.2 (Leppert et al. 1989). Meanwhile, this localization has been confirmed in other pedigrees (Malafosse et al. 1992). A gene for the a4 subunit of the Nicotinic acetylcholine receptor (CHRNA4) was localized to human chromosome 20 by Pilz et al. (1992). This localization was refined by Steinlein et al. (1994) to chromosome 20q13.2–13.3; i.e., to the same area where a gene for benign neonatal convulsions has been localized. Nicotinic acetylcholine receptors are found in many parts of the central and peripheric nervous system (for details see Steinlein et al. 1994). The subunits are coded by various genes of a gene family and they differ in their expression patterns. In the same area of chromosome 20 a dominantly inherited gene for the human low-voltage EEG was localized (Steinlein et al. 1992; see Sect. 4.3). This linkage study shows genetic heterogeneity; only about 30% of the genes for this EEG type were localized in this area. However, genetic heterogeneity was also found for benign familial neonatal convulsions (EBN); another gene for the same anomaly is located at chromosome 8q24 (Lewis et al. 1992).

The next major step of genetic analysis is identification of individual mutations leading to genetic anomalies and variants. Genes for neurotransmitter receptor units are excellent candidate genes for anomalies of neuronal function. And, indeed, in one family a potassium channel gene (KCNQ2) was located on 20q13.3, and the disease was found to be caused by an insertion of five base pairs that led to deletion of more than 300 amino acids from the carboxyl terminus of this gene (Bienert et al. 1998). In expression experiments in the frog *(Xenopus laevis)*, potassium-selective currents were shown that activated slowly with depolarization, while expression of the channel protein containing the mutant failed to show measurable currents. This example shows how identification of genes, and, especially mutants may help in elucidating basic functional failures leading to certain diseases such as epilepsy. Another potassium channel gene (KCNQ3) was localized to chromosome 8q24, in the same area in which another gene locus (EBN2) for dominantly inherited neonatal convulsions had been localized before. Here, a missense mutation was found in the critical pore region (Charlier et al. 1998).

Another autosomal dominant epileptic disease is nocturnal frontal lobe epilepsy (ADNFLE). This has been defined only recently as a distinct entity (Scheffer et al. 1994, 1995). The patients suffer from partial motor seizures, almost exclusively during drowsiness or sleep. A linkage study again led to localization at 20q13.2–20q13.3 (Phillips et al. 1995). A missense mutation in the gene encoding the neuronal nicotinic acetylcholine receptor a4 subunit (CHNRA4) was found in the affected members of this family. Serine was replaced by phenylalanine in the second transmembrane domain of the protein which is thought to be involved in the ion-conductive pore of an ion channel (Steinlein et al. 1995).

There are some more gene loci for which some evidence exists for localization of genes within specific areas of the human genome. Examples can be found in the review of Szepetowski and Monaco (1998). Positive results for linkage exists, for example, for juvenile myoclonic epilepsy (EJMI; 6p, 15q14), partial epilepsy with auditory symptoms (10q), benign infantile familial convulsions BIFC (19q12), infantile convulsions and choreoathetosis ICCA (16p12–q12), Unverricht-Lundborg disease EPM1 (21q22.3), progressive epilepsy with mental retardation EPMR (8p), Lafora disease (6q23–q25) and others.

1.4 Possible Significance of These Studies for Genetic Analysis of the Human EEG

It is not the purpose of this monograph to review genetics and analysis at the molecular level of epilepsies. Epileptic seizures are results of a break-down of the coordinated function of neurons or groups of neurons. Certain anomalies trigger common discharges of large groups of neurons; these discharges normally begin in a certain place or functional unit; then, they spread over large parts of the brain. However, for analyzing the molecular basis of the normal, and coordinated "firing" of neurons, such abnormalities may provide certain hints. They might help in analysis of normal function. For example, the acetylcholine neurotransmitter system has been suspected for some time of being involved in the production of the normal EEG (Steriade et al. 1990). The studies on molecular defects in certain forms of epilepsy may help in identifying at least plausible candidate genes for genetic analysis of variation in the normal EEG.

An important step is finding of more genetic variation with monogenic inheritance. It is not by chance that the first examples for a thorough molecular analysis of certain types of epilepsy were found in two rare epilepsy types with simple autosomal dominant inheritance. Monogenic modes of inheritance suggest single genes; with the great number of DNA markers available to date (see Vogel and Motulsky 1996), localization of such genes by linkage studies has become more or less a matter of routine; and once the location of the gene has become known, its identification and analysis may need patience, technical skill, and sometimes ingenuity. Once the gene has been identified and the mutation leading to mendelian segregation within pedigrees has been spotted, the altered function may be analyzed "bottom-up," i.e., from the altered DNA molecule up to the protein, and to its function. However, such a "bottom-up" analysis is becoming much more difficult, and often is a matter of good luck, if there is no clearcut evidence of a monogenic mode of inheritance. Therefore identification of such a mode of inheritance, if ever possible, should be an important step in the analysis. However, it cannot always be the first step. This first step should be to answer the question whether (and to what extent) variation in a certain phenotype in the population is genetically determined.

In the genetic analysis of the (normal) EEG these questions should be answered first. This, as any further genetic analysis, requires painstaking description and identification of phenotypes. For identification of the relevant gene or genes, the candidate gene approach is very useful. Genes should primarily be studied for which there is a certain prima facie plausibility for an involvement in EEG activity. As suggested by the results on certain rare types of epilepsies, genes coding for neurotransmitter receptors and ion channel proteins may be suitable candidates. Szepetowski and Monaco (1998) have enumerated 9 localized genes for calcium channels, 23 genes for potassium channels, 13 genes for sodium channels, 10 serotonin receptor genes, 14 GABA receptor genes, 16 genes for glutamate receptors, 9 genes for the nicotinic acetylchloine receptor, and 7 protein kinase genes. This provides an almost disturbing number and variety of candidate genes for genetic search.

CHAPTER 2

2 The Human EEG: General Aspects

2.1 History

The living brain shows a rhythmic electric activity which can be recorded from the surface of the head. This activity was first observed by Caton (1875; 1877) in Liverpool, in monkeys and rabbits. The first picture of such an activity in a human being was published by Neminsky (1913) which, however, had no major effect on thinking and conceptualization in brain research (for a more detailed report on the early history of EEG research, see Niedermeyer 1993). The real father of EEG research was Hans Berger, professor of psychiatry in Jena. Using various galvanometers, he recorded rhythmic activity from the heads of some individuals. In his first report, published in 1929, he described the alpha waves and the alpha blocking response, and in 13 further reports, up to 1937, and in a monograph (1938), he described many of the basic EEG phenomena (for detailed references, see Christian 1968). He also coined the termname *Elektrenkephalogram,* which from the linguistic point of view is more correct than the conventional term "electroencephalogram," since the three components of this term are all Greek in origin. This newly discovered EEG became popular among neural scientists, after the prominent British neurophysiologist Adrian, together with Matthews (1934), had confirmed and enlarged Berger's observations. Interestingly enough, they also found the first hint for interindividual variation in the normal EEG: While Adrian himself showed a classical alpha rhythm, no such rhythm was seen in the EEG of Matthews. He may have had a low-voltage EEG.

In the following years, most of the phenomena of the EEG in normal individuals and in various diseases were described; the EEG became one of the most prominent methods for examination of the brain. (For details of this development see Jung 1953a,b; Niedermeyer 1993).

The fact that the method is noninvasive and can therefore be applied without molesting the individuals being studied while allowing a picture of the functional state of the brain at the time of examination to be obtained is especially attractive for the clinician. In more recent years, other methods such as computer tomography (CT) and magnet resonance imagining (MRI) have come to share this advantage but the EEG has kept its place in the diagnostic armamentarium of the neurologist especially in the diagnosis of epilepsy but also in many other fields (see, for example, Niedermeyer and Lopes da Silva 1993).

Very early, some scientists realized that the EEG opened new chances for studies on genetic aspects of brain function in health and disease: The Davieses and Raney published twin studies as early as the late 1930s (Davies and Davies 1936; Raney 1939), and Lennox, together with F.A. and E.L. Gibbs, investigated normal and abnormal EEG phenomena in twins and families – mainly with the problem in mind of elucidating the genetic basis of epilepsies. Gottlober (1939) published the first family studies on the normal EEG.

2.2 EEG Recording

The EEG is recorded from electrodes placed on the scalp in a way that the impedance becomes as low as possible (see Reilly 1993). After many discussions among specialists, an international committee recommended the so-called 10–20 system for placement of electrodes (Jasper 1958), i.e., between 10 and 20 electrodes should be placed in standard positions (Fig. 2.1).

Up to 20 electrodes and sometimes even more are necessary for fine localization of foci of different origin, but for genetic studies, fewer electrodes are usually sufficient. Our own studies have generally been performed with ten electrodes and eight tracings (Fig. 2.2). EEG patterns must always be recorded as differences between two electrodes. Here, two main techniques are in use: Either, one scalp electrode and one reference electrode are being used, with the scalp electrode above the part of the brain to be studied, and the reference electrode at an electrically neutral point, for example, the ear (reference or, according to an old nomenclature, unipolar leads). The ear is not entirely neutral electrically but from a practical point of view, reference recordings give a good impression of the electrical activity in the part of the brain underneath the scalp electrode. Or the EEG is recorded between two scalp electrodes (bipolar leads). Such bipolar tracings have certain advantages for solving clinical problems, for example, localization of anomalies. For genetic studies, refe-

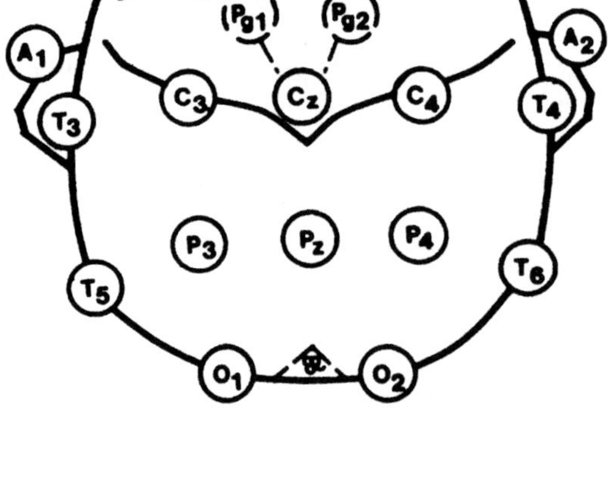

Fig. 2.1. 10–20 system of electrode placement (see also Niedermeyer and Lopes da Silva 1983, p. 73)

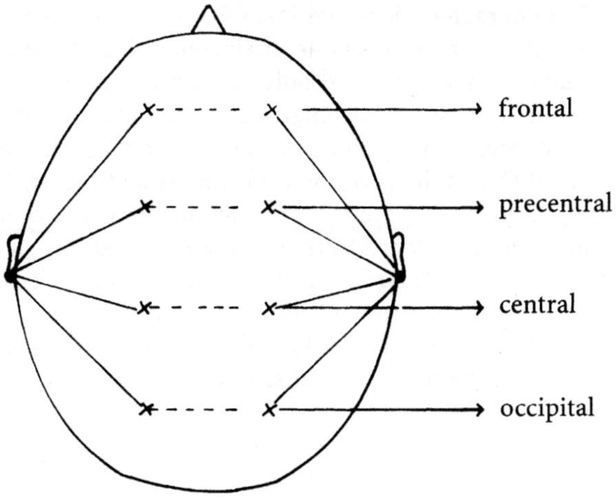

Fig. 2.2. Placement of 8 electrodes; reference leads, as used in our own EEG studies

rence leads are especially useful; these present the best over-all impression of the characteristic features of an individual EEG. In our own EEG studies we have used both reference and bipolar leads. In our analyses, however, especially comparisons between twins and characterization of EEG variants, we emphasize reference recordings. The amplitudes of EEG waves are very small (order of magnitude: μV); they must be amplified in the EEG machine. Then, they are written as curves on paper (as a rule, 3 cm/s.). Amplification used in our own studies was 50 μV = 7 mm (this is slightly more than usual in many EEG laboratories, but such an amplification is necessary for characterization of certain EEG variants); frequency screen at 70 Hz; time constant approx. 0.3. We used EEG machines from Schwarzer and Nihon Kohden.

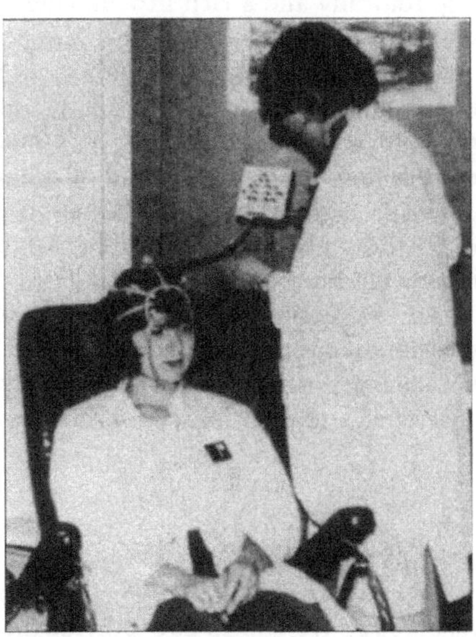

Fig. 2.3. Examination of the resting EEG. The proband sits on a comfortable chair with closed eyes. The figure shows electrode placement by the technician

The characteristic individual EEG pattern (= resting EEG) is seen when the proband sits on a comfortable chair, relaxed and with closed eyes (Fig. 2.3). Light should be dim and there should be no disturbing noise. The client should be relaxed but should not sleep. We obtained the best tracings in the morning. Electric artifacts may be caused by many disturbances, for example, poorly fixed electrodes, defects in the EEG machine, eye and body movements; the EKG and many others (see Reilly 1993). A good EEG record critically depends on experience and ability of the EEG technician. A standard EEG examination needs about 20–30 min, including various reference and bipolar leads, and provocation by a hyperventilation period of about 3 min. Ideally, the proband should have avoided larger doses of alcohol and psychotropic drugs the night before the examination, and should have slept well. An agitated, frightened proband after a sleepless night does not show a reliable EEG.

2.3 EEG Evaluation

Traditional EEG evaluation has been, and is performed by visual inspection of EEG curves, knowing certain criteria such as waveforms regarded as characteristic for certain disease processes such as epileptic seizures, certain brain tumors, and others. In a first step, tracings were classified into three categories; normal, pathological and borderline. Then, in a second step, the observer tries to answer more specific questions regarding the patient under observation. This classification was fairly successful from a clinical point of view, if the EEG specialist knew his criteria, and if he could rely on thorough experience with this method. Since many EEG phenomena are nonspecific, the EEG specialist must know the essentials of the clinical picture and, especially, the diagnostic problems to be solved. However, even a short time after the discovery of the EEG, the first attempts at a more quantitative evaluation of the EEG phenomena were made. Today, EEG records can be stored electronically and a rich instrumentarium of computerized evaluation methods is available (see Lesser et al. 1993). Modern EEG machines show the EEG on the computer display; often, paper is not necessary anymore. Some scientists may have hoped that, in the near future, EEG interpretation by the "experienced observer" might be replaced completely by computerized evaluation. So far, however, this has not become true; each method of computerized data procession of the EEG systematically neglects some information contained in the records. As Niedermeyer (1993) has put it succinctly, "EEG is by far too complex for such an automation, its interpretation requires that wonderful computer that is located between the ears."

For evaluation and interpretation of data reported in this monograph, many measurement methods have been used in addition to visual evaluation, from simple measurements with rulers to complex computer programs. The methods are described, and their limitations are shown in the respective chapters.

2.4 The "Normal" Human EEG

As noted above, clinicians subdivide the EEG patterns, as a first step, into three categories: normal, pathological and borderline. Within the second and third category, a more detailed description usually follows in relation to the specific diagnostic problem. However, "the" normal human EEG does not exist. On the contrary, there is an enormous inter-individual variation, whereas the resting EEG of the healthy (fairly young) adult tends to remain constant even over fairly long time periods. There are characteristic EEG changes with brain development in childhood and youth and others tend to occur with advancing age. Definite sex differences have also been described. However, even within groups of males or females of the same age definite and fairly constant individual differences are observed. Some observers compare these individual EEG patterns with handwriting. As mentioned above (Sect. 2.1), this variation has suggested genetic studies by the twin method to determine whether and to what degree this variation is caused by genetic differences. These twin studies are discussed in detail in Chap. 3. In addition to this very general question, however, a second question can be asked: In addition to the continuous variation in certain parameters such as frequencies, amplitudes, and the occurrence of special wave forms, are there any EEG variants that can be distinguished by additional qualitative criteria from EEGs of other individuals? As shown by careful observation of EEG phenotypes, such variants obviously do exist. This is demonstrated in the following chapters. Describing them as "normal" means that they do not indicate the presence of certain diseases, for example, specific brain diseases. However, it is possible that they show correlations, sometimes weak ones, with diseases or, more frequently, with aspects of personality and performance within the normal range or in the field that is normally described – for lack of precise designation – as borderline. Examples are psychopathy, neurosis, drug addiction, and others. It is well-known that normal variation in certain parameters, for example, genetic polymorphisms of blood groups, "transplantation" antigens of the HLA system and many others contribute to the risk of being affected with certain common diseases (for examples, see Vogel and Motulsky 1996). It is very well possible that such normal variation in certain EEG parameters and variants may contribute to brain function and performance. This problem is also explored in the following chapters.

Before correlations between certain EEG types and anomalies of any kind, be it diseases or behavioral anomalies, can be explained in a meaningful way, the question should be answered whether a certain peculiarity of the EEG represents a constitutional feature of brain function that increases the susceptibility of the brain for a certain abnormal condition, or whether it is caused by this condition; i.e., whether it is a trait or a state (to use expressions common in psychiatric research). It is well known that the EEG may be modified by many factors, both external and internal, for example, physical impact, toxic substances and metabolic anomalies (see Niedermeyer and Lopes da Silva 1993).

Before these problems can be discussed, however, some basic aspects of EEG nomenclature must be described: What we see on our paper, or on the computer screen, are waves. The following wave forms are conventionally distinguished (Fig. 2.4): α waves (8–13 c/s); β waves (14 c/s and higher); ϑ waves (4–7 c/s) and δ waves (up to 3 c/s). Figure 2.4 also shows the most important pathological wave forms. Very often, α-activity shows a maximum in occipital leads, while β waves and sometimes ϑ waves may be found more frequently in frontal and frontoprecentral leads. δ waves are not part of the normal, adult resting EEG; they are found normally in deep sleep, in very young children, and may be seen in certain types of brain pathology. α waves normally disappear, and may be replaced by fast activity, when the

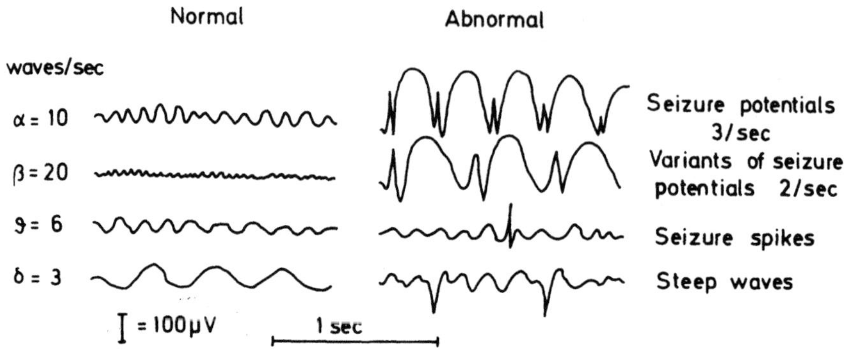

Fig. 2.4. Wave types of the human electroencephalogram (from Jung)

eyes are opened; they reappear immediately after the eyes are closed. This "α blocking" is also observed after other unexpected, sensoric stimuli such as noise. Since the EEG is often used for diagnosis of epilepsy and since many epileptic patients show a normal EEG or noncharacteristic "borderline" features during the interval between seizures, certain methods are used for provocation of more specific EEG patterns. A very useful provocation method is hyperventilation: the proband is asked to breathe deeply for about 2–3 min. This reduces the CO_2 content in the blood; in normal individuals, α waves may be replaced in part by groups of ϑ waves with higher amplitudes, and, sometimes, even by δ waves. Such EEG changes are generally more pronounced in children, but may also occur in adults. Quite as many other features of the normal EEG, this reaction shows a higher degree of inter-individual variation but even stronger reactions cannot be regarded as "abnormal." However, in some patients, wave forms characteristic for epilepsies may be elicited. Other provocation methods include photostimulation by repeated light flashes and natural or drug-induced sleep.

During sleep, the EEG shows major – and characteristic – changes, which depend on the stage of sleep to be observed (Niedermeyer 1993):

- Stage 1: "drowsiness" – α waves disappear; low-voltage slow waves appear
- Stage 2: "light sleep" – sleep "spindles"; vertex waves; so-called k complexes
- Stage 3: "deep sleep" – slow waves; k complexes, some spindles
- Stage 4: "very deep sleep" – much slowing, some k complexes, REM (= rapid eye movement); desynchronization with faster frequencies.

This description is very short and oversimplified. For a much more detailed description see Niedermeyer (1993). Moreover, there is again, as for many "normal" EEG phenomena, a high degree of interindividual variation (see Chap. 3 for twin studies; this chapter presents EEG curves of various sleep stages).

2.5 The EEG in Childhood and Youth

Human beings are born with an anatomically and physiologically immature brain. This is also reflected by brain function: for example, nobody remembers events that occurred during the first year of life. This immaturity – and the slow maturation process during infancy, childhood and youth – is also reflected in the EEG. Since the EEG provides a relatively easy and objective way to follow up physiological brain maturation, many investigators have carried out such EEG studies, either cross-sectional by comparing groups of children in different age groups, or longitudinal by repeatedly studying the same cohorts of children at different ages. The first EEG studies on children were performed by Berger (1932) and Lindsley (1936); extensive longitudinal examinations were reported by Petersén et al. (1975). Niedermeyer (1993) gave an excellent review.

Slow EEG activity (0.5–2 c/s) can be demonstrated in the fetus even at the conceptual age of 3 months. In premature children (24–27 weeks), bursts of very slow waves (0.3–1 c/s) have been observed together with short runs of faster frequencies as well as "quiet" periods. At 28–32 weeks the EEG remains discontinuous; slower activity (<1 c/s) may be prominent. ϑ- and α-frequencies may be intermixed. At the age of 32–35 weeks, differentiation starts between sleep and wakefulness; slow activity is observed, often with superimposed ripples of about 16 c/s, and occipital dominance. All these EEG results and their disturbances are important for judging the long-term chances a premature baby may have. During the first 3 months of life, the EEG changes gradually from a neonatal to an infantile pattern. At an age of 3 months, the waking baby should have rhythmical posterior activity of approx. 4 c/s, a precursor of the α-rhythm. During the following months, this activity stabilizes, and the average frequency increases. For a detailed description of these patterns, see again Niedermeyer 1993. At the age of 12–36 months, the posterior basic rhythm moves from the δ to the lowest α range; even in this age group interindividual variation regarding the speed of this development is conspicuous. Lindsley (1939) observed variation in the basic rhythm between 5 and almost 10 c/s. Moreover, EEGs at this age show varying degrees of fast and – almost in all instances – slow activity. This variation suggests the obvious question whether and to what extent such differences in the EEG maturation also reflect differences in psychological or, for example, motoric development. This problem is discussed briefly in later chapters.

During preschool age (3–5 years), the posterior basic rhythm usually reaches the α range (8 c/s). Often, the occipital α waves are interrupted by slow waves (approx. 1.5–4 c/s). As a rule, α amplitudes are higher than in adolescence and adulthood. At the age of 8–12 years, the posterior α rhythm gradually reaches a mean frequency of approx. 10 c/s, corresponding to the mean frequency in the adult. However, as a rule this α rhythm shows considerable admixture of slow activity. Slow waves of approx. 4–5 c/s often represent a subharmonic of α-frequency; this 4–5 c/s rhythm appears to have a genetic basis; this is discussed in greater detail in Chap. 8. Frontoprecentral 6–7 c/s activity may appear at approx. 6–12 years and seems to reach a maximum at approx. 13–15 years. A 4–6 c/s theta rhythm, especially in the age group below 8 years may indicate a predisposition to primary general epilepsy (Doose et al. 1973; Chap. 8). The EEG of children can be activated especially easily by hyperventilation; there is also conspicuous interindividual variation. In adolescents (ages about 12–20 years), the EEG gradually develops into the mature pattern which shows strong individual variation, which is discussed in greater detail in connection with genetic studies. According to a comprehensive study (Petersén and Eeg-Olofsen 1971; Petersén et al. 1975), the posterior α rhythm shows a mean frequency of about 10.2 c/s in males and 10.3 c/s in females; interindividual variation may stretch between 8–12 c/s. On the average, amplitude of the posterior α rhythm tends to be somewhat higher than in adulthood, but lower than at younger age. Both the admixture of posterior and precentral activity mainly in the δ range tends to diminish during this period of life.

Altogether, the EEG of adolescents becomes more and more similar to the adult pattern, until this is reached at the age of 19–20. There is one interesting difference: in the first years of this age range, low-voltage patterns do occur but are much rarer than in adults. This problem should be considered in genetic studies; this is discussed in Sect. 4.3. Altogether EEG development in infancy, childhood, and youth shows an enormous range of interindividual variation, even if obviously pathological EEG phenomena such as patterns characteristic for certain types of epilepsy are neglected. This variation offers many problems and could be approached, and in part solved, by genetic studies.

2.6 EEG Changes with Advancing Age, I

EEG development from infancy to adulthood represents, as a rule, normal processes, despite the enormous interindividual variation. Such patterns may indicate a predisposition for certain diseases such as epilepsies. Moreover, there are – sometimes even characteristic – EEG anomalies in certain, mostly rare, genetic anomalies and diseases (Chap. 8). As a rule, however, changes with advancing age can be regarded as signs of normal brain development. In aging persons, however, changes in EEG may be interpreted either as signs of "normal" development, or as symptoms of pathological processes; for example, vascular processes, but also involution of neuronal structures, and many others. Conceptually, it is very difficult, if not impossible to distinguish "normal" aging from "abnormal" or even "pathological" processes. There is only one way: Changes in EEG parameters with advancing age should be described, and correlations with otherwise recognizable abnormalities or diseases should be noted. Again, genetic methods such as the study of aging monozygotic twin pairs may help in distinguishing endogenous, genetically determined developments from external effects (see Sect. 3.4)

2.7 EEG Differences Between Men and Women

As noted above, the "normal" human EEG shows high inter-individual variation. Hence it is interesting to study whether this variation is correlated with other biological parameters. One of the most important parameters is gender. Therefore the question has been studied repeatedly whether there is a sex difference in normal EEG measures. Obviously, there is no absolute sex difference; i.e., the sex of a person cannot be determined by scrutinizing its EEG. However, there may be a sex difference in the frequencies of certain EEG phenomena or in the averages of certain measurable and quantitatively varying traits. And such differences have, indeed, been shown. Mundy-Castle (1951), comparing 85 young women and 74 men, found higher prevalence of β-activity in women; the result was weakly significant. However, it was confirmed by S.M. Smith (1954). Her work is especially interesting, because she used an early version of automatic frequency analysis, the system of Buldock and Walter. In this system, EEG waves are subdivided into 18 frequency classes. Comparing fronto-occipital tracings of 50 males and 50 females of non-specified ages, she found a higher average number of waves in 14 classes, including all classes with 12 and more waves/second in females. Hence females showed, on the average, more waves in the β band.

In one of our studies, this sex difference was examined in greater detail (Friedl and Vogel 1979). Probands were university students who were inscribed at the University of Heidelberg in 1974, and volunteered in an EEG study; mean age: 24.4 years in 290 male and 25.2 years in 198 female students (range of variation 20–35 years). An 8-channel EEG recorder from Nihon-Kohden, and reference tracings with electrodes at ipsilateral ears were used. In addition to the conventional visual analysis, a time-domain analysis was performed, using the program of the WDV company, Munich (Smith et al. 1973). This program permitted subdividing frequencies into 60 classes and amplitudes into 31 classes. For data reduction, both frequency and amplitude classes were combined to form four "superclasses" each; for frequencies, the program follows the traditional EEG classification:

$$\beta = 13.5\text{–}40\ \text{Hz};\ \alpha = 8.0\text{–}13.5\ \text{Hz};\ \vartheta = 4.0\text{–}8\ \text{Hz};\ \delta = 0.5\text{–}3.9\ \text{Hz}$$

For amplitudes, the following classes were used: 0–20 μV, 20–40 μV, 40–100 μV, and 100–200 μV. Analysis was performed on about 100 artifact-free stretches; the reliability of the method was tested in various ways. In distinction of earlier studies of this problem, precentral and occipital recordings were studied separately, since it is known that generally β and also ϑ waves tend to be more prominent above anterior parts of the brain, while in occipital areas, α waves often prevail. Table 2.1 shows some of the results. In precentral leads, both the total number of β waves and the mean β amplitudes were higher in female probands; this difference was significant only in tracings from the right-hand side. In males, on the other hand, the number of α waves was higher. In occipital leads, the sex difference as regards frequencies was more pronounced; in females, more EEG waves, and especially more β waves were counted; correspondingly, waves in the α and ϑ waves were more common in males. Moreover, there was a significant difference regarding occipital, dominant α frequencies of the left side: They were found to be higher in females. On the right-hand side, sex differences were in the same direction but were not significant statistically. Another sex difference found in the study was that females appear to show a greater number of waves with lower amplitudes in occipital leads. Hence it can be concluded that, on the average, females show more waves in the β range and, very probably, also in the higher α range than males.

Another interesting result of our study was that these sex differences regarding occipital α frequencies appear to be more pronounced on the left-hand side of the brain, while precentrally found higher prevalences of β waves were found to be more prominent on the right-hand side. In general, differences between waves at right- and at left-hand side were highly significant in both sexes; left-side precentral recordings had a greater number of waves and, especially, more β waves, while less α and ϑ waves were found. A similar, but more pronounced side difference was shown in occipital leads. This result confirms results of other authors on side diffe-

Table 2.1. Quantitative EEG parameters in males (N – 290) and females (N = 198) (Friedl and Vogel 1979)

EEG Parameter		Left-hand side, precentral					Right-hand side, precentral				
		♂		♀			♂		♀		
		x̄	S.D.	x̄	S.D.	Sex difference	x̄	S.D.	x̄	S.D.	Sex difference
Sum total,		1909.6	176.0	1932.1	181.6		1861.5	175.5	1892.7	175.9	
waves:	β- Waves	1432.6	286.8	1468.9	251.5		1347.6	293.0	1405.3	285.9	$p < 0.05$
	α- Waves	405.8	87.9	395.3	94.5		430.4	90.1	412.5	95.2	$p < 0.05$
	ϑ- Waves	70.6	37.0	66.8	34.5		79.2	37.9	74.3	34.3	
Mean	β- Waves	17.39	2.67	17.71	3.18		16.61	2.66	17.25	2.94	$p < 0.05$
amplitude:	α- Waves	31.26	5.94	31.82	6.81		30.60	5.89	31.33	6.84	
	ϑ- Waves	69.8	24.27	71.8	22.60		71.91	23.95	74.64	22.65	
Amplitudes:	0– 20	1002.1	255.6	1002.1	284.4		987.6	270.1	996.2	295.8	
	20– 40	631.8	96.0	638.2	109.6		603.2	91.3	612.3	105.5	
	40–100	270.7	158.8	285.3	182.1		265.4	159.6	277.4	177.3	
	100–200	3.7	7.6	4.9	11.2		3.90	8.11	5.36	12.59	
Mean		17.2	0.99	17.4	0.95		16.9	1.18	17.15	0.99	$p < 0.05$
frequency:	α-Index	0.274	0.07	0.266	0.07		0.291	0.07	0.277	0.07	$p < 0.05$
		Left-hand side, occipital					Right-hand side, occipital				
Sum total,		1752.7	240.2	1842.8	221.7	$p < 0.01$	1703.7	236.4	179.6	277.1	$p < 0.01$
waves	β- Waves	1129.9	418.9	1296.0	384.8	$p < 0.01$	1049.0	412.0	1223.2	395.8	$p < 0.01$
	α- Waves	551.9	162.4	489.6	149.4	$p < 0.01$	577.1	158.0	515.7	157.2	$p < 0.01$
	ϑ- Waves	70.7	42.5	56.9	31.5	$p < 0.01$	76.8	42.9	64.2	52.8	$p < 0.01$
Mean	β- Waves	18.27	4.02	18.84	4.62		18.82	4.26	19.49	4.91	
amplitude:	α- Waves	36.91	12.71	36.25	12.98		39.20	15.65	38.50	14.74	
	ϑ- Waves	55.00	21.40	54.87	20.01		59.27	21.66	63.19	26.27	
Amplitudes:	0– 20	790.4	395.0	872.8	402.5	$p < 0.05$	709.4	376.2	804.5	398.2	$p < 0.01$
	20– 40	534.8	158.2	562.2	157.4	$p < 0.05$	500.1	162.5	543.7	165.0	$p < 0.01$
	40–100	397.0	238.4	367.7	251.6		441.1	238.1	398.8	254.2	
	100–200	37.9	95.5	35.9	76.1		51.0	110.5	50.5	105.1	
Mean		16.0	1.69	16.7	1.45	$p < 0.01$	15.7	1.74	16.3	0.13	
frequency:	α-Index	0.39	0.13	0.33	0.12	$p < 0.01$	0.41	0.14	0.36	0.13	

Table 2.2a. Differences between left-hand and right-hand side leads; precentral leads

EEG-Parameter		Both sexes:	Sexes separately Males:	Females:
Sum total, waves:		36.2**	48.1	39.4
	β- Waves	59.9**	85.0	63.6
	α- Waves	-17.0**	-24.6	-17.2
	ϑ- Waves	6.8**	8.6	- 7.5
Mean amplitudes:	β- Waves	0.48**	0.78	0.46
	α- Waves	0.37**	0.66	0.49
	ϑ- Waves	- 1.92***	- 2.11	- 2.84
Amplitudes:		0.2**	0.3	0.25
	0– 20	11.8**	14.5	5.9
	20– 40	22.3**	28.6	25.9
	40–100	2.7***	5.3	7.9
	100–200	- 0.5*	- 0.2	- 0.5
Mean frequencies		0.2**	0.3	0.25
	α-Index:	- 0.011**	- 0.017	- 0.011

Positive figures: Higher values left-hand side
Negative figures: Higher values right-hand side

Table 2.2b. Differences between left-hand and right-hand leads; occipital leads

EEG-Parameter		Both sexes:	Sexes separately Males:	Females:
Sum total, waves:		24.5**	49.0	43.2
	β- Waves	40.3**	80.0	72.8
	α- Waves	-13.4**	-25.2	-26.1
	ϑ- Waves	- 2.4**	- 6.8	- 7.3
Mean amplitudes:	β- Waves	- 0.67**	- 0.55	- 0.65
	α- Waves	- 2.49**	- 2.29	- 2.25
	ϑ- Waves	- 5.92***	- 4.27	- 8.32
Amplitudes:	0– 20	56.0**	81.0	68.3
	20– 40	9.7***	34.7	18.5
	40–100	-30.2**	-44.1	-31.1
	100–200	-12.8**	-13.1	-14.6
Mean frequencies		0.17**	0.3	0.2
	α-Index:	- 0.011**	- 0.02	- 0.03

* Difference significant, $p < 0,05$; ** Difference significant, $p < 0,01$; *** Difference not significant.
For technical reasons, differences for both sexes together were computed not for the entire material but for 417 cases only for precentral, and for 348 cases for occipital leads.

rences of the EEG (Cornil and Gastaut 1947; Butler and Glass 1974; for other references see Friedl 1977). Functional differences between the two sexes in relation to their differences in EEG patterns were examined by Flor-Henry and Koles (1982). They studied 37 males and 46 females while resting and during performing verbal and spatial tasks. Using automatic analysis of power-spectra, they also found, on the average, more power in females in the β range. Interhemispheric coherence was found to be more pronounced in females but there was no relationship with handedness. In general, all these results appear to indicate a generally higher level of activation, or tonic arousal, in females. The general problem of possible correlations of EEG parameters, including β activity, is discussed in a later chapter. Nevertheless it is also important here to note that the EEG, and especially the number of β waves increases with advancing age in both sexes. Again, an earlier study from our group should be dealt with in somewhat greater detail (Vogel and Götze 1962). We classified EEGs from 3067 patients of an EEG reference laboratory, 1847 male and 1220 female, according to whether the EEG recordings contained a significant admixture of β waves. Only EEGs diagnosed as normal or borderline were included; definitely pathological recordings were not considered.

The β EEGs were classified into three categories: EEGs with frontoprecentral β groups or more or less frontoprecentral β activity; EEG recordings in which all other EEG waves are replaced by β waves; and recordings in which the β waves are mixed more or less diffusely with α (and other) waves. The first category is discussed together with other distinct, but relatively rare, EEG variants in Chap. 4; the prevalence of EEG recordings with continuous and diffusely distributed β waves showed, again, the sex difference described in the above studies; and, in addition, an increase with age in both sexes (see Fig. 4.20). On the other hand, it is obvious from Fig. 4.20 that EEG recordings with frontoprecentral β groups do not show an increase with age. They also failed to show a sex difference. As noted above, this was an early study and it was based on clinical material. In the late 1950s and early 1960s, it was not customary to supplement diagnostic EEG studies by computerized evaluation. However, the sex difference and the increase in clearcut diffuse β and complete β EEGs with age was confirmed by subsequent quantitative studies and can still be accepted.

An obvious explanation of these sex differences would be an effect of sex hormones on brain function. Such effects have, indeed, been described (see Niedermeyer 1993). However, a direct effect of hormones can hardly be the only reason since EEG differences between the sexes persist into old age. An indirect effect is very likely: During embryonic development, sex hormones, such as gestagens and androgens are known to affect brain development – with consequences for behavior (Money and Ehrhardt 1972). The problem is discussed below in connection with EEG in the Turner syndrome (Chap. 8). EEG changes after treatment with ACTH and cortisone have been described. Hyperthyroidism may lead to higher α frequencies and to an increase in fast activity, while hypothyroidism down to myxedema may lead to EEG slowing. All these possibilities should be kept in mind when problems such as sex differences, developmental aspects or genetic problems are studied.

2.8 Changes in the EEG with Advancing Age, II

The last study leads to another aspect which should be discussed at least briefly, before genetic studies can be discussed: the EEG changes with advancing age during the life of the adult (see also Van Sweden et al. 1993). A comprehensive review, and a table containing the data available at that time was given by Heuschert (1963) in his thesis on the EEG in healthy, aged monozygotic (MZ) twins. Almost all authors reported a slowing of a activity with advancing age. Friedlander (1958) evaluated routine EEGs from 814 hospital patients aged between 20 and 89 year; Table 2.3 presents the frequencies that he found with normal EEG.

Table 2.3. Percentage of persons with α waves of frequencies

Age (years)	8 c/s	9 c/s	10 c/s	11 c/s	12 c/s
20–29	3.7	29.2	48.7	14.4	3.9
40–59	12.0	35.7	38.5	9.6	4.0
60–89	25.9	46.6	20.7	5.2	1.7

However, many aged individuals maintain relatively high frequencies of their α waves up to a high age, showing no decrease in α frequencies in the course of life. There seems to be no agreement in the literature whether this α slowing indicates "normal" involution of brain structure, or is a sign of pathological, for example, vascular processes. The latter option is probably true for one observation reported first by Silverman et al. (1955) according to which focal abnormalities are seen in EEG recordings of aged probands, as a rule without recognizable clinical correlates. Studying 145 individuals above the age of 60, they found, in addition to α slowing in an appreciable part of their probands, in 25% focal disturbances. In other studies, reduced average α amplitudes have been found in aging subjects (Christian 1984). Bilateral slowing was also observed in the ϑ and δ range, and its degree appears to be correlated with diminished mental function and decreased longevity (Van Sweden et al. 1993) but, according to these authors, diffuse slow waves activity, such as the focal abnormalities mentioned above, has been observed in clinically "normal" persons as well. A table on EEG studies available up to that time in psychiatrically and/or neurologically ill, aged persons has again been given by Heuschert (1963). In some more recent studies, traditional EEG measures such as those noted above, such as the occurrence and amplitude frequencies of α, β and ϑ waves and their distribution over certain regions of the scalp have been supplemented by more sophisticated concepts such as "dimension," – a measure for the complexity of the EEG curve which is computed from the succession of very many single points of measurement and their correlations (see, for example, Lutzenberger et al. 1992). The approach is based on chaos theory and on attempts at analyzing nonlinear systems (see, for example, Goldberger 1996). Linear systems can be understood completely by analyzing their components separately; for example, by dissecting the EEG into its frequency bands. A nonlinear system, on the other hand, cannot be understood completely in this way, since its components interact; there may be nonlinear transitions leading, for example, to self-sustained, periodic waves. Complexity of such interactions can be measured by special mathematical functions. Such a method was used to study EEG changes with advancing age (Anokhin et al. 1996), the sample consisting of school children of both sexes in two age groups (7–8 years; $n = 41$; 13–14 years; $n = 41$), and healthy males of three age groups (20–30, $n = 93$; 31–45, $n = 109$; 45–50, $n = 28$). The result was a strong increase in complexity as measured by a strongly increasing average "dimension" in contrast to ϑ and α power spectra which show an increase in childhood and youth only, while during adult age, no systematic change in power spectra can be observed. However, power spectra in the β range increased, confirming earlier studies (see above). The authors interpreted their results as follows: "During individual development, a continuous formation and modification of neural cell assemblies (functionally related groups of cells distributed throughout the cortex connected by strong excitatory circuits and showing a repetitive synchronous activation) can be assumed ... Such 'functional systems' seem to underlie the content of individual experience ... An increase in the number of functionally related cell assemblies oscillating at their frequency should result in a greater number of independent generators, and ... lead to a higher value of correlation-dimension of the EEG time series." This development appears to continue throughout the whole life span (Fig. 2.5)

Age and gender dependent EEG changes must be considered when genetic effects on the EEG are studied. However, there is one important difference: Most studies on development in younger or older age are based on shifts of averages; and on

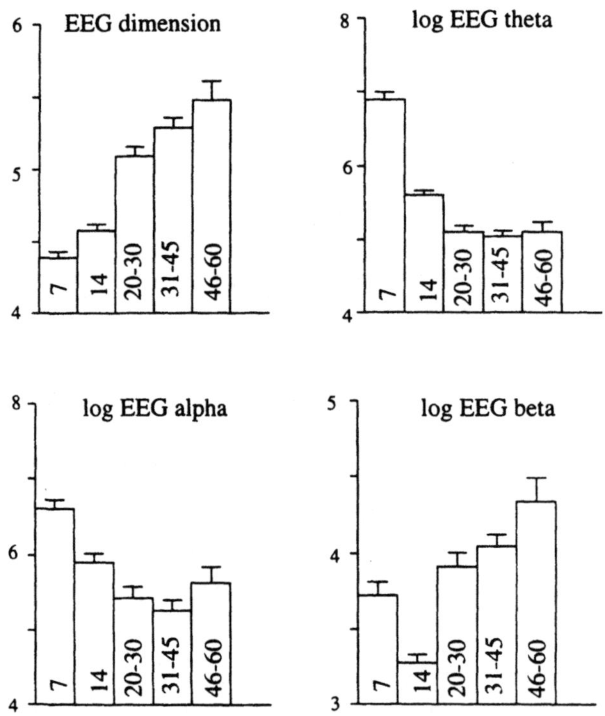

Fig. 2.5. Age related changes in EEG dimensional complexity and conventional power measures. Values are averaged across all leads. Each bar corresponds to a particular age group. (From Anokhin et al. 1996)

continuous increases or decreases in certain EEG phenomena, whether they are regarded as "normal," "borderline" or "pathological." Genetic analysis, on the other hand, tries to reduce interindividual differences to clear alternatives – ideally to alternatives between genes and alleles which, in principle, are present all over lifetime (somatic mutations, for example, those leading to immunoglobulin variants, to cancer or to break-down of mitochondrial functions are still exceptions; for details see Vogel and Motulsky 1996). This conceptual difference should always be kept in mind.

2.9 Effects of Drugs on the EEG

Drug effects on the EEG have been studied extensively; they are now forming a branch of its own within EEG research. In this report they can be mentioned only briefly, as far as their knowledge influences genetic studies and interpretation of genetic results. A review that is still worthwhile reading because of its conceptual clarity was published by R. Jung (1958). The drug most often used by human beings is probably alcohol. As shown by Propping in his twin and family studies (Propping 1977, 1978), EEG reaction may be strong in some instances but there are enormous interindividual differences both in extent and in kind of the reaction, making this alcohol reaction a paradigm for genetically determined differences in reaction of brain function to drugs (pharmacogenetics; see Vogel and Motulsky 1996). These problems are discussed in detail in the chapter on EEG and alhoholism (Sect. 7.1). Reactions to other drugs are described by Wauquier (1993) and Bauer (1993); the latter report concentrates on poisoning of the CNS. Many studies were concerned with EEG changes in general anesthesia since the EEG is often used during monitoring of surgical anesthesia.

"The initial phase is dominated by ... frontal fast activity, gradually becoming more generalized and associated with dissolution of the α rhythm. During excitation, paroxysmal activity may become discernible ... As anesthesia deepens, activity becomes slower and the voltage increases. Eventually, a burst-suppression pattern indicates the involvement of brainstem functions ..." (Bauer 1993)

Barbiturates in small doses produce an increase in β activity (approx. 25–35 c/s; shifting to 15–25 c/s), even in chronic use. Similar EEG changes can be observed after benzodiazepine; frequencies in the β range appear to be slower (14–25 c/s); while barbiturate-induced β activity is described to occur mainly in frontal and frontoprecentral leads, benzodiazepine-induced activity is said to have a more diffuse character (Wauquier 1993). For both groups of drugs, a (more or less) spindle-like conformation of β waves is often observed. Many other psychotropic drugs were also found to enhance β activity including neuroleptics, especially nonsedative ones, some antidepressants, psychostimulants such as amphetamines and those of the LSD type, nootropics, and especially anxiolytics. Sedative neuroleptics and hypnotics may also induce ϑ and δ activity (Wauquier 1993). In addition to the resting EEG, drugs may also affect EEG reactions and EEG during sleep but reviewing this literature would go beyond the scope of this report.

For designing and interpreting genetic studies, knowledge of the above drug effects is essential since researchers can be led astray by EEG peculiarities in certain probands that are incorrectly interpreted as genetic in origin but are in fact drug effects. On the other hand, certain normal genetic variants, especially those involving β activity, may be interpreted erroneously as drug effects. In medical examination of applicants for certain professions (pilots, bus drivers etc.), this may lead to suspicion of drug abuse and to unfair refusal.
A point considered only rarely in connection with drug effects, except in the above studies on alcohol effects, is the possibility of genetically determined individual variation in drug reaction. Such variation is widely known especially as regards drug metabolism, action and side effects (Evans 1993; Vogel and Motulsky 1996). It could also be more important than is known so far for drug reaction of the EEG.

2.10 The EEG and Somatic Diseases

The EEG may be affected by many diseases which are not primary brain diseases but affect brain function directly or indirectly. Endocrine diseases are discussed in Sect. 2.6. Others include liver diseases, many genetically caused metabolic diseases, some of which are discussed in greater detail together with other genetic diseases (Chap. 8), but also cardiac and vascular diseases. As a rule, such conditions lead to EEG alterations that are diagnosed either as definitely pathological or as borderline, raising suspicions for presence of brain involvement. Occasionally, however, they may lead to a wrong classification as a normal variant. Therefore genetic EEG studies require careful case histories, even in "normal" subjects.

CHAPTER 3

3 Genetic Studies: Twin Studies

3.1 General Remarks on the Twin Method

The most general method for deciding whether, and to what extent, interindividual variation in a certain phenotype is caused by genetic variation is the study of monozygotic (MZ) twins – their similarities and differences. MZ twins originate from division of one zygote, in a very early state of embryonic development. Therefore they must as a rule be identical genetically; any phenotypic differences must largely be caused by environmental differences. Here, environment is defined in the widest possible sense: anything that is not fixed genetically. However, mutations in somatic cells outside the germ line do occur; they may lead, for example, to tumor diseases or to differences of antibodies. Mitochrondria may be distributed unevenly between the two embryos. Therefore genetic differences in such traits may occur even in MZ twins. However, these are relatively unimportant exceptions from the rule that MZ twins are identical genetically: to recognize whether and to what degree a characteristic is determined genetically and to what degree its interindividual variation is modified by environmental effects, the degree of similarity between MZ twins is an important criterion. Since dizygotic (DZ) twins are thought to be affected largely by the same environmental differences as MZ twins but to have only one half of their genes in common by decent, they are used as suitable controls (for details of the twin method, see Vogel and Motulsky 1996).

A superficial observer could regard results of twin studies as more or less trivial. In one way or another, genes determine, at least affect, most aspects of our phenotypes. And for most of these phenotypic features, there is some interindividual variation. Therefore twin studies almost invariably have the result that MZ twins are more similar than DZ twins. However, this triviality immediately disappears as soon as more specific and sophisticated questions are asked; for example: How much and in which direction can a certain genetically determined phenotype be modified by exogenous factors? Which are these factors? And in which phase of the life course do they occur? The comparison of MZ twins is one of the most efficient methods for studying environmental factors that may affect human life in health and disease. This chance has been exploited by some of the twin studies to be discussed below.

However, before results of twin studies are interpreted as showing a certain degree of genetic determination of a certain phenotype, another aspect should be considered critically: The above- argument as to the similarity of MZ twins points to higher degree of genetic determination, differences between them indicates stronger exogenous differences assumes that twins, especially MZ twins are an unbiased sample of the entire population in all other aspects of their biological and psychological makeup, except of course that they are twins. However, this is not entirely true (see Vogel and Motulsky 1996). There may be anomalies during embryonic development of twins leading, for example, to certain malformations in one twin but not in the other. Therefore the twin method is not suited for studying the degree of genetic determination of malformation. One of the most sensitive organs in embryonic development is the brain. Possible effects of factors specific for embryonic development of twins should therefore be considered carefully before drawing conclusions as to genetic effects on brain development; they could also modify EEG similarity in twins. One such factor, differences in head and brain configuration, is discussed below.

In addition to such intrauterine factors, specific psychological factors should be considered, especially when EEG twin studies are used as tools in human behavior genetics. Twins, especially MZ twins, interact in specific ways not only with their parents and other family members, but with each other. Depending on the individual situation, this may lead to quite different results: Either, they might tend to identify themselves with each other becoming unusually similar, or they assume different, and sometimes complementary, roles in life. This may lead to long-lasting psychological differences.

In conclusion, the twin method, despite its conceptual simplicity, may pose very difficult methodological problems. However, it may also offer possibilities for answering specific and sophisticated questions.

Another problem is posed by the fact that twins, as other persons, normally cannot be observed continuously over their lifetime but, in most instances, only for very short times, and very often only once. For morphological traits, for example, stature, this does not affect the results since such traits develop slowly, and then in adult age remain constant over long time periods: Even with somatic diseases, this problem can be overcome easily since the case histories, for example, information on age at onset, course of the disease and complications, are as a rule documented. In mental diseases, the situation may be more difficult but can often be dealt with. The situation may become critical when either parameters of normal psychology are to be assessed by psychological tests, or if aspects of organic function are being studied. In both instances, the examination only lays hold of a very small sample from a life-long continuum. This immediately raises two questions: First, to what extent does the method used allow conclusions regarding the individual property to be studied? Does it have a sufficiently high validity? This question often comes up in psychological research, when we ask whether a certain test is valid to help assessing, for example, an aspect of intelligence. However, there is a second question: Does a necessarily short examination render sufficient information on long-term (and sometimes life-long) individual properties of the examined individuals? To use again a term popular among psychologists: Does the method to be used have a sufficiently high reliability? In studies on physiological (or, for example, many biochemical) parameters, the validity problem can be solved in most instances by proper techniques, by utilizing the available methods according to the "state of the art." In the EEG field, these methods can be learned by studying appropriate treatises (for example, Niedermeyer and Lopes da Silva 1993) and – still more important – by practical work in an EEG laboratory. The problem of reliability, however, is more critical for interpretation of similarities and differences in twins. Twins, even MZ twins, never show absolutely identical EEG records. Here, the questions to be asked cannot only be: Are MZ similar? And not even: are they more similar than DZ twins? Even if this question can be answered with "yes", the result is still not very exciting. What we need, is the answer to a much more specific question: Do MZ twins show reliable differences that go beyond the differences normally found between different examinations of the same individual? In which parameters can they be found? And if there are such differences, how can they be explained? These questions should be kept in mind when twin studies are now reviewed.

3.2 The First EEG Twin Studies

H. Davis and P. Davis (1936) were the first to study the EEG of twins. They examined the resting EEG of 8 MZ pairs at the age of 18–58 years, comparing it with five or six times repeated EEG records of 31 controls. They evaluated these records on the basis of the following criteria: (a) Presence or absence of a regular α rhythm, (b) frequency of α waves, (c) percentage of recording time at which the α rhythm was present (= α index, according to later studies; Rohracher 1950), (d) strength of α blocking when eyes are open, (e) occurrence of other, for example, β waves, (f) β frequency, (g) approximate average amplitude, and (h) difference between recordings form vertex and occiput. They concluded that recordings from MZ twins were as similar as recordings from the same individual at different times. Hence this ingenious study already asked the same questions, and provided preliminary answers for them, that have been studied again in many research programs up to the recent past. Meanwhile, the research methods have become more sophisticated, and the problems to be solved sometimes, but by no means always, more specific. Loomis (1936) described a female MZ pair at the age of 27 months. The recordings during waking and in sleep were almost identical while a DZ pair at the age of 3 years showed differrences in α activity.

The next series of MZ twins was studied by E.T. Raney (1937, 1939), a coworker of H. Jasper. He was interested mainly in a possible mirror-image asymmetry of the two sides of the brain in MZ twins; he had studied before the same problem by trying to demonstrate prevalence of one side during binocular vision. Studying the resting EEGs of 17 MZ twin pairs, he evaluated the records using three main criteria: α frequency, α index (see above) and mean amplitude.

For these parameters, he calculated the Spearman rank correlations between the 2×17 individuals of the 17 twin pairs; the results varied between 0.91 ± 0.029 for frequency and 0.61 ± 0.0108 for α% in occipital leads. He concluded that, as a rule, EEG records of MZ twins are very similar but that occasionally, EEG records of such twins may be less similar in some parameters than those of unrelated persons. Obviously, he examined his twins only once, and neglected the above fact that EEG records of identical twins, on the average, cannot be expected to be more similar than those taken from the same person at different times. As to the laterality problem, he found clearcut differences between records from the right and the left side of the brain; in 76% of the twin pairs, the EEGs behaved as mirror images, while in the remaining 24%, at least one twin did not show a clear side difference. Comparing this result with other results from his own studies in which he had tried to find mirror-image laterality of brain function in MZ twins, he found very high, and sometimes 100%, agreement. The problem of possible mirror images in aspects of brain function in MZ twins has subsequently been studied repeatedly; we return to this below.

Another EEG twin study was performed by Becker and Jung, but due to World War II and its aftermath, was not published (P.E. Becker, personal communication). Probably, the results of Höchel (1942), who compared five MZ and 5 DZ pairs regarding α and δ index and a *Wellenindex* of his own, which was calculated from frequencies and amplitudes are a part of this study. MZ pairs showed differences of maximally 2.5% in the α index. Other, early twin studies were performed by Waggoner and Baghi (1943). The most comprehensive one of these early twin studies was performed by Lennox, Gibbs and Gibbs (1945). These authors studied 55 MZ and 16 DZ pairs and a trizygotic group of triplets between the ages of 5 and 61 years. A resting EEG of 20 min and the response to hyperventilation were examined. The records were evaluated regarding presence or absence of "pathological" results, and it was noted additionally whether the records were identical or nonidentical. The authors compared their twin records with a comprehensive series of nontwins; they classified those records as identical, in which the EEG of the second twin could be regarded as the immediate continuation of that of the first one. Parameters such as frequency, amplitude, shape of waves and their distribution over various areas of the brain, and reaction to hyperventilation (see Sect. 2.4) were studied. Some 85% of EEGs of MZ twins were regarded as identical, 4% as nonidentical, and 11% as dubious. Records of DZ twins, on the other hand, were classified as nonidentical in 95%. The most remarkable result of this study was that the fraction of EEGs regarded as "abnormal" was enhanced as compared with the population average: Of altogether 148 individuals, 55% only were classified as "normal." Some 20% showed an EEG that, today, probably would be regarded as borderline; in another 20% the record was undoubtedly abnormal, and in 5% severely abnormal. The authors themselves believed that this high percentage of abnormal records could in part be due to the high fraction of young persons among their probands since, according to their experience and system of classification, about 20% of individuals below the age of 20 showed abnormalities. Moreover, they remarked that their series of twins was not entirely unbiased.

Despite these qualifications, the result that EEG records of twins may show higher rates of "abnormality" than those of singletons had to be taken seriously, especially since at that time, the Gibbses were the leading EEG specialists in the world; their EEG atlas (1950–1952) was the basic source of printed information for all EEG specialists. Moreover, this result was not entirely unlikely when the special problems of twin pregnancies were considered (Vogel and Motulsky 1996; see also Sect. 3.1). However, later studies have show that an especially high rate of abnormalities in EEG records of twins generally does not exist (see Götze et al. 1958). We return to this problem below.

In conclusion, twin studies with the EEG performed up to the late 1940s and early 1950s led to the following results, and raised the following questions:

1. The resting EEG of normal MZ twins, i.e., twins who did not suffer from any known disease – especially diseases that could affect brain function, altering the EEG pattern – is very similar if not identical. Here, "identity" can mean only that differences are not larger than those between different recordings of the same

individuals under the same conditions. Heritability, i.e., the degree of hereditary determinations (see below) cannot be higher than reliability for obvious biological reasons. This point of view was not considered in the early twin studies, except in the very first one, that of Davis and Davis (1936; only a few years after Berger had published his first reports on the human EEG). The question remained: Are EEG records of MZ twins only very similar, or are they identical? Or, to put this question differently: Are there any reproducible differences between EEG recordings of MZ twins, and if so, what are these differences, in which EEG parameters can they be demonstrated?

2. As suggested by Lennox et al. (1945) EEGs of twins, especially MZ twins, could show a higher fraction of borderline or abnormal recordings than those of singletons. If confirmed, this could have serious consequences for the usefulness of the twin method in general, and especially for aspects of brain function, including normal and subnormal intelligence, personality, but also diseases such as epilepsy. Therefore this problem needed to be studied.

3. The results of Raney (1937, 1939) suggested the possibility that the EEG records of MZ twins often showed some degree of mirror imaging. This needed to be restudied, especially in the light of studies regarding the systematic differences between the left and right sides of the brain as demonstrated by subsequent EEG studies (see Sect. 2.7). Hence the question whether there is mirror imaging in EEG recordings of MZ twins was still open.

To answer these questions as precisely as possible, we started comprehensive EEG studies on twins in the middle 1950s (Vogel 1957, 1958; Heuschert 1963a,b).

3.3 Our Own EEG Twin Studies

In our first series, we examined 208 twin pairs of the same sex between 6 and 30 years of age, among them 110 MZ and 98 DZ (among them there were two sets of triplets which offered information for two twin pairs each and were counted accordingly; Vogel 1958). EEG records were taken at rest, with bipolar and reference recordings, during hyperventilation and O_2 shortage and during sleep. To compare variation in the same individuals and, at least for a brief time period, development of the EEG in a longitudinal design, the entire examination was repeated in 15 MZ pairs about 1 year later. In a few instances, definite changes were observed, pointing to EEG maturation. We show occipital waves in two MZ sisters at the age of 12 and 14 (Fig. 3.1).

A number of measurements were taken on the resting EEG, among them α frequency, percent-time α, number of sub-alpha (δ and ϑ waves), coordination of phases between left-hand and right-hand sides and amplitudes. For evaluation of the hyperventilation reaction and the sleeping records, qualitative criteria such as occurrence and morphology of certain wave forms were used. At the time, the methods of automatic frequency analyses were still being developed in a few places, and were not available to us. Therefore a special planimeter was constructed to make measurements as precise as possible, and the results were evaluated using statistical methods. The measurements on the same sides of MZ twin pairs were compared with each other, with differences between the right-hand and left-hand sides

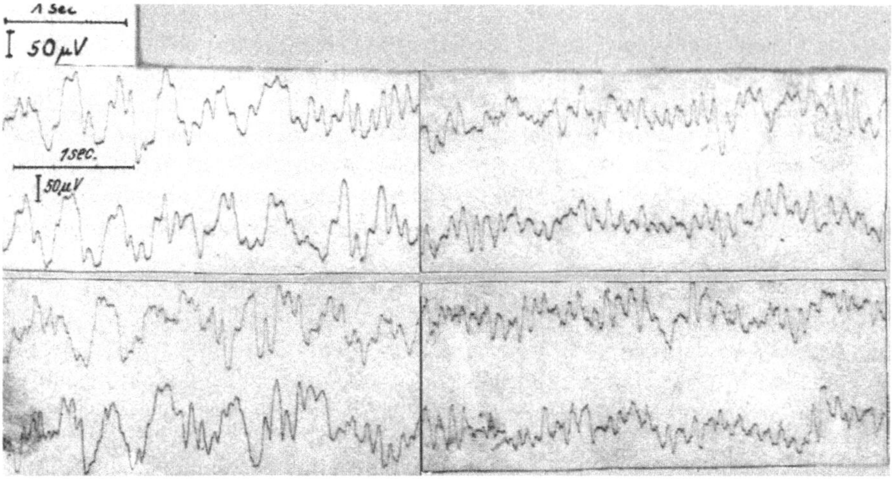

Fig. 3.1. EEG maturation: female MZ twins. Occipital α waves; reference leads. Left side, at age 11; right side, about 1 year later. (From Vogel 1958)

of the same individuals, and with measurements on EEG records of the same individuals at different times (see above). The main results were: There was no significant difference between measurable parameters in MZ twins when their differences were compared with differences between comparable features in the same individuals. However, there was one exception: Amplitudes showed a slight but significant difference between MZ twins; in contrast to the overwhelming visual similarity of their EEG recordings. We return to these results below. However, it proved soon that these measurements did not exhaust even nearly the information content of the EEG records; obviously, similarities of MZ twins went far beyond similarities of measurements. This raised the question of how the "computer between the ears" (Niedermeyer; see Sect. 2.3) can be used more efficiently. This was carried out by a blind classification experiment, for which a piece of 30 cm of a reference recording from each MZ twin was used. In 95 of 114 pairs (including 4 records from repetitions in which the EEG had changed somewhat between two examinations), matching of twins proved to be successful. With the remaining 19 pairs, the experiment was repeated leading to success in 14 instances, indicating that the 19 failures in the first experiment were not due to dissimilarities between any MZ pairs but were caused by accidental similarities between nonrelated individuals. DZ twins, on the other hand, were regarded as "similar" only in 17 of 98 pairs. Figures 3.2–3.4 present some examples.

As noted above, for evaluation of the sleeping EEG, no meaningful measurements could be performed; here, we had to rely on "morphological" criteria considering comparisons between repeated recordings in the same individuals. The results can be reported very briefly: Despite the strong interindividual variation even between children and adolescents of the same age, recordings of MZ twins could be regarded as identical; i.e., they did not differ more than those from the same persons at different times (Fig. 3.5). The 14 and 6 c/s spikes in the sleeping record were compared in a special study (Vogel 1965). Again, there was absolute concordance in MZ but

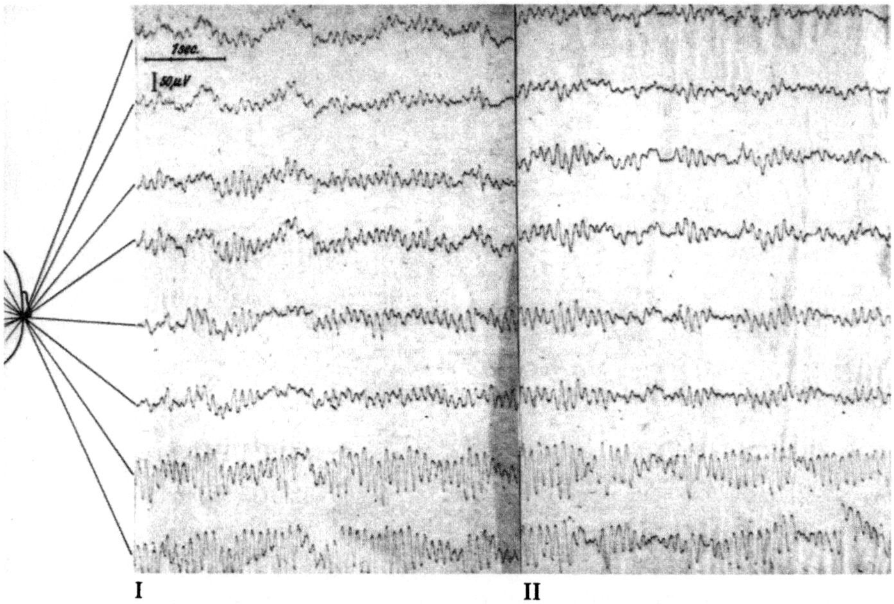

Fig. 3.2. Reference leads of a male MZ pair at the age of 15. The leads can be redarded as identical, i.e., they show no more differences than EEG leads of the same individuals at different times. (From Vogel 1958)

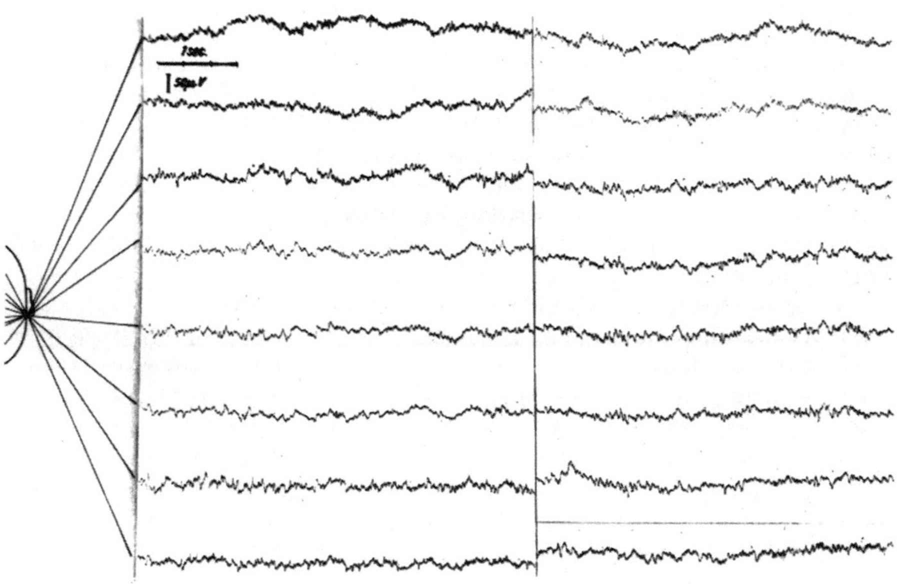

Fig. 3.3. Reference leads of a female MZ pair at the age of 27. Very little α activity, some irregular β waves and a few ϑ waves of low amplitude. (From Vogel 1958)

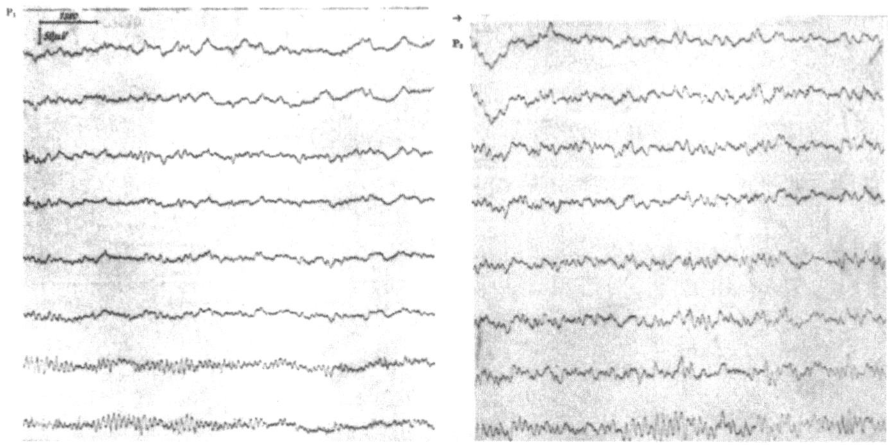

Fig. 3.4. A male DZ pair at the age of 15. There is a clearcut difference: the EEG of the second twin looks much more immature than that of the first one (P_1). (From Vogel 1958)

not in DZ twins. Studies on EEG all-night sleeping patterns were performed by Jung and Wilson (1967). They studied four MZ and two DZ pairs at the ages between 8 and 19 years. In distinction to our older studies discussed above, they also observed phases of REM (= rapid eye movement) sleep that occur during periods of dreaming. For the entire sleeping pattern, they observed concordance in MZ and discordance in DZ twins.

To come back to our own twin series, one of the 110 MZ pairs showed strong, and reproducible, differences. At their first examination, the boys were 12 years old; there was no conspicuous peculiarity in their life histories except an unusual motoric unrest. Their EEG recordings showed definite differences (Fig. 3.6): While twin 1 had a normal α record, twin 2 showed a mixture of α and ϑ waves in occipital leads, and a certain, albeit not "abnormal," increase in ϑ activity in anterior leads. This difference remained in repeated examination up to the age of 14; later we unfortunately lost contact to this pair. There can be no doubt regarding zygosity; and a careful psychological and neurological examination of both twins failed to give any hints as to possible reasons for the observed differences. Still, a small organic defect is the most probable explanation.

The question asked before could now be answered as follows:

1. In the great majority of all measurements, the EEG records of MZ twins could be regarded not only as similar but identical; i.e., the observed differences were not more pronounced than the differences between the left-hand and the right-hand side of the same individuals, or between those found in the same individual, in repeated studies under identical conditions. This conclusion was found to apply not only to the resting EEG but to hyperventilation, O_2 deprivation, and to sleeping pattern, as well. As shown by the blind classification experiment, the degree of similarity exceeds measurable parameters; it extends to so many subtle details of wave form, distribution of waves and others that the attempt at blind classification was successful in the great majority of instances. Whenever it failed, this was not caused by a lack of similarity between twins but by accidental similarity between non-related persons. However, there was one exception: the amplitude. Here, constant

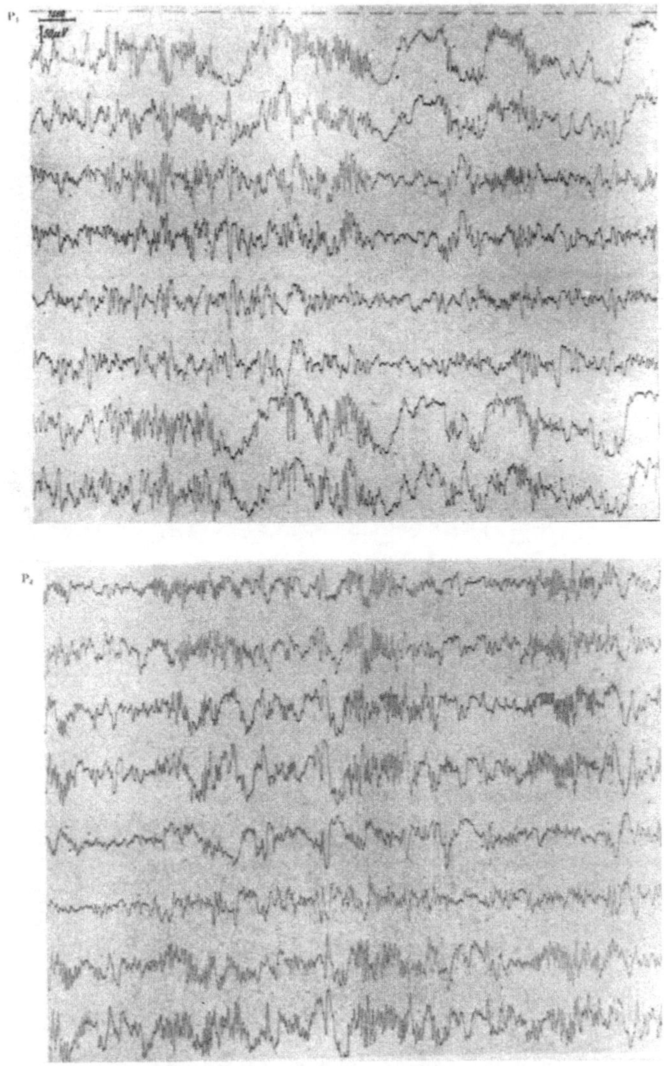

Fig. 3.5. Concordant sleeping EEG (spindle stage) in an MZ pair. (From Vogel 1958)

and reproducible differences were found among MZ twins. We explained it by assuming that they were caused by small differences in placing of electrodes in relation to the electrically active brain portions: An experienced observer (v. Verschuer) had observed before that shapes of the skulls are often different in MZ twins.

However, the one exceptional twin pair which showed a consistent EEG difference over about 18 months demonstrates that the rule "MZ EEG records are identical" may have exceptions. This is obvious in instances where the EEG of one twin shows clear signs of pathology; twin studies on epilepsy abound with examples. Other, less conspicuous examples are discussed below in the context of EEG records of aging twin pairs. In the twin pair described here, however, both twins had EEGs

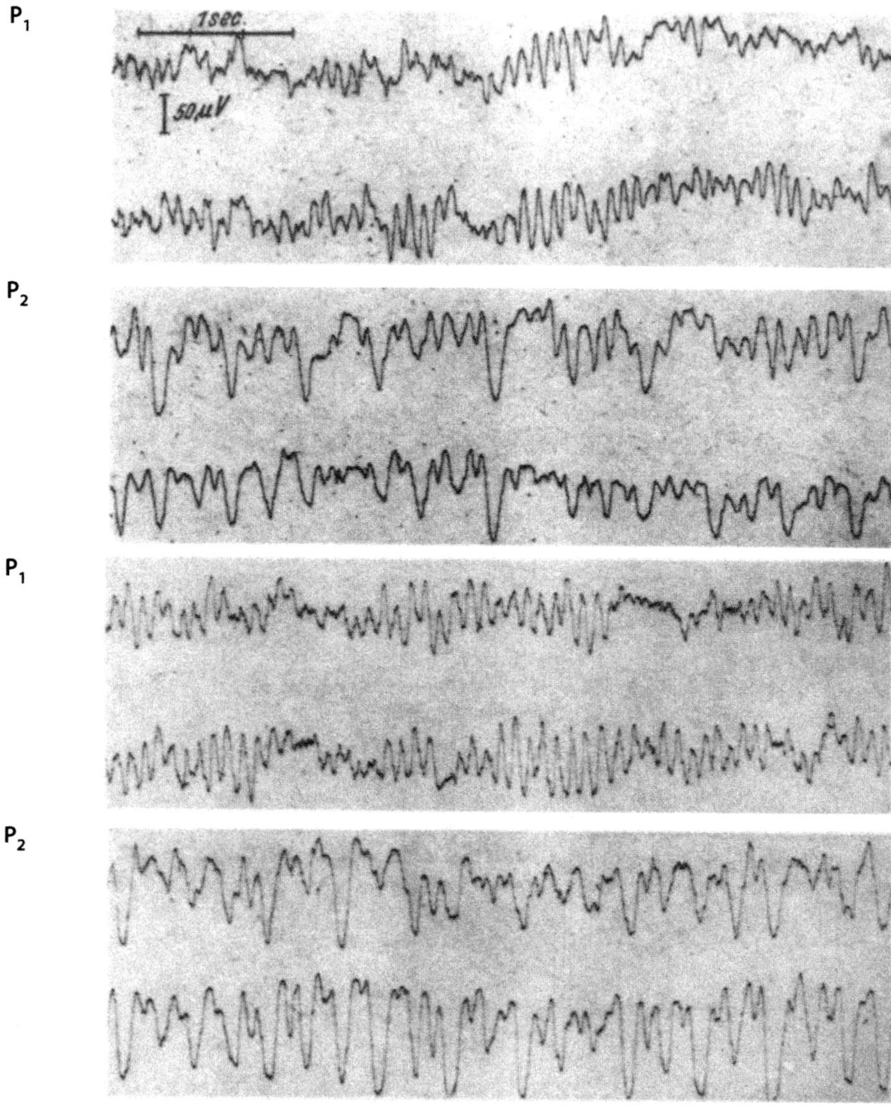

Fig. 3.6. An exception: occipital waves in a male MZ pair at the age of 11 (above) and 14 (below). There is a constant difference, twin 2 (P_2) showing a much slower and irregular activity. (From Vogel 1958)

classified as "normal" according to conventional criteria; clinically, there were no signs of clearcut brain damage. The EEG of one twin can be regarded as slightly more "immature" than that of his brother. Most likely, a small degree of brain damage may lead occasionally to a shift of the EEG record within the "normal" range. The classification into "normal," "borderline," and "abnormal" is conventional and based on statistical evidence. There may be exceptions, however.

2. The study by Lennox et al. (1945) had led to the tentative conclusion that EG records of MZ twins may be abnormal more often than record of singletons. This possibility was retested using the present twin series (Götze et al. 1958). The result was negative: Pathological results are not more common in EEGs from twins than in suitable controls.

Here, however, the age distribution of our twin series should be considered critically: In a study of 35 very young twin pairs – 17 MZ and 18 DZ – a high frequency of signs of early brain damage was reported (Keuth et al. 1965). In addition to various clinical signs, abnormal EEG results such as focal or general abnormalities, and even paroxysmal activities were described. Since all these deviations from the normal were observed much more often in the second-born than in the first-born twin, the authors regard temporary brain anoxia in the course of delivery as the main causative factor in addition to the fact that twins are often born prematurely. Unfortunately, they did not give a precise age distribution of twins at the time of examination. However, our twin series was certainly much older. A higher incidence of EEG abnormalities in 60 twins (8 MZ and 22 DZ pairs) as compared with singletons was also reported by Lipák et al. (1970) from Hungary. These twins were 5–17 years old at the time of the study. These authors also suspected frequent brain anoxia during delivery as a probable cause. Possible, there were differences in management of twin pregnancies and deliveries, or in survival of twins, between various populations. Another, and simpler, explanation may be that the twin series studied by Götze et al. was sampled in the general population, and parents having twins with clinical signs of brain damage may have refrained from volunteering in this study. The other series were ascertained in a clinical setting; they might be biased in the opposite direction: twin pairs in which at least one cotwin suffered from a certain degree of brain damage can be over-represented.

3. Raney et al. (1937, 1939) had described frequent mirror imaging in EEG records of MZ twins. This was tested using this twin sample, again with a negative result: There was neither a hint for mirror imaging, nor any correlation of EEG differences between left-hand and right-hand sides, and handedness. More recently, these problems were reexamined by Meshkova (1992) with refined methods of measurement, and in 20 MZ and 20 DZ pairs. There were intratwin pair differences in the degree of EEG asymmetry but among the MZ pairs, there was not even one "mirror" pair, i.e., opposite asymmetry of the EEG; despite the fact that there were pairs with opposite handedness. Moreover, there was no evidence of a genetic effect on intensity of EEG asymmetry.

3.4 The EEG in Aging Twins

As described in Sect. 2.8, the EEG shows certain changes with advancing age (see also Van Sweden et al. 1993). They may be caused internally, by a kind of "internal clock," being one of the signs of "biological aging", or be due to "exogenous" factors such as, for example, age-dependent vascular diseases. Studies on MZ twins may help in distinguishing between these possibilities. The study of Heuschert (1963a, b) tried to answer these questions.

He studied 26 MZ pairs at the age between 50 and 79 years – 20 females and 6 males (mean age: 64 years). In 23 pairs the EEG was repeated between 3 and 9 months later. In addition, standard intelligence tests were used to study any relations between EEG abnormalities and impairment of intelligence. The EEG records were evaluated with the methods described above (Sect. 3.3). The results can be summarized as follows:

- As in the studies on young twins, no significant pair differences were observed. The observed differences did not exceed those observed between different EEG recordings in the same individuals.
- Slowing of basic α rhythms, a certain lability of frequencies and β waves, often with a frontoprecentral maximum, were also concordant. However, α slowing – regarded as a common feature of the EEG in the aged (Sect. 2.8) – and a certain reduction in amplitudes were not present in all EEGs; some pairs were concordant having EEG patterns absolutely identical with those observed in young persons. Figure 3.7 shows as an example EEG recordings of the oldest pair; 79-year-old women.
- Borderline, and sometimes doubtful, nonparoxysmal and nonfocal abnormalities, mostly ϑ waves, were concordant as well, sometimes with slight differences in degree. Active dysrhythmic groups most of ϑ waves and focal abnormalities were clearly discordant. However, despite these differences, blind classification (see above, Sect. 3.3) was successful in almost all instances; only two pairs were confounded.
- In three pairs the EEG discordance could be explained easily by events in life history, such as apoplexy, suspected encephalomalacia disseminata, or general deterioration of unknown reason in one twin. In some instances, however, no clinical explanation for slight EEG differences between twin partners could be discovered. On the other hand, some clearly discordant life events in only one twin such as commotio cerebri, a progredient cancer of the gall bladder, and even an apoplexy did not leave traces in the EEG.

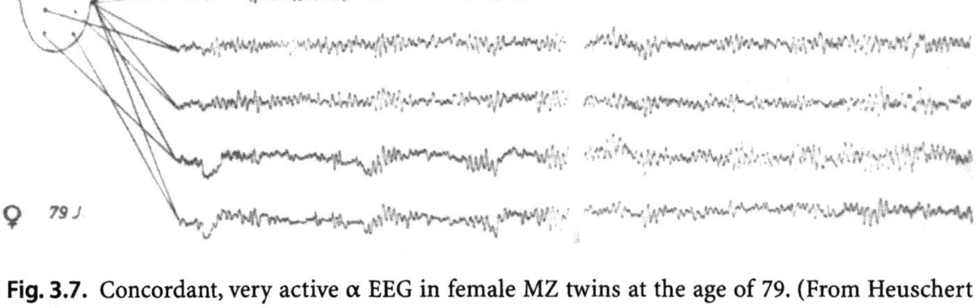

Fig. 3.7. Concordant, very active α EEG in female MZ twins at the age of 79. (From Heuschert 1963)

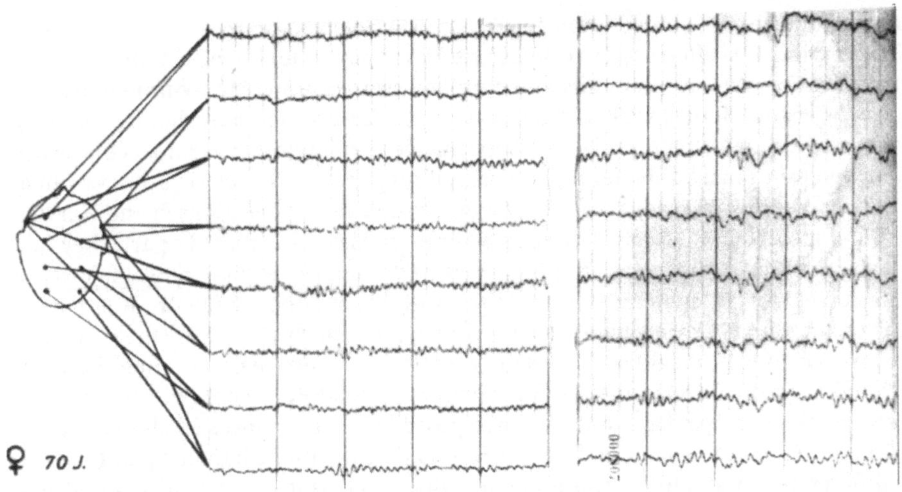

Fig. 3.8. Discordance in the EEG of one of 70-year-old MZ sisters. The EEG on the right hand side shows slightly irregular activity with theta waves mainly in the left parieto-temporal area

- Discordant EEG results such as dysrhythmic groups or focal abnormalities failed to show any relationship with differences in test performance; sometimes, the twin showing no such anomalies had the better test result, in other instances, the affected twin was the better one. As a rule, test results were related more with aspects of life history, especially intellectual challenge, than with slight organic brain anomalies. Figure 3.8 gives one characteristic example: The twin sisters were 70 years old at the time of the study. Twin II showed a temporal focus and after hyperventilation, a paroxysmal dysrhythmia, while twin I failed to have an EEG anomaly. Even in young age, twin II was regarded as the cleverer one. She remained unmarried and later became secretary of manager in a large company. Twin I became a housewife, did not have children. They had an IQ difference of 21 points, the greatest difference found in any twin pair. However, twin II, who showed the EEG anomalies, was the better one! Life-long intellectual challenge has a stronger effect on mental performance at advanced age than minor brain damage.

3.5 Studies on Twins Reared Apart

A common argument against straightforward genetic interpretation of twin studies, and, especially, of similarities in MZ twins is the following: Twins have not only their genetic endowment in common; they also share most of their environment, especially during the formative years of childhood and youth. The commonly used argument that this applies to DZ twins as well is said to be not entirely true: Because of the phenotypic likeness MZ twins may share much more of their environment than DZ twins do. Therefore similarities between them in the parameters to be studied may be due not to their common genes but to parallel effects from the environment. This argument is often used to criticize studies in psychological or psychiatric genetics. There is one way out of this dilemma, however: examine MZ twins reared apart (see Vogel and Motulsky 1996). Such twins are, of course, very rare, but it is possible to find them, and their study has helped in confirming other results achieved by more conventional twin studies, for example, in genetic research on schizophrenia.

The first EEG twin study of this kind was published by Juel-Nielsen and Harvald (1958). Juel-Nielsen (1965) described a series of MZ twins reared apart; they had been separated a short time after birth and, as the authors wrote, "in the majority of cases, the twin partners were not reunited until in adult life, frequently after having experienced very varied modes of life which had widely separated them socially from each other." In eight of these pairs, six female and two male, age range between 22 and 72 years, EEG studies were performed. Again, EEG records of cotwins were largely identical, blind classification was possible in all instances (Juel-Nielsen and Harvald 1958). A few smaller differences should be mentioned: In one pair (age 46), a difference in α amplitude was found for which no reason could be discovered; one cotwin only of a 37-year-old pair showed an isolated series of 6 c/s activity in frontal leads, also without an obvious reason. In another pair, both twins showed small 8 c/s paroxysms; one of them had just finished recently a series of electroconvulsive treatments. On the other hand, none of the twins studied had ever suffered from any kind of epileptic seizures, except for one 22-year-old man, who had suffered from febrile convulsions and enuresis in infancy. Interesting enough, this twin pair was concordant in that occipital a waves were replaced by 5 c/s waves (α equivalents?). The authors did not comment this observation specifically; this EEG variant is discussed in greater detail in Sect. 4.6.

Another series of MZ twins reared apart has been, and is still being, studied in Minnesota. The EEGs were reevaluated together with a team in Zürich which used a method of computerized EEG evaluation (Lykken et al. 1982; Stassen et al. 1988). This study is discussed together with other, more recent twin studies in which methods of computerized EEG analysis were used.

3.6 Alpha Attenuation Response

The EEG and, especially, the a rhythm reacts to sensory effects by attenuation. The best known way to show this is a blocking ("off effect") when the eyes are opened. This had already been discovered by H. Berger. A way for quantifying this effect is photic stimulation by serial light flashes. Such an experiment was performed by Young et al. (1972) in 17 MZ pairs (mean age 28 years) and 15 DZ pairs (mean age 27 years). age range 19–40 years. Again, high intraclass correlations were found between cotwins of MZ pairs while correlations of DZ pairs were much lower (but still higher than between suitable matched pairs of unrelated individuals). The results confirm the hypothesis that phenotypic variation in the α attenuation response is also largely determined by genetic variation. The authors also studied visually evoked EEG potentials; these results are discussed below (Chap. 5).

3.7 More Recent Twin Studies in Which Methods of Computerized EEG Analysis Are Used

The twin studies discussed above were performed using more conventional methods of EEG evaluation including relatively primitive methods of measurement. They also date back several years. During recent decades, however, methods for automatic and computer-aided EEG evaluation have developed (see Niedermeyer and Lopes da Silva 1993). To put it in somewhat oversimplified terms, two different ways have been tried: In one – and a more common – approach, the entire "EEG power" in a certain frequency range is determined. This power is a product of the number of waves and their amplitudes; "power spectra" cover the entire range of frequencies occurring in a specific EEG. The second approach is the "time-domain analysis." Here, the number of waves within a certain frequency range is scored; their amplitudes are determined separately. Both methods can be applied to recordings from various parts of the brain, and secondary parameters such as the "coherence," for example, between homologous leads of the two sides of the brain, or between frontal and occipital leads can be determined. For applying any of these methods, however, it is necessary to take the EEG information on tape. This registering on tape should be controlled visually, especially for the very common artifacts, and these artifacts should be marked on the tapes to avoid their erroneous evaluation as EEG potentials. In addition to these relatively simple approaches, more sophisticated methods were developed. These methods were also used in twin studies, in the hope of getting more detailed information on the ways in which genetic factors, on the one hand, and external (as well as other, internal) factors may modify the EEG. The problem to be solved in such studies was set out by Stassen et al. (1988) as follows:

> EEG time series are characterized by considerable fluctuation concerning not only the distribution of amplitudes but also the 'mixture' of spectral components. Hence the key goal of a genetic approach to EEG analysis is to decompose the information contained in the human EEG into a static component representing the individual EEG characteristics of a person and to a dynamic component reflecting reactive changes in EEG due, for example, to the immediate environment of a person or to longer persisting processes. ... Moreover ..., one had to determine (1) the 'typical'" coincidence of brainwave patterns between unrelated individuals and, (2) the typical intraindividual stability ... over time.

Probably the first study in which a computerized method of frequency analysis was used was that of Dumermuth (1968). It was the main purpose of this study to help solving the problem of quantification of EEG background activity in childhood. The method used was computation of power spectra; it has been described in detail in that report. The study was performed in seven MZ pairs, five female and two male, between the ages of 9 years, 7 months, and 22 years, 5 months, and four DZ pairs, two female and two male/female, between the ages of 10 months and 12 years, 8 months. With one exception, the MZ pairs showed almost identical records, while the members of the DZ pairs showed a high degree of individuality. In the one discordant MZ (12 years, 5 months, old), one twin presented a sharp wave focus over the midcentral region; this twin also had a slightly lower maximum of α frequency. He did not have any clinical signs of epilepsy but a brother of this pair is an epileptic with generalized spikewave paroxysms in his EEG. Both twins showed "a stable high intensity of α rhythm"; from the picture, it is well possible that they had the EEG variant called by us "monomorphic α waves." As is shown below, this variant is also found fairly often in parents of children with spike-wave complexes (Doose 1995; see also Sect. 4.7). These twins may merely have been at the limit of a spike-wave EEG, with one of them just tipping over. In this twin pair a follow-up study would have been interesting.

In the following we show first how "time-domain analysis" was used in 26 MZ and 26 DZ pairs, young healthy male adults (mean age 23–24 years). This study was planned to explore possible genetic effects on the EEG of a moderate alcohol dose (1.2 ml/kg). The EEG was recorded before, and 60, 120, 180 and 240 min after the beginning of drinking. In addition, at least 2 min of reference recording were stored on tape which was then analyzed by a program for time-domain analysis (Smith et al. 1973). Furthermore, to test intraindividual variability, 13 male volunteers were subjected to the same procedure with the only difference that the investigation in the cotwin was replaced by repetition of the experiment in the same individual (time distance: at least 8 weeks).

The program allowed for quantification of the following parameters: The numbers of EEG waves and their distribution over the usual frequency classes (β: 14–30 c/s; α: 8–13 c/s; ϑ: 4–7.5 c/s; δ: 0.5–3.5 c/s) for a time period of 120 s, distribution of amplitudes (classes: 0–20 μV; 20–40 μV; 40–100 μV; 100–200 μV). In addition, mean frequencies and mean amplitudes were calculated. Statistical comparisons were performed using methods of nonparametric statistics. Figure 3.9 shows differences between left-hand and right-hand sides between twin pairs and between repeated studies of the same individuals for numbers of various waves and for mean frequencies.

Figures 3.9, 3.10 present mean amplitudes for the various wave categories and their overall average. The result on the resting EEG can be summarized as follows:

- Number and frequencies of the EEG waves of the resting EEG are no more different in MZ twins than in repeated studies of the same individuals; a small difference in number of ϑ waves is not significant. There is also a small (not significant) difference between mean amplitudes of MZ twins and repetitions in the same person. This latter result confirms an observation by Vogel (1958); as noted above, this may be due to a difference in shape of skull and brain (Steinmetz et al. 1994).
- Differences between DZ twins were much larger in all parameters tested than in MZ twins and its repetitions of the same individual. This confirms conclusions from earlier studies.
- There were small but fairly consistent differences between left-hand and right-hand sides in the same individuals; they confirmed other studies and are not discussed further.
- As noted above, this study was performed to investigate genetic variation in the influence of alcohol on the EEG. The results were the following: on the average, alcohol led to a better synchronization of the EEG; the number of β waves decreased while the number of α and ϑ waves increased. However, the extent of

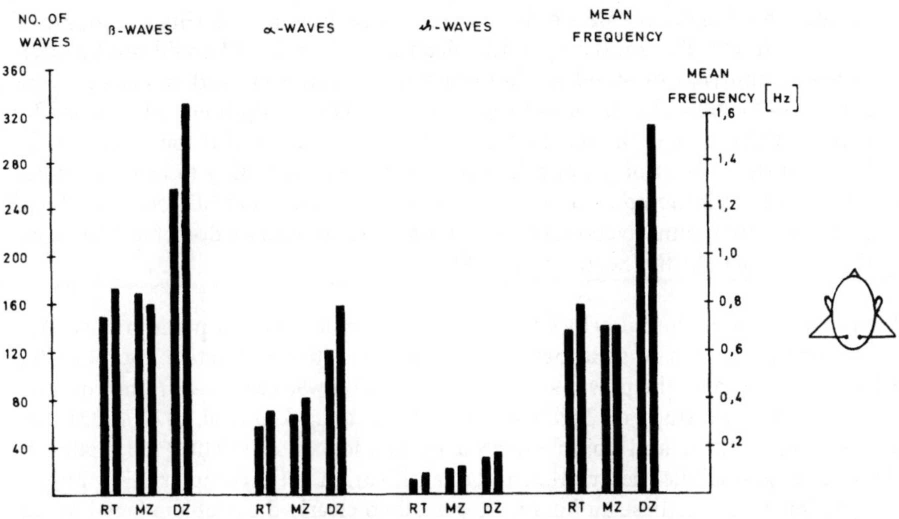

Fig. 3.9. Mean intrapair differences in mean amplitudes of beta, alpha, and theta waves and in mean frequency in the resting EEG in MZ and DZ twins and in repetitive tests in the same subjects *(RT)*. Left *(left columns)* and right *(right columns)* unipolar occipital leads. (From Propping 1977)

the alcohol effect varied enormously between individuals: it was especially strong in persons whose α rhythm in the resting EEG was slightly irregular and not very continuous. In a few other individuals, β activity increased after alcohol intake. Reaction of MZ twins was absolutely identical; their EEGs even showed a tendency to become still more similar under the influence of alcohol. DZ twins,

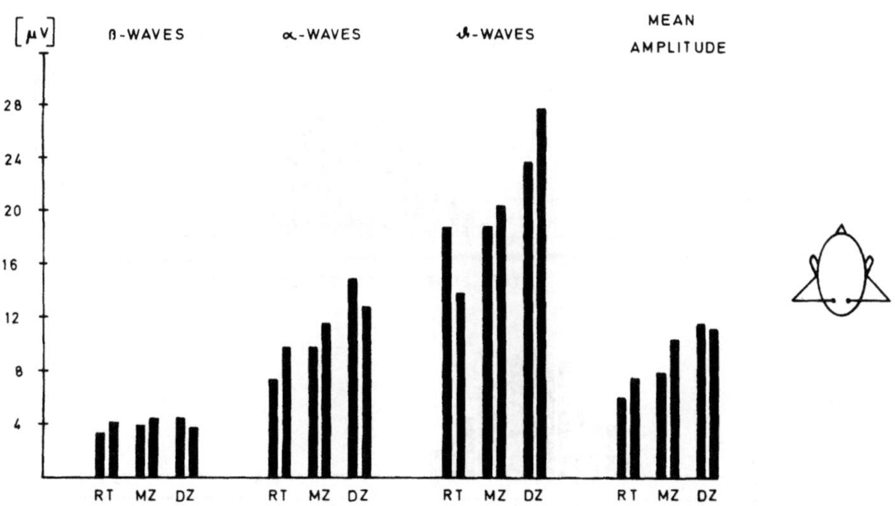

Fig. 3.10. Mean intrapair differences in mean amplitudes of beta, alpha, and theta waves and of overall mean amplitude in the resting EEG in MZ and DZ twins and in repetitive tests in the same. (From Propping 1977)

> on the other hand, became, on the average, more dissimilar during the course of the experiment. The similarity of the alcohol reaction in MZ could not be attributed to similarity of blood alcohol levels which had been studied before in the same twin sample (Kopun and Propping 1977). Obviously, they were caused by genetic differences in the reaction of the brain to alcohol. This topic is taken up below in the context of genetic factors affecting susceptibility to alcohol addiction. However, it should be noted that the latter findings, that EEG records of MZ twins tend to become even more similar after a small alcohol dose, has been confirmed more recently (Sorbel et al. 1996).

As discussed above, the study by Propping (1977) employed a computer program for time-domain analysis was. Sorbel et al. (1996) used the alternative approach for EEG quantification – the power spectra. This method was also used in the comprehensive Minnesota study on MZ twins reared apart (Lykken et al. 1974, 1982). The method was refined and complemented by Stassen et al. (1980, 1985, 1987a, b, 1988a, b) to give a fuller description and quantification of the complex EEG pattern. As mentioned above, these authors have described clearly the problem faced by the investigator. They developed such a method and first applied it in a sample of 81 healthy individuals: First, EEG curves were measured and analyzed in certain frequency bands, according to the principles of Fourier analysis. The resulting equations were then modified by attributing weights to these classes; the weights were chosen in a way that intraindividual similarities were optimized mathematically so that optimal intraindividual patterns were created, i.e., the parameters were weighted in a way that optimal distinction between individuals and computerized recognition of individuals become possible. In the 81 normal healthy individuals

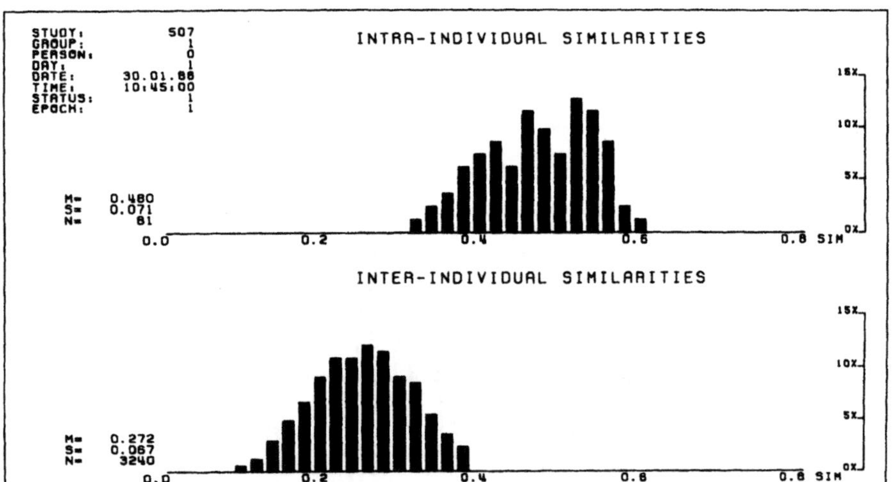

Fig. 3.11. Distribution of similarity indices at repeated studies of the same individuals (*above;* 81 subjects) and, for comparison, similarity indices found by comparison between (unrelated) individuals. (From Stassen et al. 1988)

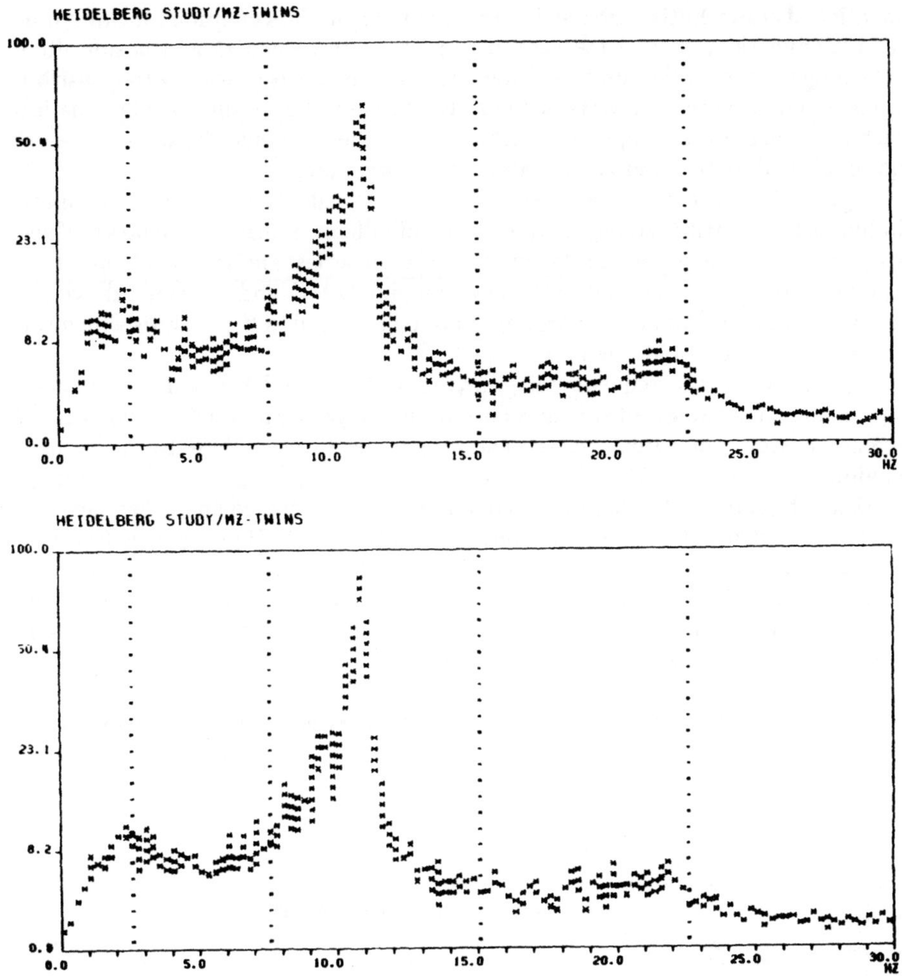

Fig. 3.12. Spectral intensities for various frequency bands in a male MZ pair, 19 years old, brought up together. *Vertical axes*, the spectral intensities are plotted on log proportional scales. Obviously, the two patterns are very similar. (From Stassen et al. 1988)

mentioned above, EEGs were recorded twice under similar conditions, the first time as a "design sample," and the second time as a "test sample," and optimization "learning process of the computer" was to lead to as few as possible wrong attributions. To put it more simply, Stassen et al. tried to repeat by a suitable mathematical technique, using the computer, to achieve what the "computer between the ears" accomplished in the blind-classification experiment (Sect. 3.3).

Figures 3.11 shows the similarity coefficients calculated in this way, intra-individual similarities (above) and inter-individual similarities (below). These similarities were now used in the analysis of twin series. The sample of adult twin pairs reared together was that studied by Propping (1977), and described above. For technical reasons, two of the pairs could not be included in the analysis which was therefore based on 24 MZ pairs.

Figure 3.12 shows frequency diagrams in a 19-year-old MZ pair; the diagram shows how many points of the (axis have been analyzed. The y axis shows spectral intensities (log proportional scale). The similarities between these two patterns is obvious.

Using the same method, the series of adult twin pairs reared apart that had been studied by Lykken et al. (1982) was reexamined (Fig. 3.13). Here again, within-pair similarity was very high; there was no difference to the result on MZ twins reared together. DZ pairs, on the other hand, were only slightly, but significantly more similar than unrelated individuals (Fig. 3.14 gives one example). The results were summarized as follows:

- There exists an almost perfect one-to-one mapping between each individual and its EEG.

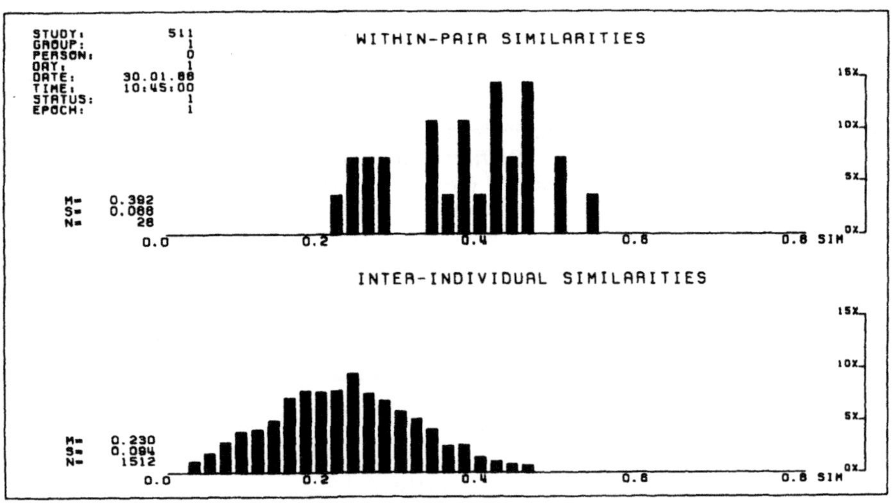

Fig. 3.13. Similarity indices computed in the same way as in Fig. 3.11 for 28 MZ pairs reared apart (Minnesota study). Within-pair similarities above; intraindividual similarities below. Twenty-four MZ pairs reared together have a very similar picture. (From Stassen et al. 1988)

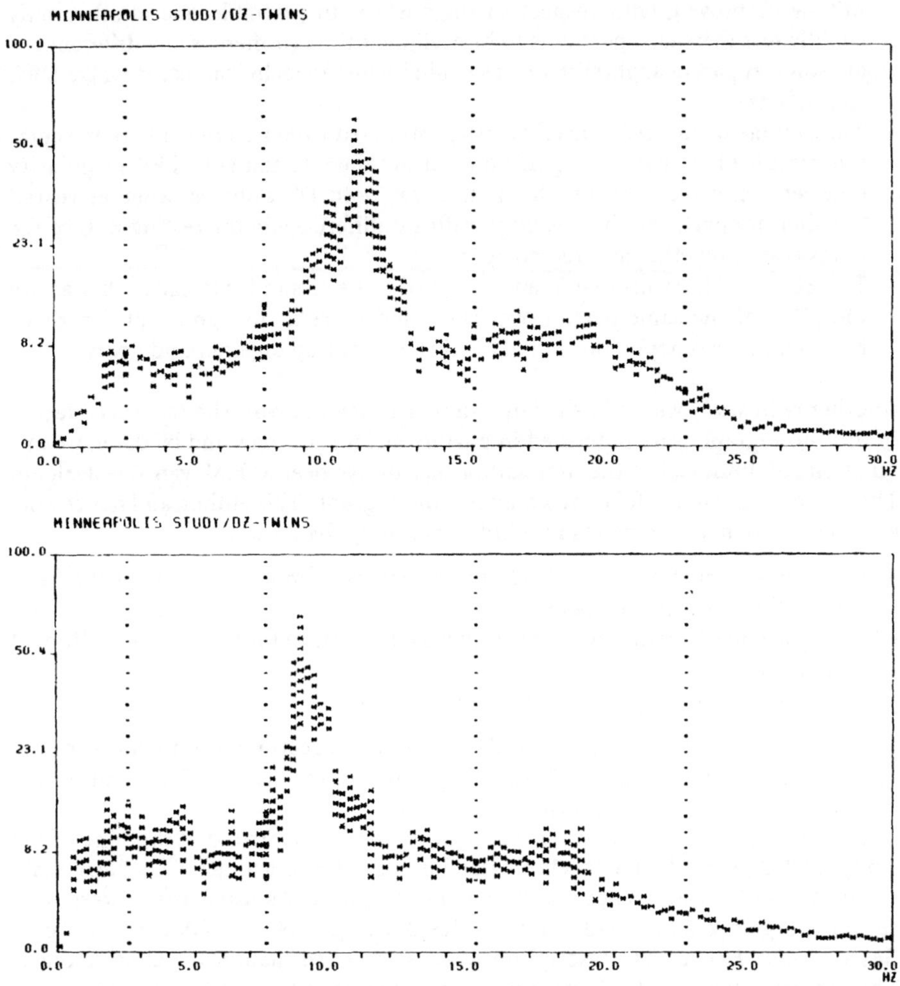

Fig. 3.14. Pair of DZ female twins, 39 years old, brought up apart. *Vertical axes,* spectral intensities plotted on log proportional scales (as in Fig. 3.12). The two patterns are much less similar than those shown in the MZ twins in Fig. 3.12. For example, the frequency of a waves is much higher in twin I *(above)* than in twin II *(below).* (From Stassen et al. 1988)

- MZ twins proved, with respect to their EEGs, to resemble one another only slightly less than each person is to himself over time (if there is any difference at all; some apparent slight differences could be due to technical disturbances such as artifacts).
- The average within-pair EEG similarity estimated from a sufficiently representative sample of DZ twins is significantly above the interindividual EEG similarity between unrelated persons; this is true for both DZ samples, whether reared together or apart, and there is no significant difference in the resting EEG of DZ twins reared together and reared apart.
- The EEGs of MZ twins reared apart proved to be as similar to each other as are the EEGs of the same person over time, and there is no significant difference between the two populations of MZ twins brought up together and apart.

Another twin study was published by van Beijsterfeldt (1996). The reports collected in this monograph were published in part in various journals and by diverse combinations of authors, but the first author has always been C.E.M. van Beijsterfeldt. Therefore we cite in the following only this monograph. This author, and her coworkers, had three main problems in mind in planning their studies:

- Estimating heritabilities for EEG power spectra in more locations of the head surface than investigated before.
- Studying coherence of EEG patterns in various parts of the brain as an additional parameter.
- Examining the P300 peak of the evoked potential.

In the following report only the studies on power spectra and on coherence are reviewed; discussion of the P300 study is postponed to Sect. 5.2. The details of the first two studies were the following:

A sample of 207 twin pairs was studied; all were 16 years old at the time of the study (of 213 pairs 6 had to be eliminated because of EEG artifacts). Fourteen scalp electrodes and two reference ear electrodes were used. As usual, the powers were summed together into broad bands: δ (1.5–3.5 c/s), ϑ (4–7.5 c/s), α (8–12.5 c/s), β (13–25 c/s). Hence EEG description was less detailed than in the above studies. The sophisticated statistical analysis using concepts of biometric genetics are not repeated here; suffice it to say that heritabilities were calculated. In addition, two hypotheses were tested: (a) Are the right and left hemispheres affected by common genetic factors, or is an additional, hemisphere-specific factor needed? (b) Is there an environmental covariance between the hemispheres? Figure 3.15 shows the electrode locations and mean distribution of powers.

The heritabilities averaged over all brain areas were: δ 76%; ϑ 89%; α 89% and β 86%. Unfortunately, they could not be compared with reliabilities estimated by repetition of EEG examinations within shorter times. However, the authors, comparing their result with that of other authors on test-retest reliability of power-spectra, came to the conclusion that "the high reliabilities and MZ correlations approach the test-retest reliability normally found for EEG powers in adult subjects. … Thus, the similarity of the EEG in a twin pair should equal the EEG similarity within a subject measured on different days."

This conclusion confirms those of earlier studies that the overall EEG similarity between young and healthy MZ twins is comparable with similarity between

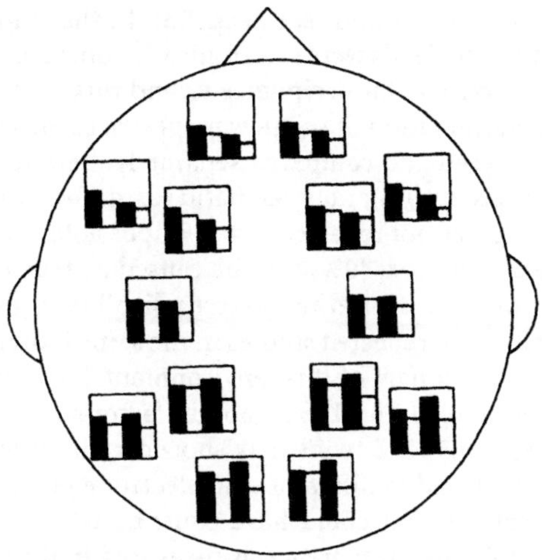

Fig. 3.15. Mean value for absolute power (log-transformed) for all electrode locations on both hemispheres (mean values for all four EEG frequency bands). (From van Beijsterfeldt 1996)

different recordings of the same individuals in the same conditions. The question that was raised in earlier studies whether there is a small but reproducible difference between MZ cotwins in amplitude cannot be answered since the method of evaluation used (power spectra) does not permit a decision. However, the study provided interesting information on EEG similarity in dizygotic (DZ) twins; their series comprised 122 DZ pairs. DZ twins are genetically no more similar than sibs born at different times; they have, on the average, 50% of their genes in common by descent. Theoretically their EEGs should therefore be much more similar than those of nonrelated persons of the same age and sex. Lykken et al. (1974), however, whose results in MZ twins regarding EEG power spectra were very similar to those of van Beijsterfeldt, obtained correlations of close to 0 regarding EEG power in 27 DZ pairs; van Beijsterfeldt et al., on the other hand, estimated correlations of about 0.5 in 122 DZ pairs. They assume that the difference is caused by the fact that Lykken et al. examined their twins after hypnosis. The present author would not put too much weight on this difference: Correlations and heritability estimates based on family data presume a continuous, and close to normal, variation in the parameters on which these estimates are founded. However, some of the EEG characteristics used for heritability estimates are not distributed at all normally and often not even continuously. There are quite a few – not very common but not really rare – EEG variants that show a clearcut alternative distribution (= a specific variant present: yes or no). Depending on presence or absence of such variants, (and due to different age distributions in the two series of DZ twins – remember, for example, the increase in β waves with advancing age) – correlations between DZ cotwins may differ quite substantially.

Another interesting parameter studied by van Beijsterfeldt et al. (1997) in their twin sample was coherence. EEG coherence measures the covariation between two electrode locations as a function of frequency; it is used to study the electrophysiological coupling between cortical regions. One aspect of coherence – phase coordination of EEG waves from left-hand and right-hand sides of the brain – was studied as early as 1958 by Vogel, albeit not electronically, but manually, with a self-constructed planimeter. High concordances regarding the degree of phase coordinations were found (see Sect. 3.3). In the study referred to here, power spectra from different leads were electronically compared; for example, frontalprecentral, frontal-central, frontal-occipital, etc., and this on both sides separately as described for the determination of the power spectra themselves. Frequency ranges from δ to β were analyzed and compared separately; heritabilities were high but not extremely high (approx. 60%); no systematic sex difference could be discovered: Since EEG recording was not repeated, it was impossible to decide which part of the remaining variance (approx. 40%) may be caused by true nongenetic variance, and which one was caused by a lower test-retest reliability of the coherence measure. Citing some literature on repeated studies in the same individuals, the authors surmised that at least the main part of this "environmental variance" may indeed be due to a lower test-retest reliability. Here, another factor should also be considered: As discussed above (Sect. 3.3) MZ twins may show certain differences in the shape of their skulls; this might lead to differences in electrode placement in relation to the underlying brain portions that could have contributed to slight but consistent differences in EEG amplitudes. Coherence as measured in the way described above may be affected by this factor.

As stated by the authors themselves, "coherence is probably a relatively rough measure of neural connectivity." For example, it does not permit, at least directly, comparison of phases of single waves. Moreover, the research design, in which the two sides were analyzed directly does not permit any conclusions regarding coherence of the two sides of the brain, much less about phase relationships. Some authors have studied EEG and left-right interhemispheric coherences in twins at the ages between approx. 5–7 years (Ibatoulinna et al. 1994; van Baal 1997).

The study of van Baal (1997) is performed by the same group that also examined the above series of 16-year-old adolescents. However, this time, children at the age of 5 years, 209 twin pairs overall, were studied; to examine brain development as manifested by the EEG, it is planned to repeat this study 18 months later. The method of the EEG recording was identical with that used in the other study; heritability in the α band was, again, high (around 80%); heritabilities in the δ and ϑ bands were lower. In general, heritabilities in this series tended to be somewhat lower than in the series of 16-year-old adolescents. Heritabilities for absolute and relative power decreased from posterior to anterior leads. Unfortunately, in this study, again, no repetitions of EEG recordings were carried out during the weeks after the first studies; therefore it cannot be decided definitely whether these heritabilities exceed reliabilities of EEG recordings at this age, despite the fact that split-half reliabilities were calculated (first half against second half of an α band at the same recording) and were found to be very high. It is well known, however, that EEG recordings of children often show irregularities and intermixture of slower potentials especially in anterior leads. Many of them are biologically real – signs of brain immaturity. However, often it is not easy to distinguish them from artifacts, for example, due to eye movements. The authors themselves remark that among the "environmental" factors that may have affected the frequency of slow waves especially in anterior leads, drowsiness in some children may have played a certain role. It is unfortunate that, in this study, the chance of looking for and recognizing, true and constant differences between the EEGs of very young MZ twins was not used. As noted above, MZ twins may show definite differences at birth (see also Vogel and Motulsky 1996) that are caused by special conditions during embryonic and fetal development of twins. It is also known that average intellectual development of twins, especially MZ twins, may lag behind during the first years of life. Moreover, certain studies suggest that MZ twins might sometimes show a higher frequency of abnormal EEG pattern than singletons. This should be taken seriously even if these studies did not use entirely unbiased samples.

Studies on EEG coherence (see above) were performed on 167 twin pairs of the same series (70 MZ; 97 DZ); heritabilities varied from 30% to 71% with a mean heritability of 49%. These values tend to be lower than those found in 16-year-old sample; this difference is difficult to explain, especially if the special biological conditions of early development of MZ twins, as well as the problems of EEG recordings in very young children are considered.

EEG power spectra in newborn twins in active (REM) and quiet sleep were reported by Nolte et al.(1968). There were eight twin pairs and one set of triplets. Birth weight of these twins ranged between 850 and 2700 g; some of these pairs showed enormous intrapair differences in body weight. All twins were studies within 4 days after birth, the triplets within the first 8 days. This report did not give any information on zygosity; obviously the main purpose was getting information on a special group of mostly prematurely born children. Power spectra showed a progressive change with increasing conceptual age; at 31-32 weeks the *tracé alternant* pattern in quiet sleep was characterized by complete blackout between bursts; with increasing age, the periods of reduced activity were replaced gradually by ϑ and δ waves. In active sleep, however, at 31–32 weeks, high amplitude slow waves were present, superimposed with rapid activity. It is a pity that zygosity does not seem to have been determined; again, any possible differences between MZ twins, especially those with different birth weight, would have been of great interest.

3.8 Specific Problems To Be Studied by Comparison of Twins

Comparison of twins, especially the MZ twins, can be used for solving a variety of other problems, in addition to the traditional question to what extent interindividual variation in a certain parameter is caused by genetic factors. For example, MZ twins are ideal controls in experimental designs: If certain experiments are performed in one twin, the other one can be used as the ideal control. In this way "nuisance" variation which often makes case-control studies so difficult, can be avoided most efficiently. Typical problems are effects of certain drugs in clinical pharmacology or efficiency of educational techniques in developmental psychology (= method of cotwin control, first proposed by Gesell and Thompson in 1929; see also Vogel and Motulsky 1996).

In the twin studies discussed in the preceding chapters, especially in those referring to aged twins, pairs were described in which one twin had suffered some brain pathology or, for example, electroconvulsive therapy before, while the other one had remained unaffected. In a few instances, the EEG of the affected twin showed deviations from the cotwin that could be related to this event, in other instances, this was not the case. A common diagnostic problem in many EEG laboratories is posed by the possible late effects of head accidents leading to commotion or concussion of the brain. Here, the EEG is often used to help in the decision whether certain complaints are related to such an accident; this decision may have legal and financial consequences. If major focal abnormalities are present, this question can be answered easily. In some instances, however, only minor abnormalities are found, or the EEG shows nothing defininitely "abnormal" by conventional criteria. Here, studying twin pairs in which one cotwin only had suffered such an accident may help in solving the problem of possible, subtle long-time EEG changes.

Dencker (1958) had published a comprehensive study of 128 closed head injuries in twins, in which unaffected cotwins were used as controls. In 28 cases, 19 male and 9 female, who had suffered closed head injuries and in their uninjured cotwins, a follow-up EEG study was performed (Dencker 1958; Sulg and Dencker 1968). At the time of this follow-up, the ages varied from 10 to 55 years; the injured twins were reexamined 2–25 years after their accidents. EEGs were classified visually, but a detailed scoring system for severity of head injuries and for EEG description was used. The most important results were:

- There was a high rate of concordance between injured twins and their uninjured partner. In 22 our of 28 pairs, the twins had practically identical EEGs; in 16 of them, no abnormal findings were observed, while 2 pairs had slightly abnormal, and 4 pairs moderately abnormal records.
- The probands showed, on the average, a slightly more pronounced tendency toward slightly pathological aberrations than their cotwins. However, in some instances, the uninjured partner had a higher abnormality score than the injured one. Unfortunately, the reports give very little details on the specific kind of differences that could be attributed to the accident. In one case, however, for which EEG curves were shown, the proband who had been injured 2 years before relatively mildly, showed lower frequency, more asymmetry in background activity and more paroxysmal discharges. However, this twin probably suffered also from a birth injury, and was more "neurotic" and aggressive. This observation and other results from this study permit the more general conclusion that the examiner should be very cautious and should consider alternative possibilities, before peculiarities of the EEG, especially relatively subtle ones, can be related to a brain accident, especially with accidents dating back many years.

Here an own observation should be presented. During the twin study discussed above (Vogel 1958; Sect. 3.3), an 18-year-old male MZ pair was observed. One of the twins had suffered a relatively severe cerebral commotion in a motorcycle accident only a few days before his scheduled examination; when his EEG was taken, he was still hospitalized. The EEG was almost completely flat; no α or β waves were seen. Flattening of the α rhythm, generally for a short time, is known among EEG specialists as a sign of cerebral commotion or contusion. Hence the observer could have concluded that the brain damage was much more severe than the clinical picture seemed to show, had not the uninjured cotwin been examined at the same time. He proved to have an absolutely identical low-voltage EEG (Fig. 3.16). The diagnosis of this EEG variant was later confirmed in both twins, when they were restudied together with their family.

Here, a legal problem should be noted, in which the present author was asked for his expert opinion by a social court *(Sozialgericht)*. This case has not been published so far. A 12-year-old girl suffered a severe traffic accident which led to incon-

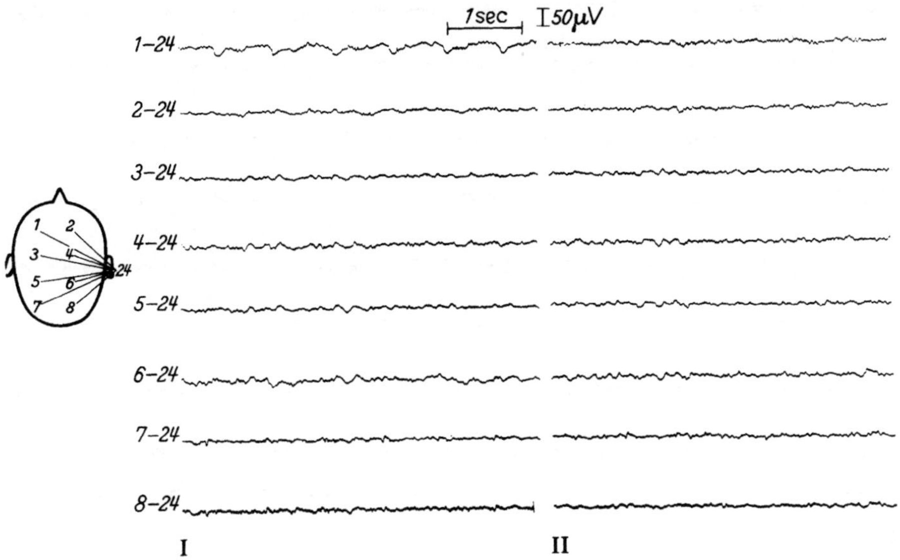

Fig. 3.16. Low-voltage EEG in a male, 18-year-old twin pair. (Own observation)

ciousness, apallic syndrome and tetraplegia for several weeks. In later years the girl recovered up to a certain degree but remained wheelchair-bound and, at the age of 24, suffered from cerebral signs such as impairment of short-time memory; her IQ (Raven test) was average. The EEG which had been severely pathological after the accident still showed frequent generalized groups of ϑ and, in part, δ waves which were especially strong at the right-hand side in temporal and parietal leads (Fig. 3.17). The proband was again able to work half a day, carrying out simple office work (such as feeding data into the computer). At noon, she was exhausted. As with all school children, she was insured for accidents on her way to school. The insurance company agreed to pay an annuity that would cover the income difference between her half-day job and a full-day employment of the same lowly kind. The young woman asked for a higher annuity, asserting that, without this accident, she would have been able to obtain a better education and to take a job with a much higher salary. To prove this she pointed to her MZ cotwin who had finished highschool, college and a business school, got a diploma as a trained social worker (comparable to a MA degree), and held a well-paid position. Examination of the two sisters had the following results: Both showed closely parallel development up to the accident; they had very good grades in school. Development of the unaffected sister later proceeded undisturbed; her decision to become a social worker was affected by the fate of the cotwin. Psychological tests had an excellent result; in the Raven, she scored better than 98% of the standard population. Her background EEG, with slight irregular α activity, looked similar to the background EEG of her injured sister but she did not have a group of ϑ and δ waves. In my expert statement I wrote that, without the accident, the injured woman would very probably have been quite as successful as her cotwin. The observed differences were clearly caused by the accident. The court decided, and the insurance company agreed, that financial compensation for the victim used the cotwin's achievement as criterion. Similar situations are not so

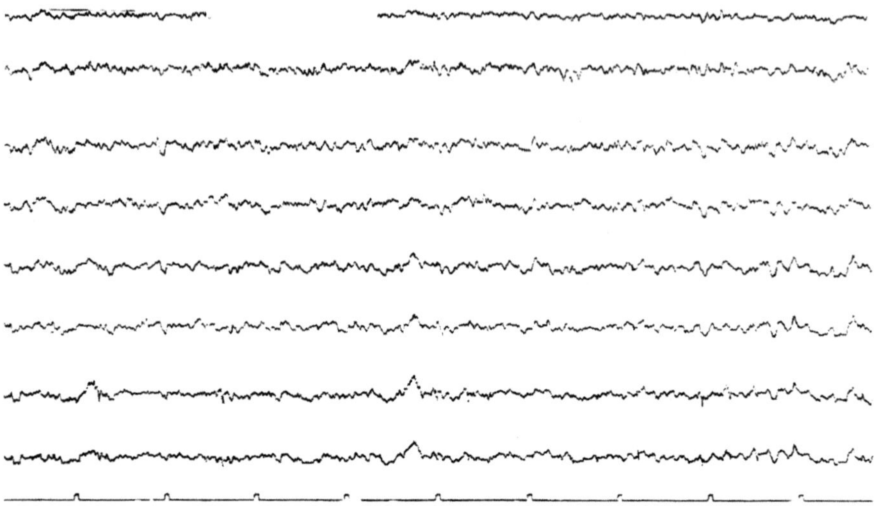

I

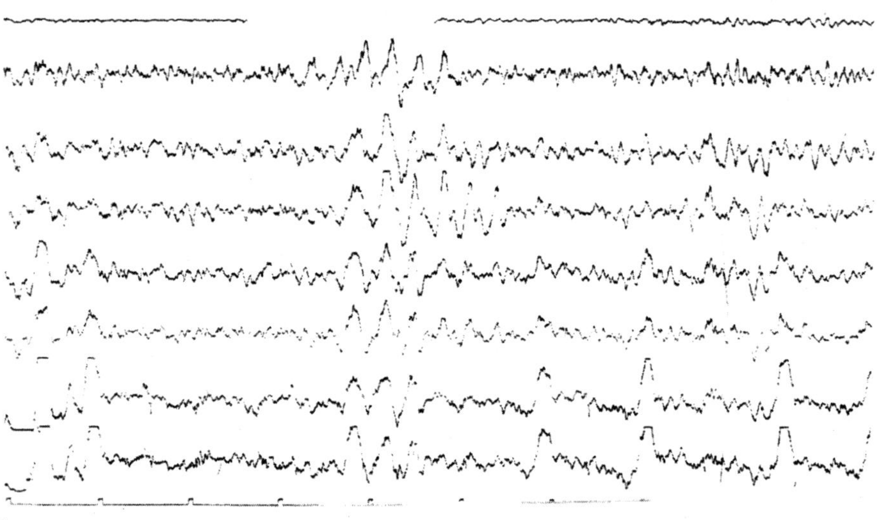

II

Fig. 3.17. Female MZ twin pair at the age of 24. Twin II had a severe traffic accident at the age of 12. She is still suffering from a variety of neurological symptoms. For details see the text. (Own observation)

rare; lawyers should use comparisons with MZ cotwins much more often in the rightful interest of their clients.

A brain trauma in one of a pair of MZ twins is one discordant, environmental difference in the life history that could lead to a permanent difference in EEGs of twins. Being reared separately in different familial environments may cause another kind of permanent difference – often not spectacular but, in the long run, effective. However, even when twins have lived together in the same families, and under, at least superficially, similar effects from the same family members, they might show definite and permanent differences in aspects of their personalities; psychodynamic reasons for such differences can sometimes be found when the psychosocial "microclimate" in such families is analyzed in a subtle way (Schepank 1974, 1996). Such "analysis of discordance" of MZ twins is an efficient method for studying the interplay between genetic and environmental factors in normal and in abnormal human development.

As shown by the above twin studies, and corroborated by those discussed in this section, the EEG normally represents an aspect of brain function that is, at the same time, very variable between individuals and strongly affected by genetic variation. Therefore it has been used to clarify relations between brain physiology and psychic functions – normal and abnormal. However, before possible relationships between EEG and aspects of intelligence and personality or mental performance in health and diseases are interpreted in a causal way, the question must be raised whether certain long-lasting psychological peculiarities may have an effect on the EEG. Such effects have, indeed, been observed for short time periods. For example, every EEG technician knows that, due to a certain psychological tension, α activity may be reduced when EEG recording begins; in some instances, this may even feign a low-voltage EEG. There are also some reports in the literature; Goldstein (1975), for example, in a longitudinal study of one proband, demonstrated a relationship between EEG amplitude and degree of anxiety. In many other reports, EEG changes during affective states are described (see, for example, Becker 1972). Here, however, we are interested mainly in possible permanent changes in the EEG, i.e., those that may have established themselves independently of the present state of mind.

Again, a way for testing this possibility is a study of EEGs in twins discordant for the personality aspect to be studied. If this aspect may affect the EEG for a longer time, at least partially discordant EEG patterns in MZ twins are expected. A group of psychic anomalies is diagnosed as "neurosis." These are long-lasting disturbances of the emotional life of the individual that, on the one hand, do not fulfill the criteria for a mental disease but, on the other hand, lead to so severe disturbances of individual life that the patient needs help from a trained psychotherapist.

A twin study on a large sample of twin pairs, one cotwin of which had been diagnosed as neurotic was performed by Schepank et al. (1974, 1996). The twin probands had been selected from a series of 26,799 patients seen in a clinic for psychotherapy between 1950 and 1969. The degree of neuroticism was defined by a specially devised score extending from 0 to 24 points. It was based on degree of somatic and psychic impairment; sociocommunicative impairment; vital hazard. From a much larger series of twin pairs, EEG studies were performed in 17 pairs of the same sex, 10 MZ and 7 DZ, between 12 and 63 years of age (Vogel et al. 1980). A visual comparison according to the customary clinical criteria showed, in MZ twins, again complete EEG concordance even in instances where neurotic development and life histories were extremely different. In addition, EEG records were evaluated using a – slightly refined – method of time domain-analysis used in another series of twins by Propping (1977). Concordance in all measurable parameters was as strong in the 10 neurotic (and, in part, psychologically discordant) MZ twin pairs, as in the 25 healthy MZ pairs studied by Propping. Among the DZ twins, the same degree of average EEG discordance was found, as in the control series of healthy DZ twins. Hence differences in development and severity of neurosis in MZ twins were not reflected in EEG differences that could be caused by this neurotic development. This does not mean, however, that certain EEG variants do not show any correlation with psychological anomalies commonly regarded as "neurotic". This problem is discussed in Chap. 6.

3.9 Conclusions from EEG Twin Studies

The comprehensive – and, with slight variations, often repeated EEG twin studies – allow the following conclusions:

- The interindividual differences of the normal resting EEG in children, adolescents and young adults are largely genetically determined as shown by practically identical records in MZ twins studied under identical conditions: The same result is found in MZ twins reared apart; therefore EEG identity in MZ twins cannot be caused by common environmental effects.
- This result is independent of the method of EEG evaluation, whether visual inspection, or various methods of measurement on paper records, or more sophisticated computer evaluations are used. As shown by the success of blind classification, similarity of EEG records in MZ twins goes beyond measurable attributes; the resting EEG is a highly characteristic individual trait. A small, but in some studies consistent difference of average amplitudes may be due to differences in the shapes of skulls in MZ twins.
- A high degree of similarity is also found in reactions to hyperventilation, photic stimulation, and sleep-including REM sleep.
- Maturation of brain function as measured by the EEG shows characteristic phases but strong individual differences between children of the same age groups. These differences are largely genetically determined.
- The EEG is known to undergo slow changes with advancing age, up to senility. These changes also show a high degree of interindividual variation. Some aspects of these changes, such as showing of a waves or reduction in amplitudes, are concordant in MZ twins and are therefore largely caused by genetic effects; others, such as some intermixture of slower waves, or slight focal abnormalities, may be discordant. They may have been caused by certain "events." Such events may sometimes have gone unrecognized.
- The EEG may be used to study reaction of the brain to defined external factors. For example, MZ twin pairs have been studied one cotwin of which had a brain trauma. Long-term comparative observation of both twins, the traumatized and the untraumatized one, often permits a precise assessment even of minor traumatic effects. In instances where a certain exogenous factor is known to exert very different effects, comparison of MZ twins may allow determination of whether and to what extent such differences are affected by genetic differences. The effect of alcohol is one example. Here, considerable individual differences in the EEG reaction have been found which are genetically determined as shown by complete concordance in MZ twins. These results have become important for our understanding of genetic effects on susceptibility to alcohol addiction.

- Before twin studies are used to draw conclusions regarding the degree of genetic determination of a certain trait, it must be clarified that the twin method is adequate for studying the trait in question. This would not be the case if this trait would be affected by the fact that the individuals to be studied are twins. For example, there are reports asserting that borderline or abnormal EEG results may be more common among twins than in the general population of singletons. Studies on unbiased samples of twins, both children and adults, seem to contradict this assertion. It is well known, on the other hand, that twins are often born prematurely, that certain malformations are more common than in the general population, and that their intellectual development may lag behind somewhat. Therefore early EEG anomalies and occasional delays in EEG maturation would not be too unlikely, at least in some instances. The one discordant MZ pair in our own EEG series is possibly an example. Hence this problem should be kept in mind, especially when the EEG is used in studying very young children.

In conclusion, the twin method in general and also its application to problems for which the EEG may be helpful is a useful method for studying a variety of problems in genetic variation in brain function. Contrary to the opinion of some "modern" research workers, it is not intrinsically dull. Its potentialities have not even nearly been exhausted. However, as with all methods, it should be used critically and, above all, imaginatively.

CHAPTER 4

4 Family Studies on the Normal EEG

Twin studies permit conclusions whether and to what extent interindividual variation in a certain trait is caused by genetic variation. They do not give any hints as to the kind of this variation, the modes of inheritance, and the gene (or genes) involved. For analysis with this goal in mind, family studies are required. Here, "classical" human genetics offers two different approaches. One of them, used for continuously varying and quantifiable traits, consists in measuring such a trait, and calculating correlations between defined categories of relatives. From these calculations, conclusions are possible regarding the degree to which variation in a certain trait is caused by genetic variation. Correlations expected if a certain part of a trait's variation, measured by its variance, goes back to genetic variation, have been calculated based on Mendel's laws together with certain assumptions (Fisher 1918; see Vogel and Motulsky 1996). Conventionally, this fraction is expressed by a measure called heritability which is defined as $h^2=V_G/V_P$ (h^2 = heritability; V_G = genetically determined variance; V_P = entire genetically, and nongenetically determined variance). This approach to genetic analysis has been called the "galtonian approach," since it was proposed by F. Galton in the 19th century (Vogel and Motulsky 1996). In principle, its analytical power is much higher than that of a simple comparison of MZ and DZ twins. In fact, measurable traits in twins are often analyzed further by heritability estimates. As noted repeatedly in Chap. 3, this approach has also been used in the analysis of quantifiable EEG data, such as average α frequency or the α index.

The second, alternative approach is that proposed by Mendel: The first things the investigator is looking for are clearcut alternatives of the phenotype: in the ideal case, a certain trait is either present or absent. Hereditary diseases are classical examples: the individual is either affected with achondroplastic dwarfism or is not affected. In these instances, a more thorough genetic analysis is possible: a certain mode of inheritance can be established (in achondroplasia it is autosomal-dominant). This means that a mutation in a certain gene is responsible for the clearcut phenotype and there are now techniques available to identify this gene. (In achondroplasia it is the transmembrane portion of a receptor protein determined by a "fibroblast receptor gene" on chromosome 4; Shiang et al. 1994). However, achondroplasia also allows another observation: the most visible aspect of the achondroplasia phenotype is small stature, easily distinguishable from the normal range of stature in our population. Stature, however, is a typical example for a trait that has been analyzed by comparison of twins and relatives, and calculating heritability (heritability is very high at least under present living conditions; see Vogel and

Motulsky 1996), Our conclusion is: Continuous variation analyzable so far only by the galtonian approach – measurement and heritability estimates – may occur concomitantly with variation in which the mendelian approach is possible, discontinuous variation, analysis of modes of inheritance.

Achondroplasia is a rare trait. However, alternatively distributed traits may also be common; genetic polymorphisms such as blood groups, transplantation antigens, and serum protein variants have been known for quite some time. Polymorphisms of the DNA structure have become known in more recent years; they are now excellent tools for identification and analysis of genes (see Vogel and Motulsky 1996). This "classical" way of genetic analysis – from phenotype down to the gene (or genes) – has been supplemented more recently by an alternative approach, from the gene and its variants up to the phenotype. When the first examples had been discovered, it was called very appropriately "reverse genetics," since the usual way of analysis was reversed. It is now commonly named "positional cloning," because it requires first cloning of a gene (or genes). So far, positional cloning has not become possible in genetic analysis of EEG phenomena, but the "classical" mendelian approach has been applied successfully. Yet before such studies together with their results can be described, it is necessary to explain in which situation the two alternative approaches – quantitative genetics and mendelian analysis – can be used, and which are their shortcomings and pitfalls.

The galtonian approach is appropriate for analysis of measurable traits, especially if the trait in question shows a unimodal distribution (i.e., a distribution with one maximum) in the population. As far as it goes, it often gives clearcut results and allows for meaningful comparisons. It is its most important disadvantage that it does not permit a deeper analysis of the genes involved in the determination of the phenotype under study and, especially, their mechanisms of action. One of the most common pitfalls in using this approach is its application for genetic analysis of traits that may be measurable but in which measurements describe aspects of but do not exhaust phenotypic variation. The mendelian approach, on the other hand, in principle allows an analysis down to the genes and to the mutations involved. In fact, establishing a mode of inheritance is the first step of this analysis. Therefore the geneticist always tries to describe, and often define a phenotype, so that alternative distributions can be made visible in a way that the mendelian approach can be used. Its main pitfall is that it is applied in instances where it is inappropriate. Mendelian analysis requires careful and critical appraisal of the phenotype.

4.1 Family Studies of the Normal EEG: First Attempts and Various Approaches

To the best of my knowledge, the first family study on the normal EEG was published by Gottlober (1938). He examined 15 families consisting of both parents and at least two children at the age of at least 14 years. As appropriate at this early state of EEG studies, the EEG records only consisted of one occipital reference (uniplar) record of 30 cm from each individual. He asked a group of three colleagues to attribute the records of the children to those of their parents; criteria used were shape and extent of α activity and general similarity. Neither EEG type nor aspects of basic rhythm permitted clearcut attribution; the author had the impression that EEGs of daughters were more similar than those of their fathers and the sons' EEG records tended to resemble those of their mothers. Hence this study was unsuccessful; EEG recordings and analysis were inadequate due to the very early state of general knowledge of the human EEG. Still, Gottlober's work should be considered as a pilot study. In their twin report from 1945, Lennox et al. mentioned that EEG records from sibs of the same sex tend to be more similar than those of sibs of the other sex. More recent family studies using the "galtonian" biometric approach are discussed in Sect. 4.11. First, however, studies are described in which simple mendelian modes of inheritance were shown.

4.2 EEG Variants and Their Genetic Analysis

As discussed above, a mendelian analysis is preferable if feasible. This raises the question: Are there any traits or variants of the normal human EEG that permit such an analysis? Such variants are, indeed, known. Some of these are described here. In all these instances it is necessary first to characterize the phenotypes as precisely as possible. It would be ideal if this could be done using precise numerical values. Unfortunately, however, this is not entirely possible. Only approximate measurement data are available; they may help but must be supplemented by visual characteristics. This necessarily introduces an element of judgment based on "experience of the investigator" into classification of such variants; the "computer between the ears" (Niedermeyer) is an excellent research tool but often it is difficult to communicate its results (fortunately, it is difficult, but not impossible). Below we describe first variants of α activity and their genetic analysis. Variants involving β waves are then discussed. Descriptions are based mainly on visual criteria, but data from quantitative computerized analysis are presented wherever possible.

4.3 The "Low-Voltage EEG" and Its Borderline Cases

Even in the first phases of EEG research, records in which α activity, especially on occipital parts of the brain, either seem to be absent completely, or almost completely, or showed very low amplitudes. One of the first reports on the EEG, in which Berger's discovery was confirmed, came from Adrian and Matthews (1934). In this report, Adrian confirmed presence of the α rhythm in his own EEG but in Matthews' EEG it was not found. Probably, Matthews had a low-voltage EEG. In the following decades, many authors have considered EEG types with little or no α activity either in normal individuals of various ages, or in persons with various diagnoses such as psychoneurosis, schizophrenia and other mental and behavioral disorders, and in epileptics (Vol. 6A of the EEG-handbook; 1976). Among 14 reports between 1943 and 1966, prevalences among adults of various ages and sex vary between 0 and 22%; single values tended to cluster between 6 and 10%. This variation may be caused, in part, by the various groups of anomalies included in this tabulation but probably is caused mainly by differences in classification. Below we describe first our own classification, briefly discussing determination of prevalence based on it, and then our genetic analysis. Subsequently we discuss a study of borderline cases and their families.

The low-voltage EEG studied here is characterized as follows:

a) The occipital α waves are lacking completely or there are only traces in a few places, and they show a very low amplitude.
b) The entire EEG in leads from all areas of the brain may look completely flat. More frequently, however, irregular activity with very low amplitude may be seen, especially in frontoprecentral and temporal leads. In adolescents between about 12–20 years, it may be somewhat more active; it often consists of irregular flat ϑ waves, similar to those often observed in adolescents who have an α EEG. In older individuals, and especially in women, fast β waves of very low amplitude may be present.
c) When eyes are opened, the low voltage EEG shows no visible reaction, i.e., there is no off-effect. Immediately after closing of the eyes, however, a few α waves can appear for a short time; they disappear after one or a few seconds being replaced again by the low-voltage pattern.
d) In some instances, but not always, α waves may be produced by hyperventilation; they disappear approx. 1–2 min after the end of hyperventilation. In addition, persons with low-voltage EEG may but must not show slower waves as other normal individuals (Fig. 4.1).

This EEG type should not be confused with EEG records with many α waves of very low amplitudes but with a typical off-effect. Distinction of this EEG type from the true low-voltage EEG requires recording with amplification of (at least) 7 mm/50 μV. Recording with lower amplification leads to confusion. Another source of error is high psychic tension of the proband; it may lead to transitory disappearance of α activity and hence to erroneous assumption of a low-voltage type. Therefore it is recommended to carry out the recording in a relaxed atmosphere and to disregard the first minutes of recordings whether visual inspection or tape recording is planned. In the great majority of instances, the low-voltage EEG can be recognized

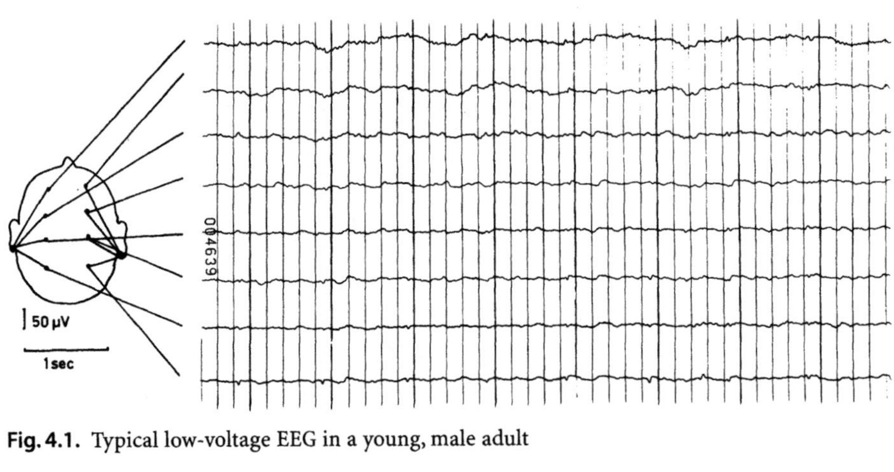

Fig. 4.1. Typical low-voltage EEG in a young, male adult

$$I = \frac{\text{Number of } \alpha \text{ waves in 10 sec}}{\text{Basic } \alpha \text{ rhythm} \times 10}$$

Fig. 4.2. *I*, (α Index)

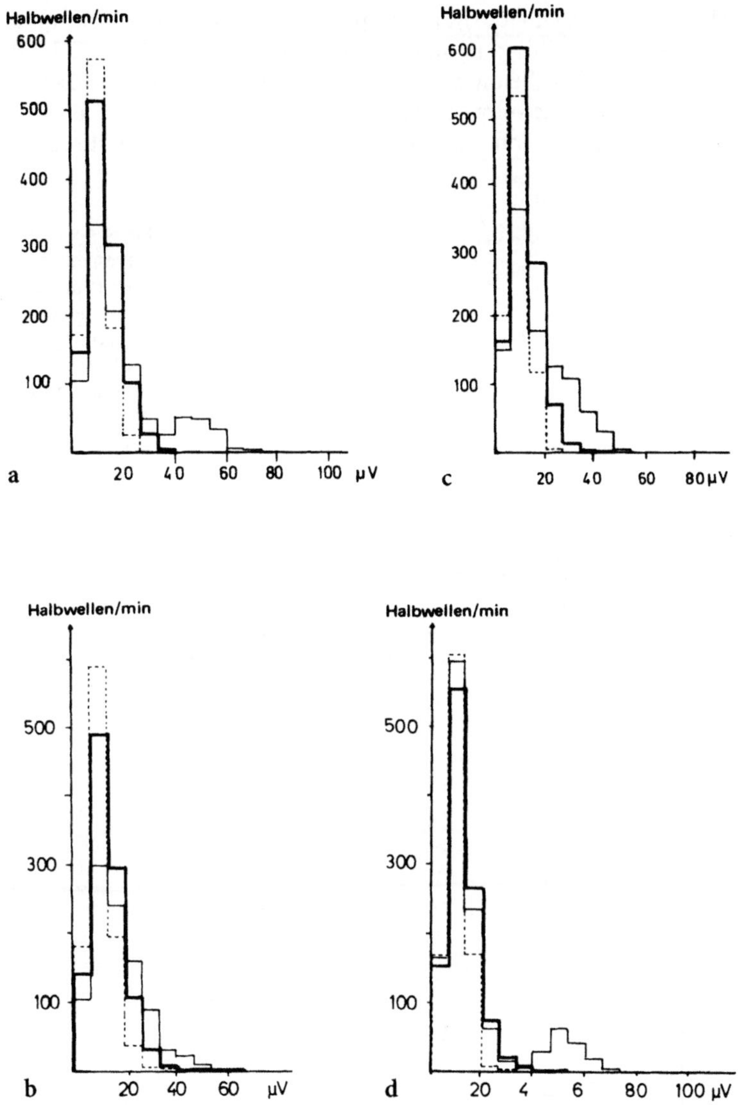

Fig. 4.3a–d. Distribution of half waves/min to various amplitude classes in adult males with low-voltage EEG. **a, b** Left and right precentral. **c, d** Left and right occipital. A method for amplitude interval (time-domain) analysis was used. *Thin lines,* most extreme individuals; *thick lines,* mean of 47 subjects. (From Vogel, Krüger and Schalt 1981)

easily provided that recording is carried out properly. However, there are always quite a few "borderline" cases whose correct classification may be difficult. For a genetic analysis, it may therefore be useful to try some measurement methods. All these measurements were performed in reference records. The simplest method to be used is the α index (= percentage time α). (Fig. 4.2). A more sophisticated method is distribution of amplitudes in time-domain analysis (Vogel et al. 1981a,b; Figs. 4.3, 4.4). In these figures distribution of amplitudes is compared with that found in probands with monomorphic α waves, the most different EEG variant (see below, Sect. 4.7). Obviously, the amplitude distributions appear quite different.

Application of discriminant analysis to EEGs of 243 adult males, including variants described below and probands with more or less average EEGs, gave relatively good but not fully satisfying discrimination. We concluded that really satisfactory discrimination required more sophisticated measurement and analysis.

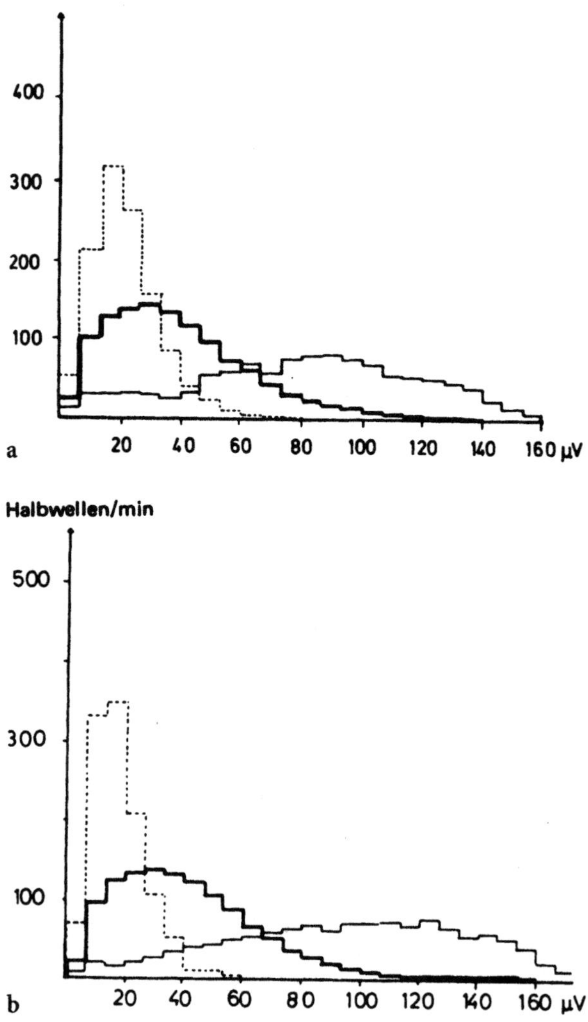

Fig. 4.4a, b. Distribution of half waves/min to various amplitude classes in adult males with monomorphic α-waves. **a** Left side. **b** Right sides. Occipital leads *Thin lines,* most extreme individuals; *thick line,* means of 46 subjects. (From Vogel, Krüger and Schalt 1981)

Recently, this goal seems to have been achieved (Dünki et al. 1996). The result is "... a simple two-gene mendelian scheme to explain inheritance of the clinical low-voltage EEG group. In this ... scheme, the low-voltage property does not occur when dominance of a certain allele ... is absent."

The family studies were based on simple visual evaluation of EEG records. Therefore misclassification of some "borderline" cases may have occurred. Three series were studied: A German series published by Vogel (1962; some of these families were included in Vogel and Götze 1959); another German series collected for a linkage study, and a large family from Azerbaijan. The two latter series were described by Anokhin et al. (1992). In all three series, the α index was measured by hand, and a bimodal distribution was obvious. It is remarkable that it was found not only in the two German series but in the Azerbaijanian series as well. Segregation analysis was performed using the methods now available (Vogel and Motulsky 1996; Appendix 2), using the genetic model of simple, autosomal-dominant mode of inheritance. Earlier studies (Vogel 1962) had shown that the low-voltage EEG only manifests gradually during the second decade of life. Therefore individuals younger than 19 years were not included in the analysis. Most of the families analyzed were nuclear families consisting of two parents and a varying number of children. A few large families were broken down to nuclear families for analysis; in a few others, only one parent was available for analysis. In estimating segregation ratios, the way of ascertainment had to be considered. Some sibships were ascertained by one parent. In these instances, no correction of segregation ratios is required. Other families were ascertained by one sib with the low-voltage EEG. Here, ascertainment bias had to be corrected. The cases did not occur that a sibship was ascertained independently twice or even more often; therefore the model of "single selection" (see Vogel and Motulsky 1996) was applied. In instances where only one parent could be examined, and this parent showed a low-voltage EEG, it was assumed that the nonexamined parent did not have a low-voltage EEG.

In all families studied, at least one parent showed a low-voltage EEG; in a few families, both parents showed this trait. Table 4.1 shows the expected and estimated segregation ratios. Expectations are not 0.75 for the mating LV × LV, and 0.5 for the LV × α, as expected from Mendel's law but somewhat higher since the trait is not very rare (see below). Therefore a certain fraction of homozygotes (LV/LV) had to

Table 4.1. Segregation analysis of the LVEEG. Families sets: the sample studies in the EEG linkage project (for details see Steinlein et al. 1992); sample of families studied by Vogel (1962); the two samples pooled together. "?" denotes unknown parent phenotypes. SFE and SFO indicate the expected and observed segretion frequencies, respectively: SE is the standard error of segregation frequency estimate. *t* and *P* are Student's statistique; the corresponding *P* value (two-sided); NS = not significant (Anokhin et al. 1992)

Sample	Mating type	SFE	SFO	SE	*t*	*P*
New data	LV/alpha; LV/?; ?/alpha; ?/?	0.709	0.400	0.050	2.26	0.02
	LV/LV	0.759	0.300	0.187	2.45	0.02
Vogel 1962	LV/alpha; LV/?; ?/alpha; ?/?	0.509	0.477	0.075	0.43	0.25
	LV/LV	0.759	0.750	0.153	0.06	0.85
Pooled	LV/alpha; LV/?; ?/alpha; ?/?	0.509	0.420	0.040	2.33	0.02
	LV/LV	0.759	0.625	0.129	1.03	0.3

be assumed. The empirically found segregation ratios (0.420 for the mating LV × α; 0.625 for the mating LV × LV) are somewhat lower than their expectations. The reason is unknown. Possibly a few individuals with low-voltage EEG have been misclassified as having an α EEG. As noted above, the low-voltage patterns only develop during the second decades of life; possibly, this development needs somewhat more time in some individuals. There was no effect of gender within these families: both sexes were present in equal frequencies among LV and among non-LV siblings. A problem to be studied in future, however, is the development of the low-voltage pattern during childhood and youth. We have seen quite a few individuals with a clearcut low-voltage pattern at the age of 15. However, what about younger children? As discussed above (Sect. 2.5) EEGs of children and adolescents show a high degree of interindividual variation. There may be enough space for special EEG types, possibly with few a waves and many ϑ waves of relatively low voltage, that could later develop into low-voltage EEGs.

Whenever a phenotype shows an autosomal-dominant mode of inheritance, the next step of analysis is localization of the gene (or genes) involved within the genome. This is carried out by a linkage study: genes whose location in the genome is known are used to determine whether the gene to be examined is close to one or more of these genes. Here, "genetic polymorphisms" are most suitable, i.e., genes for which as many as possible, but at least two alleles are common in our population. Such linkage studies require relatively sophisticated statistical methods which were, however, available in the 1950s. At that time, it was the main problem that not enough polymorphisms were available, not to speak of polymorphisms for which the genes had been localized. Meanwhile, and with the advent of DNA studies, this has changed thoroughly. Now, we have an almost unlimited number of DNA polymorphisms; therefore linkage studies in traits with simple mendelian modes of inheritance have become a matter of patience more than of ingenuity (by the way, this is quite different for conditions, where the mode of inheritance is not established).

4.4 Linkage Study

For the alert human geneticist, the way of further analysis, and especially the necessity of linkage studies, was obvious as early as the late 1950s (Vogel and Helmbold 1959). Available polymorphisms such as blood groups were examined in the low-voltage families known at that time; not surprisingly, no linkage was found; exclusion of linkage was achieved for the Rh blood group locus. Linkage with less than 20% recombination could be excluded significantly. This, admittedly somewhat trivial, result has stood the test of time. The problem of linkage could be taken up again only in the late 1980s when DNA polymorphisms became available. The first such polymorphisms were the "restriction fragment length polymorphisms" (RFLPs). Their handling was still difficult and time-consuming. Meanwhile, other types of polymorphisms have become available: especially the so-called microsatellites (for details see Vogel and Motulsky 1996; for strategies of linkage studies see Ott 1991). However, the linkage study for the low-voltage EEG was performed using 73 RFLPs and, in addition, 22 "classical" markers such as blood groups, serum pro-

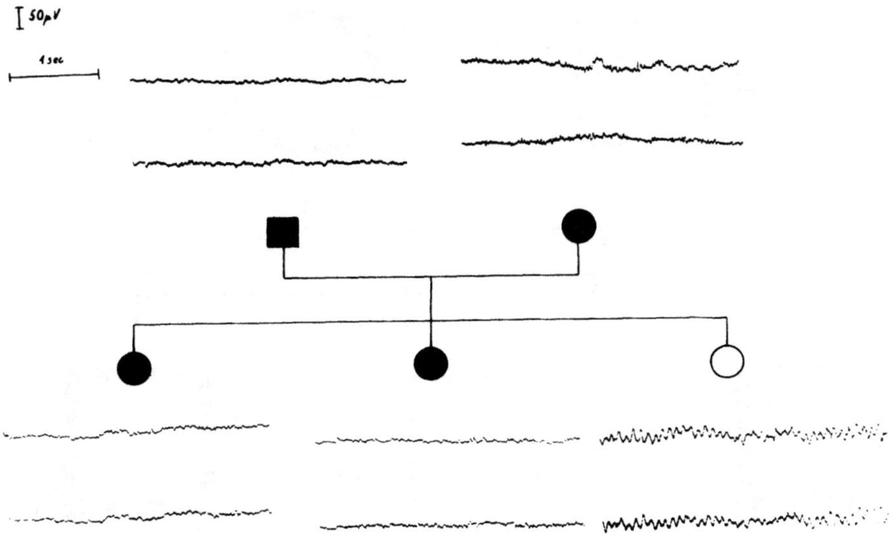

Fig. 4.5. Family with two parents having a low-voltage EEG and three daughters, two of which show this EEG type

tein variants and enzyme polymorphisms (Steinlein et al. 1992). Seventeen families with altogether 190 individuals were examined. A standard computer program for computing lod scores was used. Since it cannot be expected that all families in which the LV EEG segregates are caused by mutations at the same gene locus, an additional program for testing genetic heterogeneity was applied (Ott 1983). One of the RFLPs, the marker CMM6(D20M19), located on the distal part of chromosome 20q showed linkage without recombination in seven of the families. A marker may not be "informative" for linkage, when all individuals in whose meiosis this marker and the gene locus under scrutinizing could segregate are homozygous for it; in this case, it is impossible to decide whether and how frequently crossing over has occurred. However, in the case studied here, all families except three were informative; some other markers known to be located close to CMM6 also offered some evidence of linkage but were not sufficiently informative to offer definite evidence. Hence there was convincing evidence that a gene locus for the LVEEG is located near the end of the long arm of chromosome 20 – one of the smaller human chromosome, close to the marker CMM6 (Figs. 4.5, 4.6).

The next question to be answered was: is this gene responsible for the LVEEG in all examined families, or only in some of them? In other words, is there genetic heterogeneity? A brief view of the lod scores found for the families studied strongly suggests heterogeneity (Fig. 4.7). Figure 4.7 shows the lod scores for the informative families separately. Some of them, for example, that of family 2, are strongly positive, pointing to linkage. Others, however, such as those of families 17 and 22, are strongly negative, excluding linkage in these families. The above heterogeneity test yielded a highly significant result. Hence genetic heterogeneity can be regarded as confirmed. The fraction of all LV families caused by mutations of a gene at this locus was estimated to be approx. 30%. This means that in this German population in

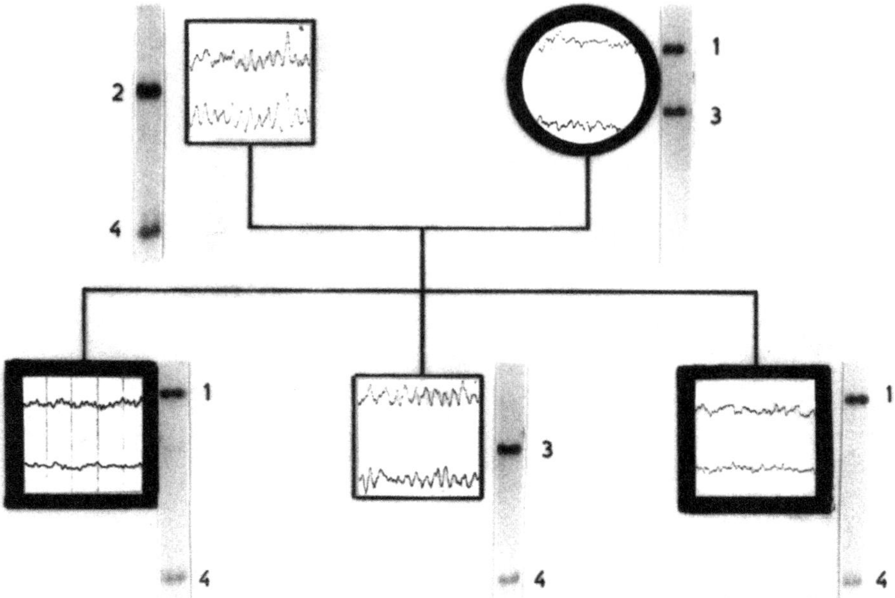

Fig. 4.6. The low-voltage EEG (occipital leads shown) segregates with the band 1 of the high polymorphic marker (MM6CD20S19)

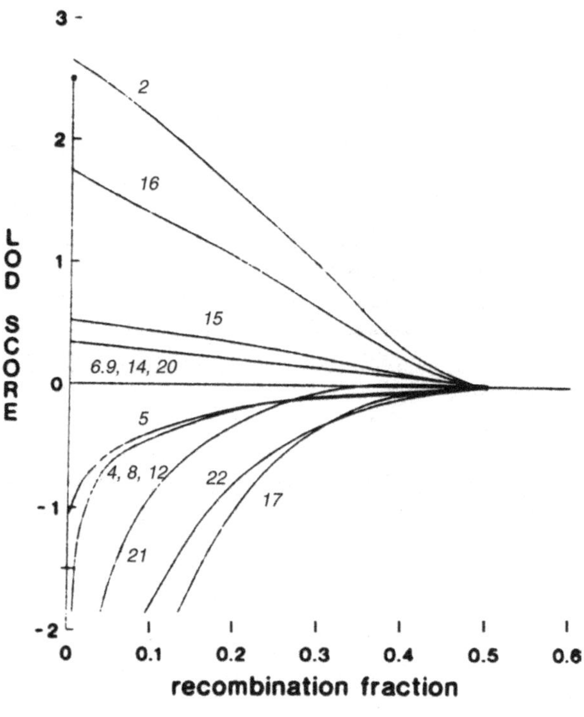

Fig. 4.7. Results of two-point linkage analysis between the low-voltage EEG locus and the marker (MM6CD20S19). The lod score values at different recombination fractions are plotted separately for individual families (number inside the graphs). Only families informative for the corresponding markers are shown. A few curves represent several families with identical results. Some families have highly positive lod scores (= evidence for linkage), whereas others show negative scores (= evidence against linkage). This apparent contradiction points to genetic heterogeneity which was confirmed by statistical analysis. (From Steinlein et al. 1992)

about 70% of families in which the LVEEG segregates mutations at other gene loci are responsible for this phenotype. So far, these loci have not been found.

The gene locus on chromosome 20 (20q) is especially interesting for still another reason: there is a special type of epilepsy, benign neonatal convulsions (BFNC), with autosomal-dominant mode of inheritance; the gene mutations of which lead to this epilepsy type have been localized within the same chromosome segment (see Sect. 1.3). The first, and obvious, hypothesis is that various mutations within the same gene are responsible for these two phenotypes that, after all, both involve changes in regulation of electric discharges of certain groups of neurons. However, this hypothesis has not been confirmed.

How common is the low-voltage EEG as defined above in the population? This problem could be studied in 4622 young German males (Air Force applicants) and in 3372 Japanese males of the same age group (train drivers in Tokyo; Vogel and Fujiya 1969). There were 4.2% typical and 2.25% borderline cases among Germans, and 4.57% typical and 2.14% borderline cases among the Japanese. These frequencies are, within the limits of chance variation, identical. To the best of our knowledge, studies from other populations using similar criteria are not available. This identical prevalence in two racially very different populations is surprising; so far, a convincing explanation cannot be given. Another practical aspect should also be discussed: Which environmental factors may lead to an EEG type without or with very little α waves? Psychological tensions are discussed above; another such effect is the fresh, closed brain trauma (commotio cerebri). EEG records in patients having suffered open damage of basal portions of the frontal brain often show especially low amplitudes. With the genetic studies of the LVEEG in mind, this problem was studied in greater detail in 101 patients who had suffered a closed brain trauma (Vogel et al. 1961), leading to the following results:

- The α depression after a closed brain trauma may be so strong (in 10 patients of these series) that the EEG resembles an inherited α wave free LV record. Even ϑ waves in frontoprecentral and temporal leads do not confirm a postraumatic anomaly; as noted above, they may be present in an LVEEG especially in young persons. Small and doubtful focal anomalies do not contradict presence of the inherited LV variant; they may also occur in carriers of this variant.
- α depression of a lower degree a short time after the accident is very common; much more common than general slowing of α waves or appearance of ϑ and/or δ waves.
- α depression may but must not be combined with other EEG anomalies. Occasionally, focal anomalies appear only in later records, after abating of the general depression.
- There is no clearcut clinical correlate of a general α depression. As a rule, however, these traumas are not very mild leading to unconsciousness and other severe clinical signs. However, it does not indicate a bad prognosis.

This result points to a difficult problem of differential diagnosis: when a flat EEG is found after a brain trauma, it is difficult to decide whether the consequence of a trauma, or a harmless hereditary variant is present. Repeated EEG studies over several weeks may provide an answer, but it is not known exactly how long the α depression may last; it may occasionally last even several months. In suitable cases, i.e., if parents are available for study, study of these parents may solve the issue: if the hereditary variant is present, at least one of them should also have an LVEEG. If only sibs can be studied, the situation is more difficult: Each sibling has a chance of 50% of showing this EEG type. An MZ pair with concordant LVEEG, one cotwin of which had had a brain trauma a short time before his scheduled EEG study is discussed above (see also Fig. 3.16). In conclusion, study of parents or siblings may help in clarifying a difficult diagnostic situation.

In this connection, the isoelectric EEG which occurs premortally in comatose patients should at least be mentioned; for the experienced EEG specialist it offers hardly any severe diagnostic problems. Flat EEGs that continue to exist after a long time and do not react to various activating methods (eye closure; hyperventilation; photic stimulation and various psychotropic drugs) were observed in patients with severe brain disease leading, for example, to cerebral atrophy (see, for example, Synek 1969). The problem of α depression in Huntington disease, which also leads to brain atrophy, is discussed in Chap. 8.

As noted repeatedly, it is not always possible to distinguish the real (almost) α-free low-voltage EEG from other EEG types, especially those showing many α waves but with very low amplitudes. One way for improving the possibility for distinguishing these EEG types is using a slightly increased amplificaton when the EEG is recorded (at least 7 mm/50 μV). The relatively high number of borderline cases found in our study on normal German and Japanese males (see above; Vogel and Fujiya 1969) is caused by the fact that the EEGs had not been recorded by us, and that the amplification used was somewhat lower. However, even under optimal conditions of recording, some cases remain that cannot be classified definitely by visual inspections. In such instances, Reinke (1966) performed a family study. Starting from young male probands (Air Force applicants), 24 families were examined, with the following results: One proband showed a clearcut α EEG when restudied. During the first EEG recording, he may have been tired or very tense; it was not possible to ascertain this. A few probands were now showing a clearcut low-voltage EEG. In a third category of patients, α waves with very low amplitudes resembled superficially a low-voltage EEG and family studies failed to give the typical picture of a dominant mode of inheritance. Finally, there were a few instances, where it could not be decided by visual inspection whether an LVEEG was present but again family studies failed to show the typical mode of inheritance. In such instances, which are truly borderline, only a family study can decide whether the proband belongs to the true LV group. The fraction of these borderline cases, however, is much smaller than prevalence studies based on EEG records taken by others (see Vogel and Fujiya 1969) seemed to indicate. Still, this situation is not really satisfactory. Hopefully, application of a recently developed, computer-aided method of classification may permit a completely reliable classification (Dünki 1996); although the number of individuals in which clearcut classification was achieved, is small, and the LV persons all came from families in which this EEG variant showed a clearcut autosomal-dominant mode of inheritance. A classification program by which a definite diagnosis of the true low-voltage EEG can be achieved either by off-line computerized analysis of tapes or even on-line would be ideal. This has not been achieved so far, but the study of Dünki et al. (1996) shows in which direction the solution could be found.

4.5
Fast (16–19 c/s) Alpha Variants

According to customary definitions, waves within this frequency range should be named β waves. However, in some instances, they show all features of α waves, except, of course, frequency. Their distribution over the skull is exactly identical with that of α waves (Fig. 4.8); and they are blocked by opening of the eyes. When eyes are closed, some but not all probands show a few waves in the typical α range (9–13 c/s). There are also individual differences in amplitudes, and here, intrafamilial variation is smaller than variation between families. Among 1985 young German males (Air Force applicants), 12 cases were found (0.6%). The confidence interval ($p = 0.95$) lies between 6.2 and 20.96. The corresponding figures for 3372 Japanese males (Tokyo train drivers) was found to be 14 (0.42%); with a 95% confidence interval 7.65–23.49 (Vogel and Fujiya 1969; see also Vogel 1966). In this study, 24 sibships in 22 families, complete and incomplete, were examined. In four instances, both parents of the propositus could be examined, and in each of them, one parent showed the trait. In three additional families, only the mother could be studied; the father had died. In two of them, the mother showed the trait. Altogether, it was transmitted five times by the mother, once by the father, and once probably by the father; among the sibs, both sexes were represented in carriers as well as in noncarriers. In segregation analysis, only individuals above the age of 19 were included, since this variant cannot be diagnosed reliably in younger persons. Segregation analysis was performed taking into account ascertainment (for details see Vogel 1966). The result was: $P = 0.499 \pm 0.097$.

Hence all data suggest an autosomal dominant mode of inheritance (Figs. 4.8, 4.9). Since the trait is rare, practically all sibships are expected to have one heterozygous and one "normal" homozygous parent; the expected segregation ratio for a simple autosomal dominant mode of inheritance is very near to 0.5. Hence there is an ideal agreement of the estimated ratio with this expectation. In one family, this fast α variant occurred together with frontoprecentral groups of β waves (see Sect. 4.9). The two traits were shown to segregate independently (Vogel 1966).

Another family (Fig. 4.10) was ascertained via the 58-year-old father who showed a typical low-voltage EEG. His wife had 16–17 c/s fast α variants. The two sons, 22

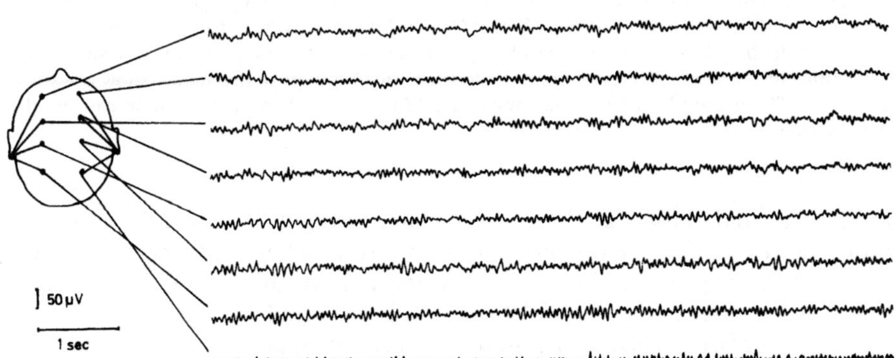

Fig. 4.8. EEG in a 37-year-old healthy male with about 15–16 c/s fast α variants

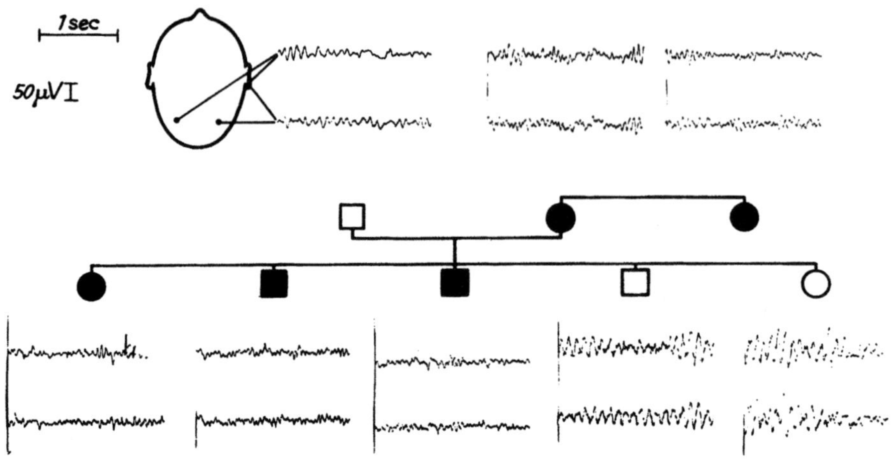

Fig. 4.9. A family with autosomal dominant inheritance of about 16–17 c/s fast α variants

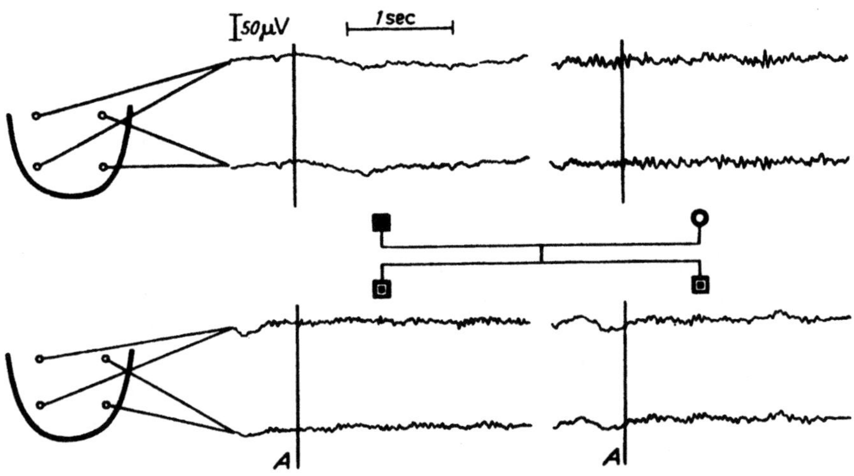

Fig. 4.10. A family in which two autosomal dominant EEG traits are segregating. The father has a low-voltage EEG, the mother shows about 14 c/s fast α variants. The two sons have inherited both variants; they have a low-voltage EEG. Immediately after closing the eyes *(A)*, some subjects with a low-voltage EEG show a few a waves. The two brothers in this family show a few fast α variants. The mutant leading to the low-voltage EEG is epistatic over the mutant causing the fast α variant

and 24 years old, showed a clearcut low-voltage resting EEG. When the eyes were closed, however, 16–17 c/s occipital waves were seen in both of them. They disappeared completely after 1–2 s. As was discussed above, the same frequently happened with a waves in the LVEEG. The LVEEG in this family appears to be epistatic to the gene for fast a variants. As most β waves are not suppressed in the LVEEG, this observation offers an additional argument in favor of the conclusion that the 16–19 c/s occipital waves are variants of α and not of β waves.

Contrary to the first impression, diagnosis fo the 16–19 c/s variant is not entirely straightforward. For example, there are EEG types that are completely covered by β waves which, however, do not show all properties of α waves. These are described below.

4.6 The 4–5 c/s Rhythm

In this variant, which, after incomplete earlier reports, was described first completely by Vogel and Götze (1959), the resting EEG, when the proband is relaxed, shows regular occipital or occipitotemporal 4–5 c/s waves instead of α waves. These waves are blocked, as are α waves, when the eyes are opened. Amplitudes were found to vary between about 20 and 120 μV (Kuhlo et al. 1969; Fig. 4.11). They differ from superficially similar waves in children in their behavior after closing of the eyes. They do not reappear immediately. First, α waves can be seen which are replaced again by 4–5 c/s waves after some seconds (Figs. 4.12, 4.13). Besides, the 4–5 c/s pattern can be disturbed by small stimuli such as clasping of hands, crackling the EEG paper etc. The 4–5 c/s waves are then replaced immediately by normal α waves which then, after a very short time, give way again to the 4–5 c/s pattern (Vogel and Götze 1959). Photic stimulation also leads to disappearance of this pattern which, however, may return after a longer period of stimulation. A short time before the start of natural sleep, on the other hand, when α waves normally increase in amplitude, the 4–5 c/s disappear, and α waves are seen. Afterwards, these α waves also disappear, and sleep begins (Kuhlo 1967).

The topical distribution of the 4–5 c/s rhythm is not completely congruent with that of the posterior α rhythm; in a series of 40 cases, this variant was seen only occipital or occipital and parietal in 11 instances; in 29 cases, it was occipital and temporal. In three cases, it was asymmetrical (Kuhlo et al. 1969; see also Pitot and Gastaut 1956).

The only known series of normal probands is the series of Japanese train drivers reported by Vogel and Fujiya (1969). Among 3372 young males, there were four

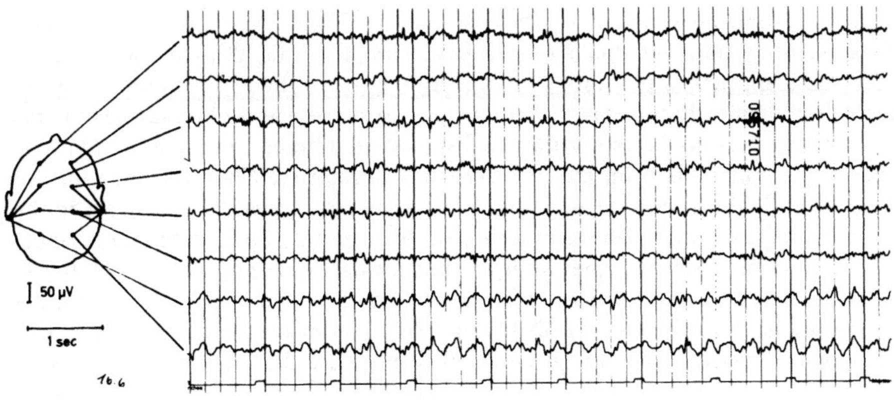

Fig. 4.11. Slow (3–4 c/s) α variant within a young women

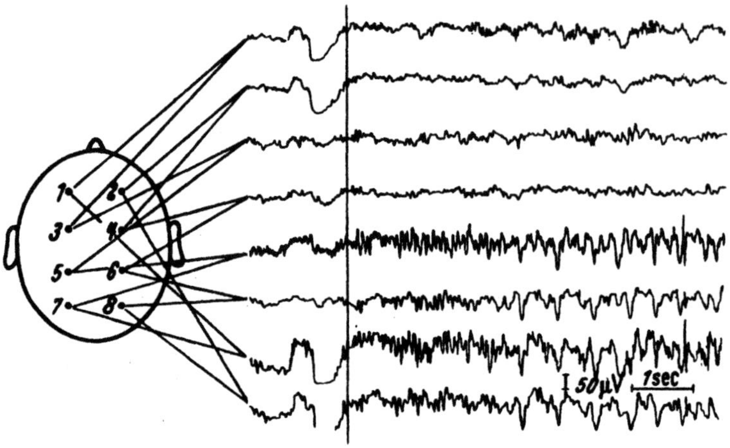

Fig. 4.12. In subjects showing the slow α variant, α waves appear for a short time after the eyes are closed; after 1–2 s the slow (about 4 c/s) pattern reappears

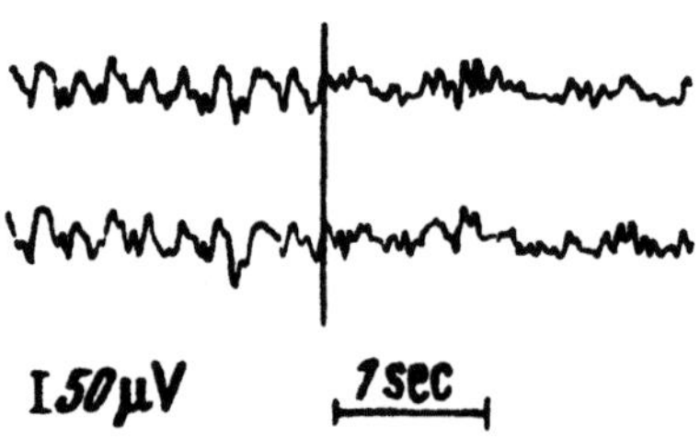

Fig. 4.13. Slight disturbances such as clasping of hands or crackling of paper makes the slow variants disappear for a short time

carriers (0.12%). Kuhlo et al. (1969) found 11 cases among 14,764 tracings of the Freiburg EEG laboratory (corresponding to about 11,000 individuals) – and 12 cases among 23,000 tracings of a Stuttgart laboratory (corresponding to about 15,000 persons). Prevalence is estimated by these authors to be between 0.025% and 0.075% in their laboratory population, i.e., among individuals having some medical indication for their EEG examination. At first glance, this estimate seems to be somewhat lower than that from the series of Japanese studied by Vogel and Fujiya (1969). Upon closer scrutiny, however, this is not the case: First, the trait, although occurring in both sexes appears to be more common among males than in females; of the 40 cases described by Kuhlo et al. (1969), there were 28 male and 12 female (MZ twins taken as one person). Secondly, the age distribution differed from that found in the reference populations from the two German laboratories. While the age range of these 40 individuals varied from 12 to 54 years, mean ages were 23.18 years in the Freiburg and 26.15 in the Stuttgart series. The average age of patients in these laboratories is certainly much higher, although reliable data were not available. Of the 40 cases studied 13 came from a Berlin laboratory in which Vogel carried out his examinations. Here, data are available for 1962. The mean age of 4371 examined individuals (excluding the age group 0–10 years where the variant cannot be diagnosed) was 42.94 ± 0.25 years. Among Japanese train drivers, average age, although not known precisely, was certainly much lower. Besides, all of them were males.

Hence, even if precise age distribution of the populations from which these data were coming is not available, there is some indirect evidence pointing to the possibility that this variant may disappear some time during mature life. However, in the series reported by Kuhlo et al. (1969) this could not be observed directly: While in 21 patients, only one recording was possible, 8 were examined at least twice, with an interval of 1–17 months between the first and the last records; in 7 individuals, the interval between first and last recording was 1–3 years, and in four persons, 6–10 years. The issue was later clarified, however, by another study which included longitudinal data (Heintel et al. 1984). In the Stuttgart laboratory discussed above, 54 trait carriers were observed between 1953 and 1984. The oldest was no less than 84 years of age, the youngest 11 (the latter patient had already been examined at the age of 6.58 years; and at that time the 4–5 c/s variant was not present). In this series, the sex ratio was 1:1; a predominance of males that has been observed previously (Kuhlo et al. 1969) could not be confirmed. The average age was 38.24 years compared with 52.46 years in the entire population study. Dominant EEG frequencies varied between 3 c/s and 5 c/s; most individuals had a 4–5 c/s, a few a 3–4 c/s rhythm. The age distribution of trait carriers did not indicate slowing with advancing age. In two individuals, disappearance of this variant was observed directly: A male showed it at the ages of 11 and 17 but not at 27. In another male, it was seen at 15 and 25, but not at 42 years; small groups of 3–4 c/s waves were present instead. In two other individuals, however, the variant had not disappeared after 27 and 8 years, respectively; it was still visible at the age of 51 and 72. Hence this variant may but must not disappear some time at middle age. Two, and possible three, MZ twins were observed over the years; all of them were concordant.

Vogel (1958) described twin girls who were 15 years old at the time of their first examination in the year 1954. They were found accidentally in a study of normal twins. The 4–5 c/s variant was still present in 1962. However, 22 years later, in 1984,

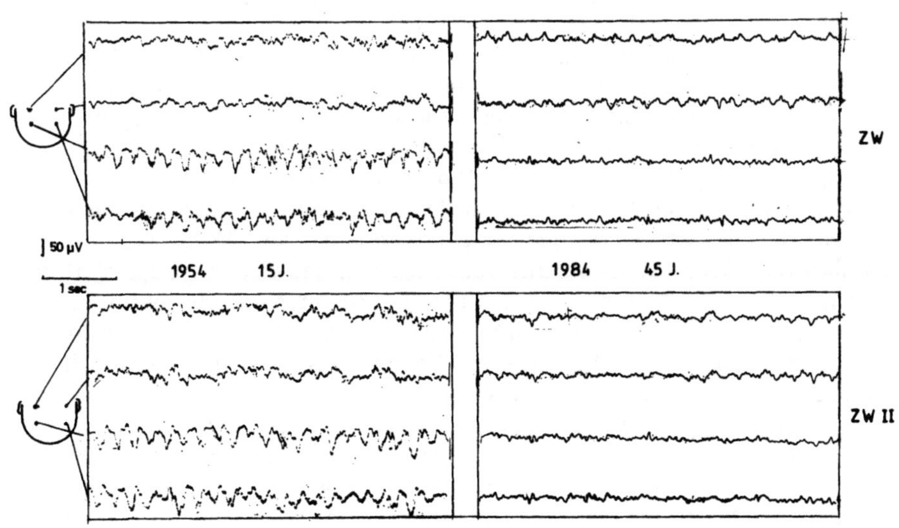

Fig. 4.14. Central and occipital waves in a female MZ pair at the age of 15 (left-hand side) and at the age of 45. The 4–5 c/s pattern disappeared especially in occipital leads. In the mid-20s it had still been present

the EEG of both twins had changed appreciably (Fig. 4.14; Heintel et al. 1986). In occipital leads, where there had been the maximum in earlier examinations, the 4–5 c/s waves had now disappeared completely; irregular and fast (approx. 13 c/s) α activity predominated. A slightly irregular and flat 4–5 c/s rhythm was seen exclusively in central leads; here, activity had not changed very much during 30 years. As at the age of 15, EEGs were still completely concordant at 45 years; despite quite different life experiences (one twin was divorced and had one child; the other one was married and had two children). Another MZ twin pair was described by Kuhlo et al. (1967). The tracings of the twins were completely identical in all aspects, including intensity and distribution of the 4–5 c/s rhythm. Among the MZ pairs reared apart who have been described by Juel-Nielsen and Harvald (1958), there is one pair which, according to the published EEG, could easily have this variant, although the authors do not comment specifically on this pair. In any case, the EEG of this pair is concordant as well. In conclusion, these, admittedly very limited, twin studies suggest a genetic basis of this variant.

Family studies, however, gave a much more contradictory result. The first families were described by Vogel and Götze (1959). Four families were observed; of the eight parents six could be examined; two fathers had died previously. These persons did not show the variant; the father in one family, 52 years old at the time of examination, had a regular α pattern but showed rarely short groups of 2–4 4–5 c/s waves predominantly in temporal leads. Despite its slightly different localization, this pattern is not so different from that seen in the twin pair described above. The father of this twin pair had died before; their 57.0-year-old mother and two sibs, one sister 30.6 years old, and one brother 24.9 years old, did not show the trait. There were two families, in which both parents could be examined. In one of them, with the 51.5-year-old father who showed some 4–5 c/s waves predominantly in temporal leads, there were four sons between 17.1 and 13.5 years of age (Fig. 4.15). Three of these, the first, the second and the last one, showed the 4–5 c/s variant. The second son was the proband. In the remaining two families, there were, in addition to the proband, five sibs, four boys and one girl. In four of them, this variant was certainly absent; in one (6.3 years old), classification was impossible. In another proband who was 48 years old at the time of his examination, the wife and the 17-year-old daughter were studied; neither showed this trait. Additional family studies have been performed in Freiburg and Stuttgart; in these families, no additional cases were discovered.

Müller-Küppers and Vogel (1965), on the other hand, had discovered another sibship. Two sibs – one women (27 years old) and one man (26 years old) – were described (Fig. 4.16) as carrying this trait. The father had died at the age of 51; the mother, 56 years old, showed a normal α EEG. Up to 1968, 40 carriers of this variant (9 fathers, 13 mothers, 23 brothers and 17 sisters) had been examined. In addition to the above families, no further relatives with the 4–5 c/s variant, and especially no further sibs carrying this trait were discovered.

Shortly thereafter Neundörfer (1970) studied another series of cases. Nine probands were patients either from a hospital of the German army, or from a University hospital, and, in addition, five members of a family who were ascertained through one of these probands, could be examined. In 19 other family members of these probands, the trait was not present. Of the 14 carriers, 10 were male, 4 were female. Figure 4.16b shows the pedigree. It is unusual since the proband had married the sister of another trait carrier; all four children, one son and three

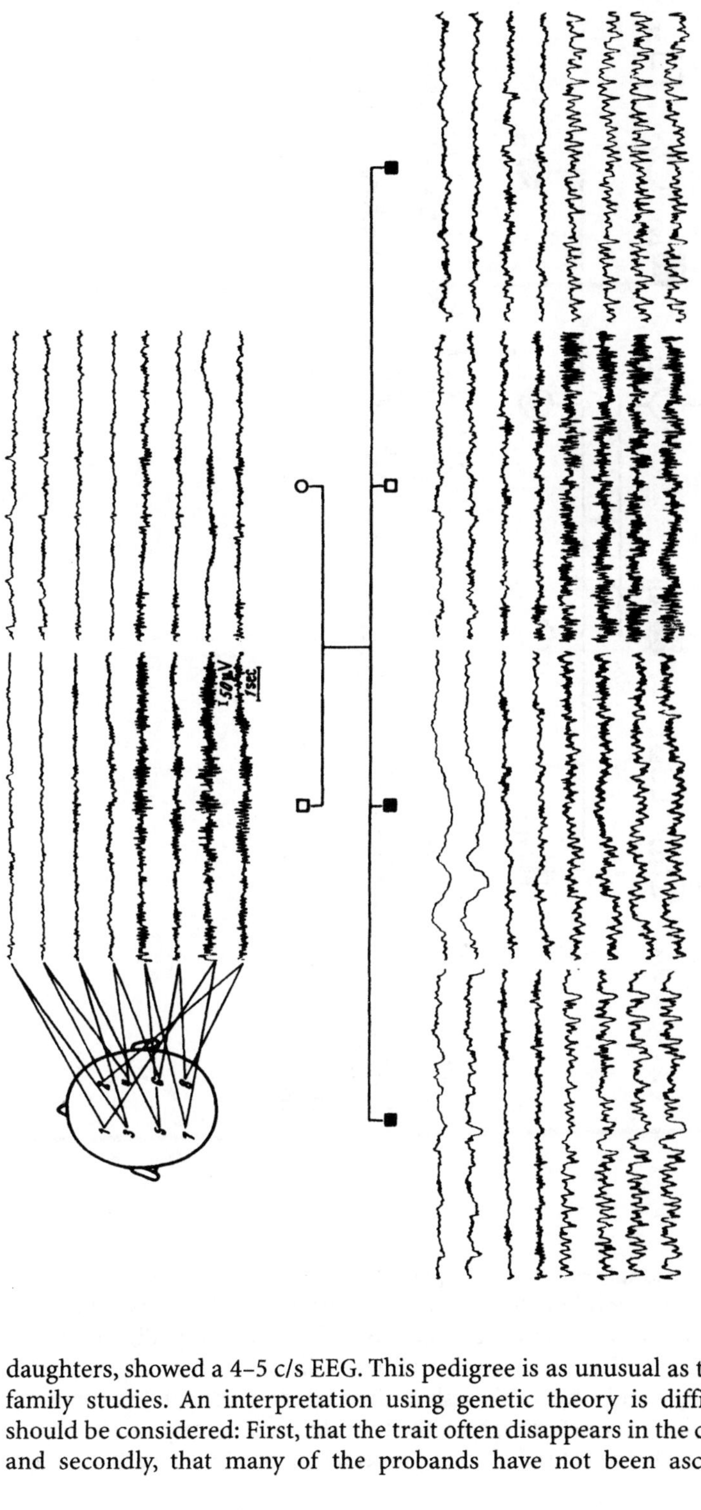

Fig. 4.15. A family observation: Both parents showed a normal α EEG. Of their four adolescent sons, three showed the 4–5 c/s slow α variant (in the second son, the EEG is disturbed somewhat by electrical artifacts due to insufficient cooperation of the proband who suffered from behavioral disturbances)

daughters, showed a 4–5 c/s EEG. This pedigree is as unusual as the other results of family studies. An interpretation using genetic theory is difficult. Two aspects should be considered: First, that the trait often disappears in the course of adult life, and secondly, that many of the probands have not been ascertained from an

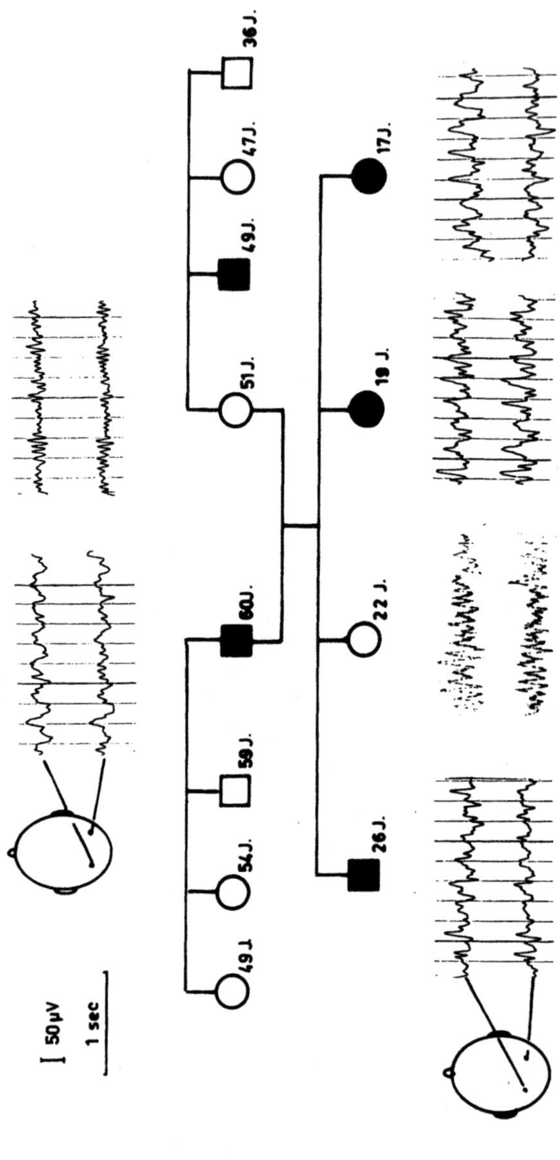

Fig. 4.16a. Another pedigree with the 4–5 c/s variant. Here, the trait was found by chance in two unrelated families. (From Neundörfer et al. 1970)

unbiased population sample but from samples of persons who had been as patients in a certain clinic. In my opinion, the most likely mode of inheritance is autosomal dominant, with incomplete penetrance in elderly individuals (in pedigrees, often parents of trait carriers). The great number of probands whose first-degree relatives, especially brothers and sisters, fail to show this variant is difficult to explain by this model. Either, in many heterozygotes, the trait disappears early in life, or the same phenotype can also be caused by environmental factors. In one early descrip-

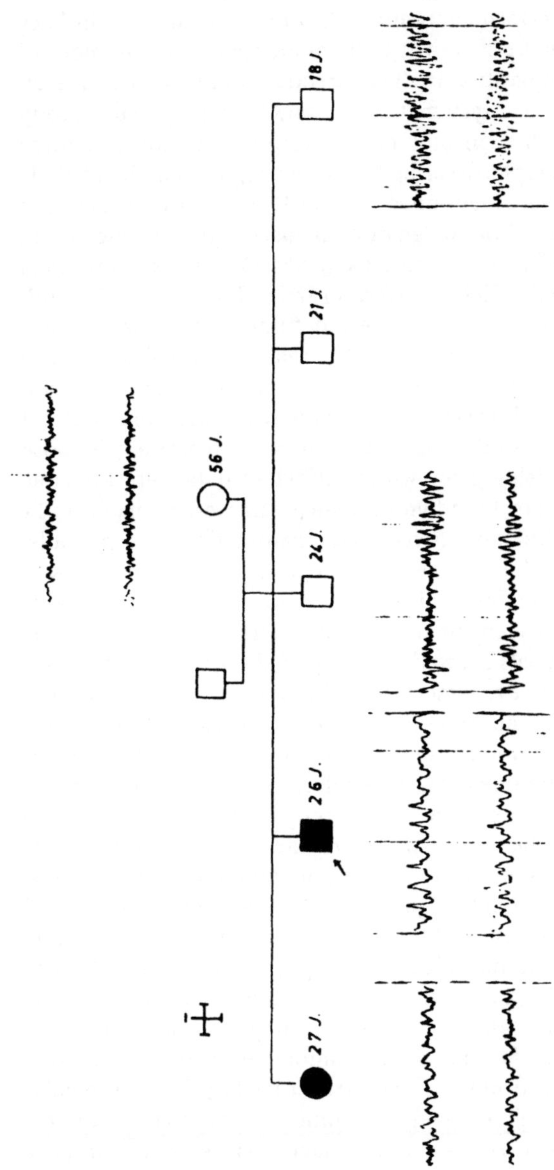

Fig. 4.16b. A third pedigree with the 4–5 c/s variant. The father had died; the fourth child, a son at the age of 21, refused to be examined. (From Müller-Küppers and Vogel 1965)

tion, Pitot and Gastaut (1956) proposed the hypothesis that it could be caused by cerebral trauma; more recent studies (Heintel et al. 1984; Kuhlo et al. 1969; Neundörfer 1970), however, have provided little evidence in favor of this hypothesis. The problem remains unsolved; large-scale epidemiological studies and family studies starting from unbiased series of individuals ascertained independently of clinical and EEG diagnosis are necessary.

While the other EEG variants described in this chapter are not associated with any obvious clinical and psychological phenotypes – less obvious correlations with aspects of feeling tone, mental performance, and behavior are dealt with in later chapters – the 4–5 c/s variant has been shown to be associated with a number of such anomalies. Observations suggestive in this direction were published even before these variants had been studied systematically. Cases belonging to this group were very probably contained in the (incomplete) descriptions of some of these authors. Pitot and Gastaut, for example, described *crises nevropathiques* in a female trait carrier. "Mental symptoms" were mentioned in 12 of 17 adult cases by Petersén and Sörbye (1962); eight of them showed "emotional instability." Dongier et al. (1965) observed "hysterical traits" in 30 of their 34 subjects. Of the cases described above, the probands from Stuttgart (Heintel) were examined systematically with psychodiagnostic methods. Of 13 probands 11 were definitely abnormal psychologically; these were many more than expected, if the relatively small fraction of psychiatric cases among the patients of this laboratory is considered. Certain intellectual defects were found in this series (Heintel and Schneider 1969), but not in the other series. The problem was studied somewhat more systematically in those individuals from Berlin and Heidelberg for which sufficient data were available (Müller-Küppers and Vogel 1965). For 13 individuals, such data were available; in 11 of them, a thorough psychological and psychiatric examination was possible, among them only three women (including one MZ twin pair). Two brothers showed a reduced intelligence, the other persons had an average or above average intelligence; in these, a discrepancy between intelligence and performance in life was noteworthy. Many of these individuals showed a variety of abnormalities in personal development; in four of them, a severe mental and behavioral anomaly was present. Since all probands (except the above twin pair) were ascertained as patients examined in a diagnostic EEG laboratory, it could be suspected that these anomalies were simply caused by an ascertainment bias; therefore we compared their frequency among such cases with another series of 93 probands with a low-voltage EEG who had been ascertained in the same way. Among these, there were 4 persons showing similar psychiatric anomalies, while 89 did not show such clincial signs. The difference (4/12 vs. 4/93) is strongly significant. However, the psychological signs – also the milder one found in some of the other 4–5 c/s carriers – were quite different. The genetically determined modification of a physiological variable does not lead to a well-defined psychological phenotype. This modification changes the ways of reaction and regulation in a completely unknown way at the level of neurophysiological function. However, so far, the manifest anomalies (up to criminality and mental disease) have been seen only in male trait carriers; the two females studied, on the other hand, were well-adapted. A common denominator may be a retarded psychological development with infantile behavior, as well as disturbance in human contacts and ability for social interactions; this anomaly can be described as "schizoid." The sex difference in psychological make-up of the trait carriers probably explains both the high prevalence of males in the observed pedigrees and the isolated cases.

The problem of this highly interesting EEG trait should be studied again in carriers from an unbiased series of EEGs, adults of both sexes and from a really average population sample (not pilot applicants! Not University students!). EEG examination should be performed with great care and in a relaxed and friendly environment since the 4–5 c/s pattern can be disturbed easily. Such series are difficult to obtain, and the conditions for proper study are hard to fulfill.

4.7 Monomorphic Alpha Waves

This EEG variant is characterized by unusually regular α waves which show relatively high amplitude and, more important, are to be seen not only in occipital leads but also over the frontal and parietal parts of the cerebral cortex. Otherwise, they behave as normal α waves. Admittedly, this characterization is somewhat diffuse; distinction of this EEG variant from the more average types of α EEG is not straightforward but an important criterion is regular α activity in frontal and parietal leads. This EEG type appears to be very similar to that described by Jung (1953) as pure α EEG and by Cobb (1963) who described it as characterized by sinusoid, monorhythmic α waves (Fig. 4.17). Dieker (1967) who published the only available, comprehensive family study, proposed a measure that was introduced in 1943 by Motokawa; this was called *Kontinuität* and was defined as follows: K = (number of α waves with amplitudes above the mean)/(number of continuous groups of these α waves. This measure indicates how frequently α waves with similar amplitudes follow each other continuously (Fig. 4.18). K was then multiplied by the percentage -time α, giving a new measure which was called *Persistenz* (persistence; p). This value p was found to give a fairly good measure of the regularity of α waves. In conclusion, diagnosis of this EEG variant mainly depends on two criteria: distribution of regular α waves, especially their presence also above the frontal and parietal parts of the cortex; and regularity of α waves as shown by long sequences of waves with similar amplitudes.

Prevalence of this trait (visual classification) was determined in 4622 German Air Force applicants (young males). It was found in 178 (3.85%). Among 3372 Japanese train drivers, it was seen in 144 (4.27%; Vogel and Fujiya 1969).

Having shown by reassessment of an old twin study (Vogel 1958) and by reexamination of some of these twin pairs that this variant is again concordant in MZ twins, Dieker performed a family study. The EEG records were taken from the above series of German Air Force applicants; all of them were relatively young men in a

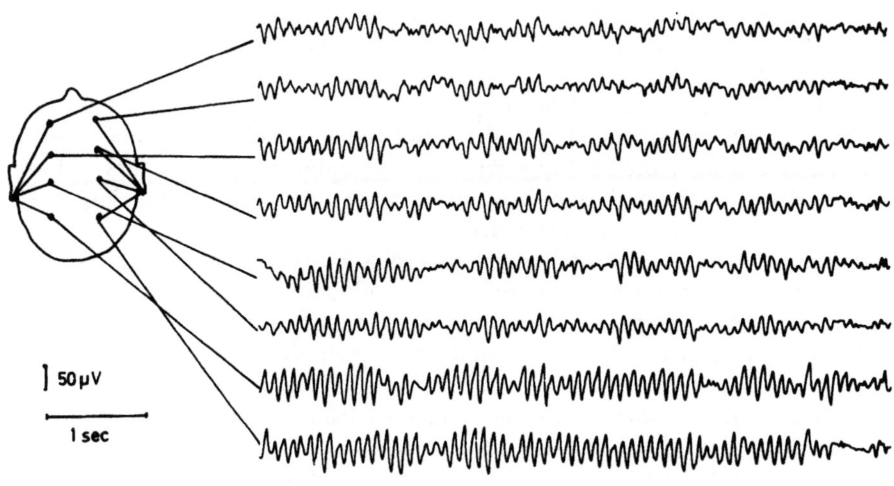

Fig. 4.17. EEG with monomorphic α waves. Reference (unipolar) leads. A 22-year-old man

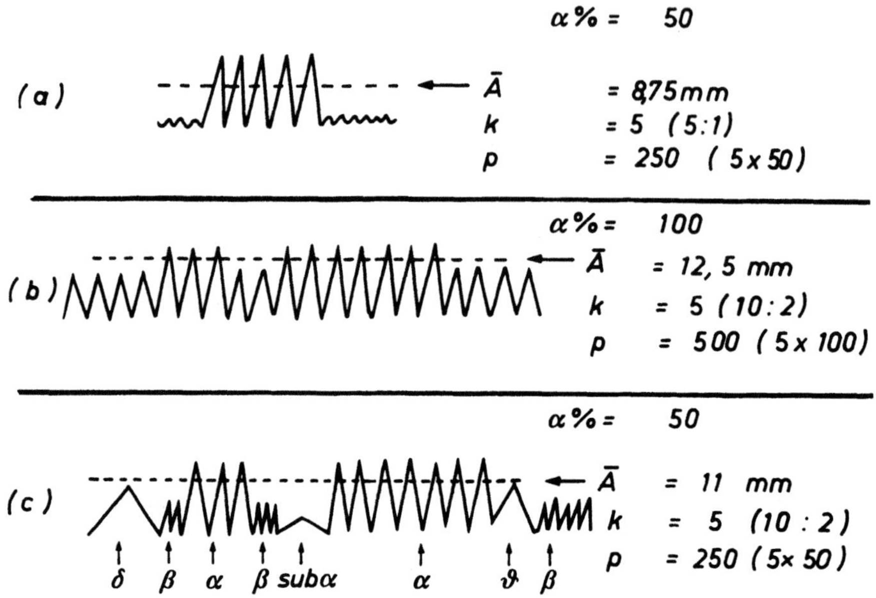

Fig. 4.18. A measurement of *Persistenz* (persistence, *p*). A measure of "continuity" of α waves had been introduced by Motokowa. It was defined as: Number of α waves with amplitudes higher than the average α amplitude, number of uninterrupted sequences of such waves. Dieker refined this measure by dividing this measure by the α index. This new index was called "persistence". It is indeed a useful measure for regularity of α waves. (From Dieker 1967)

good state of health. A total of 35 families encompassing 146 persons (including the probands) were examined. In addition to the persistence (p) measure described above, the α index (Rohracher) was determined. Moreover, the EEGs were classified visually into five categories: 1 = normal, i.e., irregular α waves; 2 = less irregular EEG; 3 = fairly regular α EEG; 4 = regular EEG; and 5 = very regular (monomorphic) α EEG. This classification was complemented by noting whether regular α activity was confined to the occipital area or whether it extended toward frontal and parietal areas.

The family studies had the following results:

The majority of individuals studied could be classified into two categories: Either, they did show the EEG type with monomorphic α waves, or they did not show it. Here "persistence" as defined above proved out to be useful (Fig. 4.18), $p = 300$ being taken as the limit (Fig. 4.19).

In 24 of 28 families in which both parents could be examined, at last one parent showed monomorphic α waves; in 6 families, both parents had this EEG type. In four families where only one parent could be examined, two parents did have this trait, while the other two did not. In another four families, no parent had a persistence above 300. In one fo them, the father showed a very regular α EEG but with very low amplitudes. However, he was completely bald-headed; it is known to the EEG specialist that bald-headedness may increase impedance, lowering amplitudes of EEG waves. In another instance, EEG recording was disturbed severely by outside noise. In a third family, regular α activity in the mother (55 years old) was disturbed

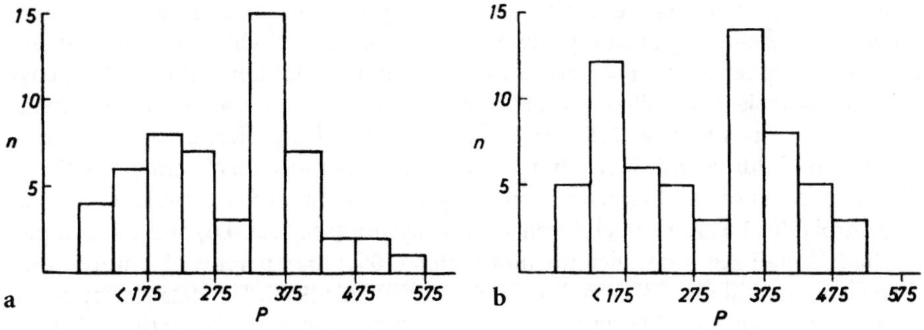

Fig. 4.19. **a** Distribution of "persistence" in sibships of probands with monomorphic α waves. **b** distribution of "persistence" among parents of probands with monomorphic α waves. Both graphs suggest (but do not prove) a bimodal distribution. (From Dieker 1967)

by numerous diffuse β waves of high amplitude, and in a fourth one, paternity was strongly disputable. Segregation analysis gave the following results: Complete families – mating type +×+ (both parents with monomorphic α waves): E = 0.7574; $p = 0.60 \pm 0.2191$; difference not significant. Mating type +×- (one parent with monomorphic α waves): E = 0.5074; $p = 0.5294 \pm 0.0856$; difference not significant. Incomplete families: E = between 0.7574 and 0.5074; $p = 0.66 \pm 0.158$. Hence the result of segregation analysis is compatible with the hypothesis of an autosomal dominant mode of inheritance. Still, the above difficulties in diagnosis of the phenotype and the fact that, in three four families, the patient carrying this trait was difficult to diagnose, raise some doubt. This problem should be reexamined using some biometric methods of EEG evaluation, for example, that developed by Dünki (1996).

Possible assortative mating: One unexpected result should be mentioned: In view of the prevalence of this trait in the population, the number of families in which both parents show this trait is very high. Taking into account population prevalence and the higher expectation for carriers of a monomorphic α wave in the mating type +×+, as compared with the mating type +×–, expectation for the type +×+ can be calculated as 1.17 of 27 families, but 6 were found. Despite the small numbers, the difference is significant ($p \approx 0.05$). Unless there was some undetected bias in diagnosis or classification, real assortative mating is, at least, possible. The result could be neglected as unexplained, had there not been a similar result in the EEG type with diffuse β waves (Sect. 4.10).

The EEG with monomorphic a waves has raised special interest recently, since this EEG variant in parents appears to predispose to spike-wave discharges in the offspring (Doose et al. 1995). Doose, who had worked for decades as head of the neuropediatric department of the University of Kiel (Germany), collected 750 pairs of parents of epileptic children. In 257 of these families, parents were examined, and these children could be classified precisely with regard to clinical and EEG features based on, in most cases very often, examinations. For the sake of comparison, groups with clinical or EEG characteristics were selected; distinction between probands showing generalized spikes and waves (SW complexes) proved to be especially informative. As controls for the parent group 156 healthy adults were examined. The most important results were: The alpha I type very similar to the monomorphic α waves described above but probably comprising a few more records was found significantly more often in parents of children with primary generalized epilepsy (18%) compared with parents of children with focal epilepsy (8%) or controls (9%). When the EEGs of the children were used for their classification, the results were as follows: Alpha I was found significantly more often in parents of children with focal sharp waves and generalized SW complexes (26%) than in parents of children with focal sharp waves without SW complexes (8%) or in controls (9%). Parents of children with ϑ rhythm (see Sect. 4.6) and SW complexes had Alpha I EEGs significantly more often (18%) than parents of children with ϑ rhythm but without SW complexes (8%) or controls (9%). The data clearly reveal an association of this EEG type in parents – which is very similar to the EEG variant described by us as monomorphic α waves – with SW complexes in their epileptic children. In 10% of children with SW complexes both parents had such an alpha I EEG, while in the group of epileptic children without SW complexes, there were no instances, where both parents had this EEG type. EEGs without regular α activity – a large and probably heterogeneous group – were underrepresented among the parents as compared with the control group.

There is an old report in the literature according to which a low-voltage ("= flat") EEG seemed to offer a certain protection against epilepsy in the trait carriers themselves (Adams 1959, 1968). In our own studies, we found in our Berlin material among 53 probands with a low-voltage EEG, who were selected from patients of a diagnostic EEG laboratory, 9 (17%) with epilepsy corresponding to the fraction of epileptics in this laboratory (Vogel 1962); therefore there was no hint for a protective effect. However, this does not exclude the possibility that genes determining the EEG type of the parents may affect susceptibility for epilepsy, or at least certain types of epilepsy, in their children. Epilepsy is not a disease. It is a symptom, or group of symptoms (a syndrome), which might be caused by many factors, both genetic and exogenous. Interindividual variation in the normal EEG and its genetic analysis may help in disentangling the effects of some of the genes involved.

4.8 The EEG with Prominent Beta Waves

While, with few exceptions, every human EEG contains α waves, only a certain fraction shows a significant participation of higher frequencies (>13 c/s). Following a suggestion by H. Berger, they are called β waves. In some instances, they dominate the whole resting EEG, while in other persons, they are present together with other frequencies, especially α waves. When power spectra are analyzed – and also with other methods of computerized EEG analysis – a certain amount of frequency in the β range can be seen in all EEGs. However, sometimes they constitute a very minor component of EEGs only, and do not stand out at visual inspection. In the electrocortigram (ECG), on the other hand, i.e., when activities are recorded directly from the surface of the brain, many more fast frequencies are visible. Therefore it is not advisable to talk about EEG records "without β waves"; there can only be more or less of them. Therefore selecting from the entire group of EEG records from normal individuals having a significant admixture of these waves naturally involves an element of subjectivity. Still, some rules can be established. As shown in somewhat greater detail in Sect. 2.7, admixture of a significant amount of β waves to the EEG of the adult is more common in females than in males, and it increases with age in both sexes, but in women more than in man. This has been discovered by visual inspection of EEG records from a great number of individuals but was confirmed by various methods of computerized EEG evaluation (Sect. 2.4). Normal MZ twins have shown complete concordance as for other aspects of the normal EEG, also for types and degree of β activity. The following describes studies using visual inspection of a great number of EEG records.

Vogel and Götze (1962) studied prevalence of the β EEG in relation to age, sex, and other variables among 4970 patients of an EEG laboratory. Among them were 423 persons whose EEG in the resting stage with closed eyes showed a clearcut β activity at least in some parts of the cortex. The clinical and EEG records were evaluated for a great number of criteria. Here we discuss only age and sex. The frequency of this group of EEG types is seen in Fig. 4.20. Figure 4.20 includes only normal and borderline EEG records; EEGs with clearcut pathological features were not included (and, of course, records from intoxicated patients, for example, after suicide attempts, were excluded, as well). Most striking is the difference between the sexes especially in older age groups: EEG with prominent β rhythm are, again, most frequent in elderly women. In these women, EEGs with very intensive β activity – up to exclusive coverage of the entire EEG – are also more common than in any other group (Vogel and Götze 1962). A certain raise in prevalence with age is seen in men, too. As shown in Sect. 2.8, the EEG in general becomes more complex with advancing age (Anokhin et al. 1996). Even more instructive was a classification of these records into three types: (a) Groups of frontoprecental β waves. Occipital α

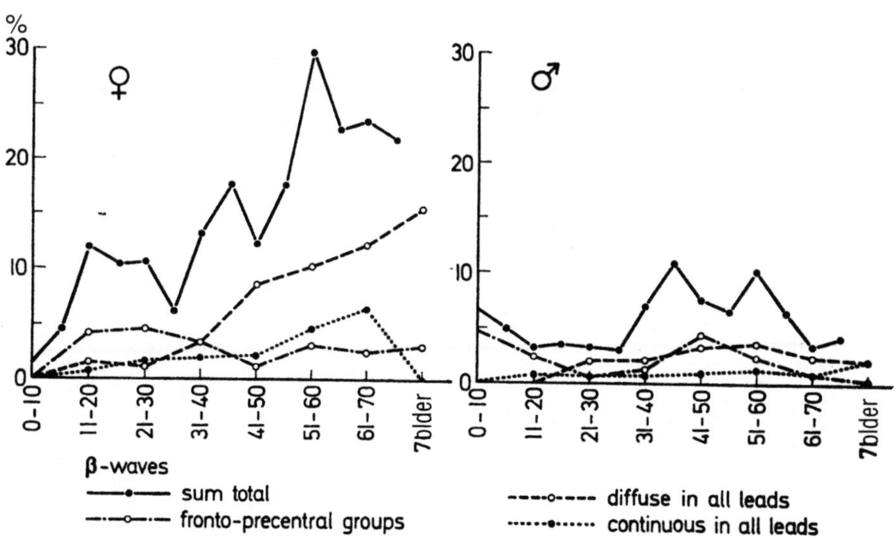

Fig. 4.20. Frequencies of the EEG with clearcut β activity at least over some part of the cortex. The entire sample of subjects was 4970. They were patients of a routine EEG laboratory but patients showing pathological EEGs were excluded. Within the entire sample, there were 413 persons with a β EEG. Its prevalence depends on age and sex. The graph also shows the types of β EEG present (for details see the text)

waves are present. (b) Continuous β waves in occipital and frequently also in precentral leads. No or almost no α waves are present. (c) Diffuse β waves mixed with α waves.

Type 1 (frontoprecentral β groups) shows about the same prevalence in both sexes and in all (adult) age groups. Type 2 (continuous β waves) shows a small sex difference in favor of women and a small increase with age. Upon closer scrutinity, some of the EEGs attributed preliminarily to this group were occipital fast α variants described before (Sect. 4.5). The major part of the age and sex difference proves to be due to type 3 (the EEG with diffuse β waves).

4.9 EEG Variants with Groups of Beta Waves with a Maximum in Frontoprecentral Leads

These β waves occur predominantly in frontal and sometimes also in precentral leads (Fig. 4.21). In a first subtype of this variants, groups of about five to ten β waves with a very fast frequency (approx. 25–30 c/s) are seen. These waves are delimited against the remaining frontal record; they may be relatively rare within the EEG; in the course of recording of about 15–20 min, only a few such groups might be present. Occipital leads show a normal α pattern. In a second subtype, groups of β waves with a maximum in frontoprecentral records are much more common, frequency is often lower, and amplitudes are often much higher. In some instances, β waves in frontoprecentral leads are present almost continuously.

Prevalence of such β groups: The first one of the subtypes described above (rare β groups with high frequency) was found in 9 of 1984 German Air Force applicants (0.45%), and in 4 of 3372 Japanese train drivers (0.12%). The second subtype (common β groups, of lower frequency and, as a rule, higher amplitude; sometimes almost continuous β activity in anterior leads) was found in 23 (1.47%) of 1984 German Air Force applicants, and in 23 (0.68%) of 3372 Japanese train drivers. Hence both types together were found in 32 of 1984 German males (1.63%) and in 27 of

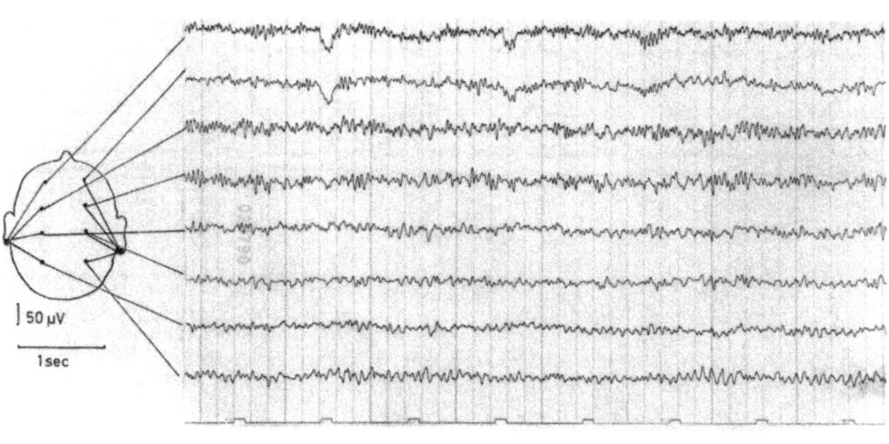

Fig. 4.21. EEG of an adult male with numerous spindlelike groups of β waves in anterior leads

3372 Japanese (0.8%). Hence the trait may be about twice as common in Germans as in Japanese, although the numbers are very small.

Fourteen German families, complete and incomplete, with 24 children were studied. In four families, both parents of the probands were examined, in all of them, one of these parents showed this variant. Persons showing this trait had 14 children, 6 of them showed it as well. In addition, there were three siblings of probands which also showed the trait; one sib with a Down syndrome could not be classified. The segregation rate within these sibships was estimated to be: $p = 0.559 \pm 0.121$. All data are compatible with a simple autosomal dominant mode of inheritance (Fig. 4.22, 4.23).

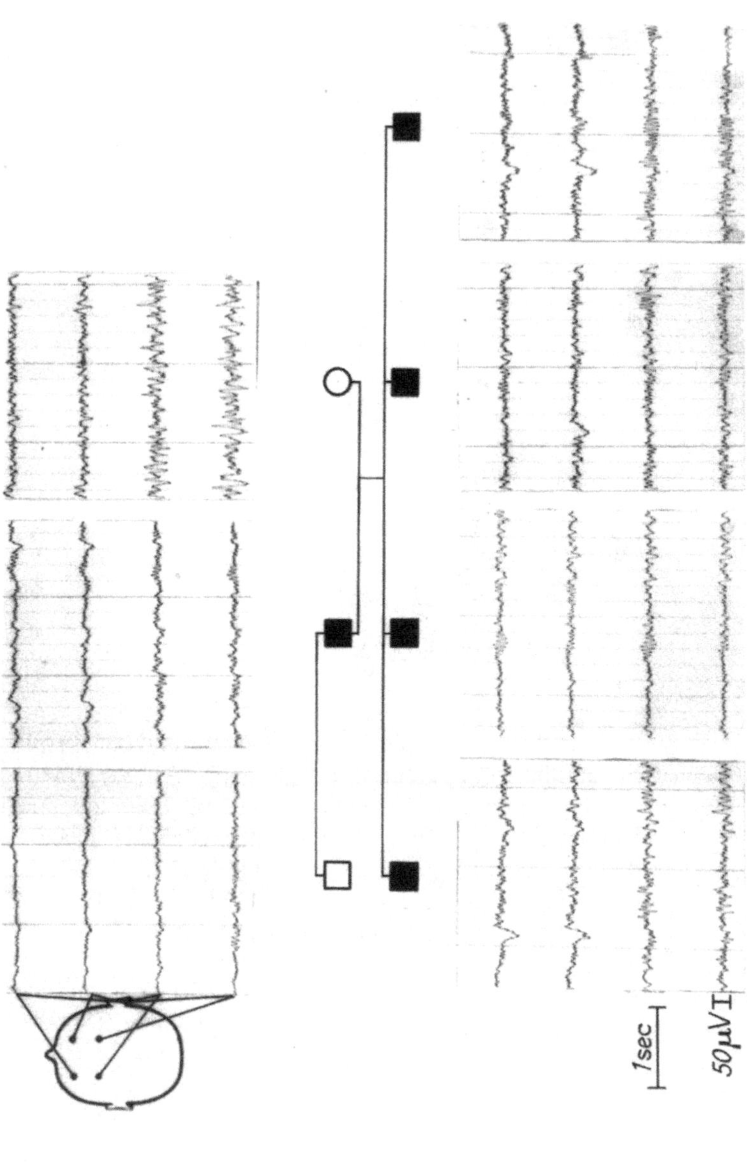

Fig. 4.22. Pedigree of a family with spindlelike groups of very fast β waves in frontal and precentral leads. As with other, similar pedigrees, this pedigree suggests an autosomal-dominant mode of inheritance

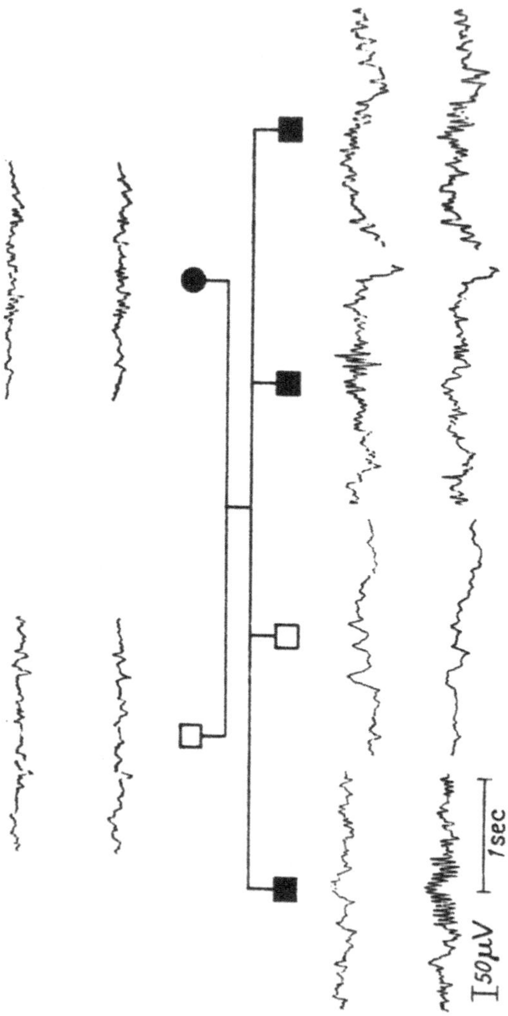

Fig. 4.23. Spindlelike groups of frontal β waves in a mother and three of the four sons

For the second subtype, 16 families (14 complete; 2 incomplete) could be investigated. In 13 of the complete families, both parents of the probands were examined. In two of them, both parents showed this trait and in the remaining 11 families, one parent showed it. Of two families in which only one parent was available for examination, this parent showed this EEG trait: Segregation ratio among 41 sibs was estimated: $p = 0.556 \pm 0.0956$. Obviously, this figure, together with the other features of the pedigrees, is compatible with the genetic hypothesis of an autosomal dominant mode of inheritance (for details of the families, see Vogel 1966).

When the population frequencies given above are compared with those in Fig. 4.20 it proves that the two EEG types found in the two series of healthy males cannot be all EEG records with β wave groups in anterior leads; there must be more. Among the young men of the Air Force material, there were 14 who showed a tendency to frontoprecentral β groups which were, however, combined with diffuse β waves in other parts of their EEG. Also in older age groups many EEGs with diffuse β waves show a certain tendency toward formation of groups in anterior leads. However, these groups are not as well demarcated as in the variants analyzed here, and β frequencies are not as stable. As a rule, the experienced investigator is able to see the difference but in some instances, especially in elderly women, errors of classification are possible.

While in healthy persons, this EEG variant - both subtypes - is clearly dominantly inherited, patients with severe brain damage sometimes show it for apparently external reasons. In our series of normal men (Air Force applicants) such incidences were not observed. However, five cases were reported by Vogel (1962) when a series of EEGs from a diagnostic EEG laboratory was analyzed. All of them suffered from epilepsy which had a clearly exogenous cause in two. Two of the five patients, the oldest ones of the group, suffered severe brain atrophy. One of the Air Force probands (not included in the analyzed material) showed clearcut frequent frontoprecentral groups, while both parents and his sibs did not show this trait. In this proband, the groups appeared immediately after α activity had disappeared, and was replaced by irregular ϑ waves. The obvious interpretation is that this proband started to sleep, showing the typical spindles at an unusually early stage of sleep.

EEG records more or less similar to those belonging to this group are also seen after taking some psychotropic drugs, for example, barbiturates (Wauquier 1993; Bauer, 193). For physicians working with patients who may take such drugs either for therapeutic reasons or because they are drug addicts, it is necessary to know the corresponding normal variants; otherwise, serious errors are possible. As noted above, many of the studies reported here were performed at the Central Medical Institution of the German Air Force (Flugmedizinisches Institut der Luftwaffe). All applicants for the Air Force must undergo among other examinations an EEG examination which was to be repeated after certain time intervals in the flying personnel. Some carriers of a hereditary variants of frontoprecentral β groups run into serious difficulties since physicians accused them to be secret drug users. We could help them by demonstrating results of our family studies to their military superiors and organizing urine studies for drug metabolites, of course, with negative results. Similar diagnostic problems, although not with such severe consequences, could arise in other situations.

4.10 The EEG with Diffuse Beta Waves

The next EEG variant to be considered is the EEG with diffuse beta waves. It does not constitute a homogeneous group but isolation and description of subtypes have not been achieved so far. As noted above, this group of EEG records is more common in women than in men, and its prevalence increases with age in both sexes, although stronger in women. Figure 4.24 shows an example. In the family studies reported by Vogel (1962), all types of β EEGs were analyzed together. Varying prevalences in different categories of first-degree relatives and their sequence mothers >sisters >daughters >fathers >brothers >sons is mainly, if not exclusively caused by the group of carriers of diffuse (sometimes even continuous) β waves.

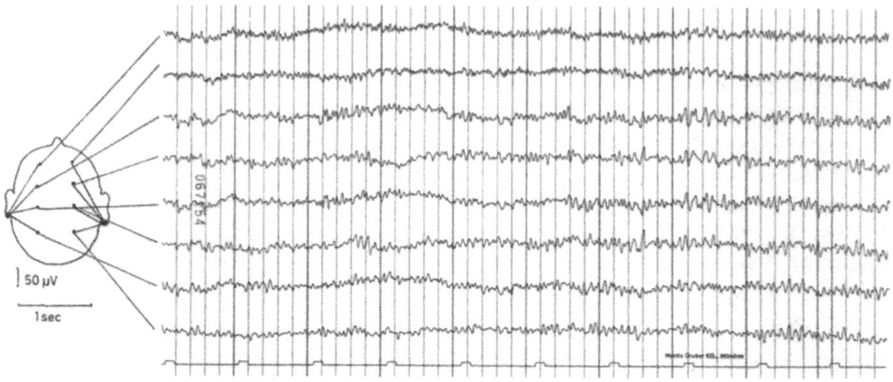

Fig. 4.24. EEG with β waves that are diffusely mixed with α waves in a 49-year-old healthy male

Prevalence of this EEG type was determined again in young German male Air Force applicants and in male Japanese train drivers (Vogel and Fujiya 1969). Among 3554 Air Force applicants, there were 118 (3.32%) with this EEG type; among the Japanese, 136/3372 (4.03%) showed this trait; the difference is not significant statistically. Twenty-nine families in which the proband was a man, and in most cases a young man, were studied. Table 4.2 shows the results (from Vogel 1970; data from Reinke 1966).

Hence individuals with β EEG are much more common than in the population (Fig. 4.25). However, the figures do not suggest any specific hypothesis; we must content ourselves with the very general model of multifactorial inheritance in combination with a threshold (for a general discussion of this model, see Vogel and Motulsky 1996). However, comparison of these data with those in our 1962 material (Vogel 1962) has led to some interesting results (see also Vogel 1970):

- In the more recent data (Reinke 1966), there is the same sequence of frequencies in first-degree relatives: Mothers >sisters >fathers >brothers.
- When the male probands with diffuse β waves are subdivided into those aged over 30 years and those aged under 30 years, prevalence of β EEGs is higher in first-degree relatives of the younger group. This means that, in this group, disposition for developing a β EEG is higher.

Table 4.2. EEG with β waves in close relatives of β probands

Degree of relationship	n	β waves	%
Fathers	22	13	59.9
Mothers	25	20	80.0
Sisters	28	18	64.2
Brothers	25	6	24.0
Daughters	1	0	–
Sons	2	1	50
Total	103	58	57.4

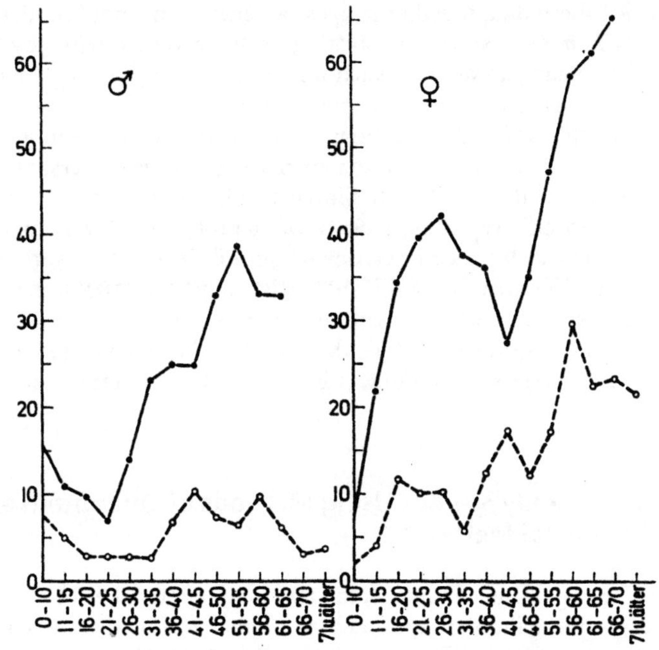

Fig. 4.25. Frequency of EEG with β waves among near relatives (parents and siblings) of β probands, according to age and sex. The small number of observations in each group required the calculation of gliding means. *Filled circles,* relatives; *open circles,* population average

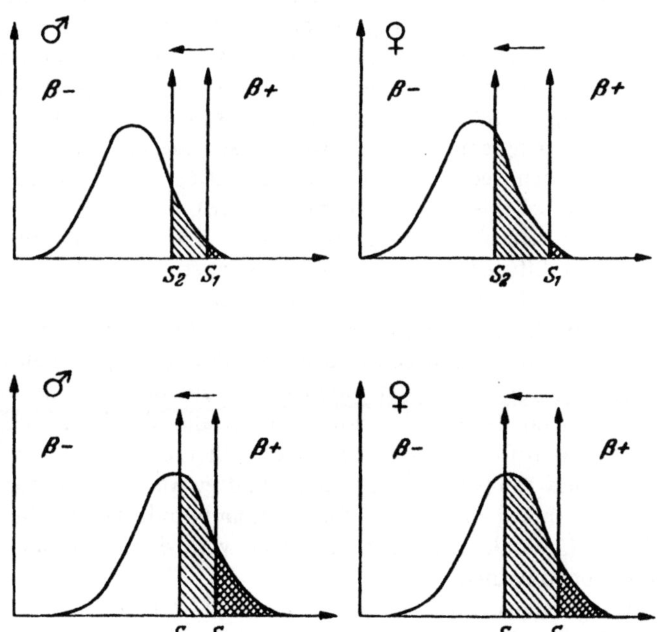

Fig. 4.26. Hypothesis for the genetic determination of the EEG with diffuse β waves. Multifactorial inheritance with a threshold which migrates depending on age and sex (S1 → S2; left-hand side of the graphs males, right-hand side females). In close relatives of probands, distribution of genetic susceptibilities, symbolized by normal distribution curve is shifted to the right, leading to a higher fraction of individuals with β waves (right-hand sides from the thresholds S1 and S2). (From Vogel and Götze, 1962)

All these data together suggest a genetic threshold model with different threshold in both sexes, and shifting of the threshold with advancing age (Fig. 4.26). The heuristic value of such a formal description may be doubted, but a better genetic model is not possible to date.

- Possible assortative mating: In connection with the monomorphic α waves, an unexpectedly high fraction of matings between persons of the EEG type has been noted (Sect. 4.7). A similar result was also found for the β EEG in general (no specific type; Vogel 1962). Of 56 probands 17 were married to a person with a β EEG, while of 54 persons without β EEG, only 5 were married to a β bearer. The difference is significant statistically ($p = 0.006$), If there is no undetected mistakę in ascertainment or diagnosis and no hidden environmental effect (which is quite unlikely) – this could be due to some psychological property of β wave carriers. This problem is discussed in greater detail in Chap. 6.

4.11 Other Family Studies Using Methods of Quantitative, Biometrical Methods

In the beginning of Chap. 4, the two main approaches of genetic analysis of family data – the galtonian approach of biometrical analysis – correlation studies and estimates of heritabilities, on the one hand, and the mendelian approach of analyzing modes of inheritance, on the other hand, were compared. The latter has the great advantage that it opens up a direct path to the genes, and to basic mechanisms. However, uncritical assumption of a simple mode of inheritance is bound to lead the research worker astray; it is less risky to carry out a biometric analysis whenever there are reasonable doubts as to the mode of inheritance. One other way is computing expectations based on various models regarding modes of inheritance, and comparing empirical data with these expectations (for a critical discussion of this approach, see Vogel and Motulsky 1996; for suitable computer programs, see appendix 2 of this book; Fischer et al. 1996).

In Sect. 4.10, a study of family data for various types of the β EEG, especially the EEG with diffuse β waves has been described for which no simple mode of inheritance seems to exist. For this group of EEGs, a certain accumulation within first-degree relatives was reported. The first correlation studies on quantitative EEG parameters were reported by Vogel and Götze (1959). In their families with low-voltage EEG, they compared parents who did not have this EEG trait with their children who also did not show it. Hence all individuals included in this comparison had an α EEG (in some instances with admixture of β and/or ϑ waves). Correlations between parents and (adult) children were: $r = 0.70$ for α frequency; $r = 0.46$ for the α index; and $r = 0.70$ for mean amplitude. Despite the low number of individuals (26 children), all three values were significant statistically. Heritabilities were not computed.

Comprehensive studies were performed by Anokhin (1986). This author examined the resting EEGs of 45 families "from a population characterized by ethnic homogeneity and relative similarity in environmental conditions." Six standard reference derivations were used. The computer program permitted to compute power spectra for 60 s in each individual. Two parameters were calculated in each of the six leads: absolute power values for ϑ, α, $\beta1$, and $\beta2$ bands (altogether 24 points), and relative power values obtained by dividing the absolute values within each frequency band by the total power of a particular lead. These values were used to set up correlation matrices between parents and children and between sibs (56 parent-offspring pairs; 40 sibships two to five persons per sibship). Without going into greater detail, the results may be summarized as follows. Absolute powers: the correlation between parents and children r_{op} was for general amplitude: 0.2; for the balance of low and high frequencies: 0.3; and for the anterior-posterior gradient of amplitude: –0.15. Correlations between siblings were: $r_{sb} = 0.46$; 0.24; and 0.05. Relative powers: Degree of prominence of α waves (parents-offspring): $r_{op} = 0.38$; relative contribution of slow waves to the EEG: 0.13. Sib-sib correlation; prominence of α waves: $r_{sb} = 0.41$; contribution of slow waves: $r_{sb} = 0.18$.

The author concluded that general amplitude and prominence of α rhythm show a high heritability; heritabilities are low for the anterior-posterior gradient and are not very high, for example, for the relative contribution of slow waves. An especially striking result is the high correlation between sibs in comparison with a much lower correlation between parents and children regarding general amplitudes; it is interpreted by the author as pointing to dominance effect. The author concluded from his study that a major part of the appreciable interindividual variation in the EEG is genetically determined. Hence such family studies confirmed, in principle, the results of twin studies.

In another family study, Stassen et al. (1998) compared the EEGs of 121 male MZ and 141 DZ twin pairs (age 14–16 years) with those of 216 fathers (42 ± 5.3 years) and 136 mothers (42.9 ± 4.2 years). They used a control group of 144 healthy volunteers with repeated measurements of 14-day and 5-year intervals to quantify constancy of EEG patterns over time (reliability). The EEG parameters studied by this group have been described before in Chap. 3. The authors concluded from their detailed quantification of various EEG parameters that "most parameters ... possess distinct trait-like qualities, as indicated by large interindividual differences, great stability over time and high within-pair coincidence in monozygotic twins." With respect to the genetic component of brain wave patterns, they found for major parameters "a heritability estimate of $h^2 \approx 0.75$ independently derived using two different methods: through an analysis of parent-offspring similarity and through an analysis of the difference in within-pair similarity between monozygotic and dizygotic twins. These heritability estimates were consistent across lateral EEG channels." The reliabilities of EEG measures in repeated recordings from the volunteer group were in the same order of magnitude as the similarities of MZ twins, confirming earlier results by Vogel (1958). Concordance in the speed of EEG maturation was also confirmed by comparing MZ in adolescence with those in adult age. For comparing parent-child similarity in adolescents (= the 14- to 16-year-old twin sample) with this similarity in adults, a control sample of 46 children (33 sons and 13 daughters) and their 19 fathers (mean age 59.3 ± 5.5 years) and mothers (mean age 55.1 ± 3.6 years) was used. Heritabilities estimated from midparent values for the EEG parameters evaluated were in about the same order of magnitude as those derived from the twin studies. Correlations between parents and sons in adolescence tended to be much lower than those between adults and their parents. "In particular, the values associated with ... 'absolute power' and 'relative power' were significantly lower among adolescents ..."

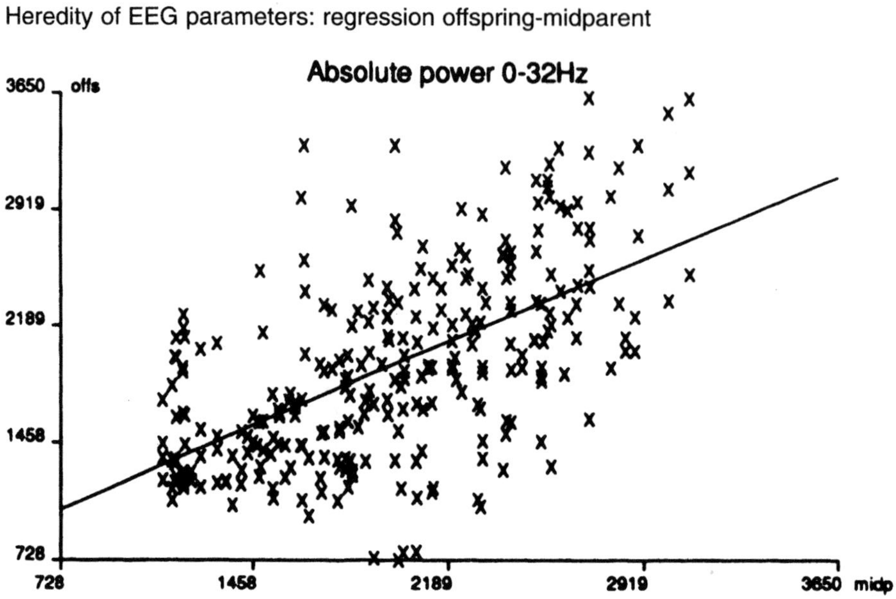

Fig. 4.27. Regression of EEG parameter "absolute power 0.0–32 Hz" of the offspring on the respective "midparent" value derived from the parents. The regression analysis was carried out separately for each of the channels F_3/F_4, C_3/C_4, P_3/P_4, and O_1/O_2. The slope of the regression line "offspr"r(midp)" is an estimate of the heritability coefficient h^2. (From Stassen)

In the opinion of the present author, this is not really surprising, considering the higher EEG, especially α, amplitudes during adolescence. Figure 4.27 gives an example of regressions between midparents and children for absolute power in the entire frequency range from 0.0 to 32 c/s and for the entire sample. The study shows how twin and family studies may be combined. The authors conclude that the normal EEG has definite "trait" character which makes it useful for studies in psychiatric genetics. This aspect is discussed in greater detail in Chap. 8.

4.12 EEG Variants and Dopamine β-Hydroxylase Values in the Blood

Variation in the EEG is caused by corresponding variation in molecular and biochemical processes in the brain – mainly neurotransmitter ion channels and enzymes regulating their metabolism. Obviously, these processes are difficult to study in the living human being; the living brain is not directly accessible to biochemical analysis. However, some of these metabolites and their enzymes can also be found in the periphery, for example, in the blood. Here, they may be accessible for analysis. Such studies were performed by Propping et al. (1979, 1980). While for MAO and proteins of the red blood cell membrane, no difference between carriers of EEG variants could be discovered, there was a significant difference in blood levels of

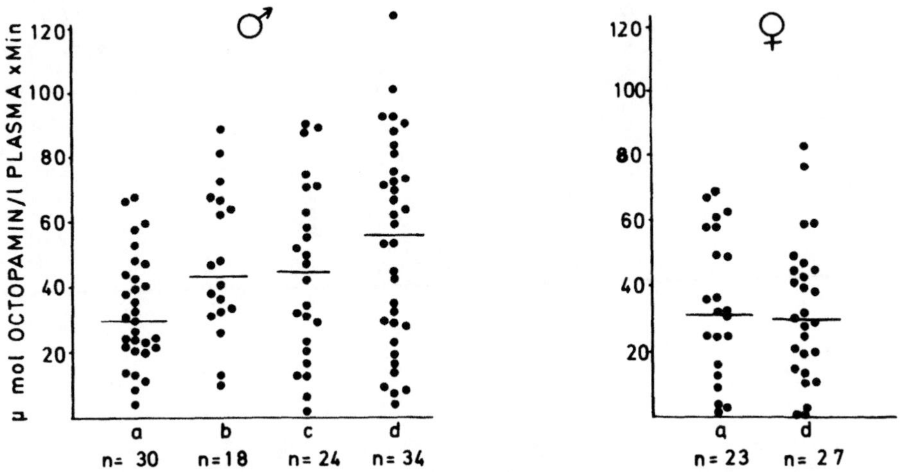

Fig. 4.28. Activity of the enzyme dopamine β-hydroxylase in the blood of probands with various hereditary EEG variants. (a) Low voltage EEG; (b) badly synchronized α EEG; (c) diffuse-β EEG; (d) monomorphic-α EEG. The difference between males with monomorphic α waves, on the one hand, and the low-voltage EEG, on the other, is obvious (and significant statistically). In females no difference could be detected. (From Propping et al. 1979, 1980)

dopmaine β hydroxylase (DBH), one of the key enzymes of catecholamine metabolism (Fig. 4.28). The low-voltage EEG, on the one hand, and the EEG with monomorphic α waves, on the other, occupy the two extreme positions, while the other EEG types are found in-between. DBH in the blood does not come from the brain; it apparently has its origin in the sympathetic cord. Hence this difference points to a more general physiological difference between EEG types. However, while differences between the means is significant (and was confirmed by a study on other probands; Propping et al. 1980), distributions of individual values overlap strongly. For unknown reasons, this difference between EEG types was found only in males, while in females even probands with the low-voltage EEG and those with monomorphic α waves showed almost identical means and distributions. Earlier twin studies of the same group had shown that individual variation in the level of DBH, as that of other catecholamine enyzmes in the blood, is strongly genetically determined (Winter et al. 1978).

CHAPTER 5

5 Event-Related (Evoked) EEG Potentials

5.1 Principle and Methods

(For more details of principle and methods, see Lopes da Silva 1993.) So far, genetic studies on the resting EEG, and in part on EEG changes during sleep and under the effect of provocation methods, including hyperventilation, photic stimulation, and drugs such as alcohol have been discussed. However, the EEG shows characteristic changes also under the effect of a variety of sensible and sensory stimuli. The best known is the off effect; i.e., the blocking of α activity after opening of the eyes. However, even when eyes are closed, sensible and sensory stimuli such as touching the hand, and, especially, light flashes or sudden sounds such as clicks cause visible reactions in the EEG. Due to the spontaneous "background" activity, these reactions are normally more or less hidden; their identification is difficult if not impossible. However, this difficulty can be overcome by a trick: The stimulus is repeated many times, for example, 50–100 times, in regular or irregular distances. The computer is programmed in a way that recording starts a short time before the stimulus and ends a somewhat longer time after it. All recordings are summed up. The stimuli are random in relation to the EEG background activities; hence these background waves tend to cancel out, and reaction to the stimulus manifests clearly (Fig. 5.1). This sounds relatively simple but recording and quantification of EEG signals offers

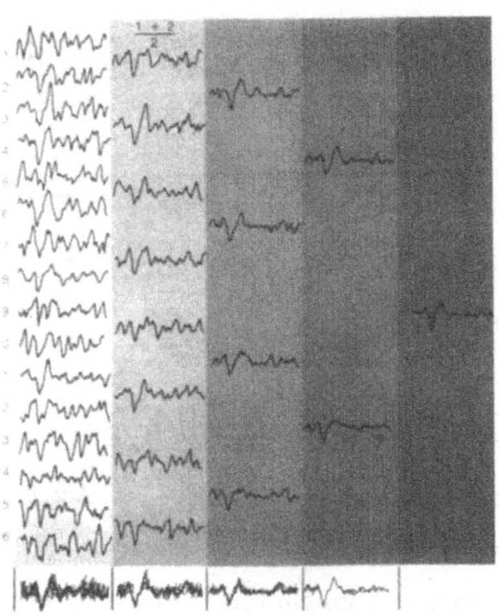

Fig. 5.1. Principle of the computation of averaged evoked EEG potentials. Frequent repetition of the experiments leads to leveling-out of the "spontaneous" EEG background. (From Birbaumer)

many problems (see Lopes da Silva 1993; Regan 1972; for an early summary of principles, see Dawson (1954), who was the first to apply this principle to the EEG). It cannot be the purpose of this monograph to go deeper into the various ways of eliciting and measuring evoked potentials (EPs; see the various chapters on this topic in the textbook of Niedermeyer and Lopes da Silva 1993). This technique is being used increasingly for many diagnostic purposes – not only in neurology but also, for example, in ophthalmology; all these applications cannot be described here. This discussion is confined to genetic problems. However, some applications in psychiatry and psychology are discussed since they are related to aspects of genetics.

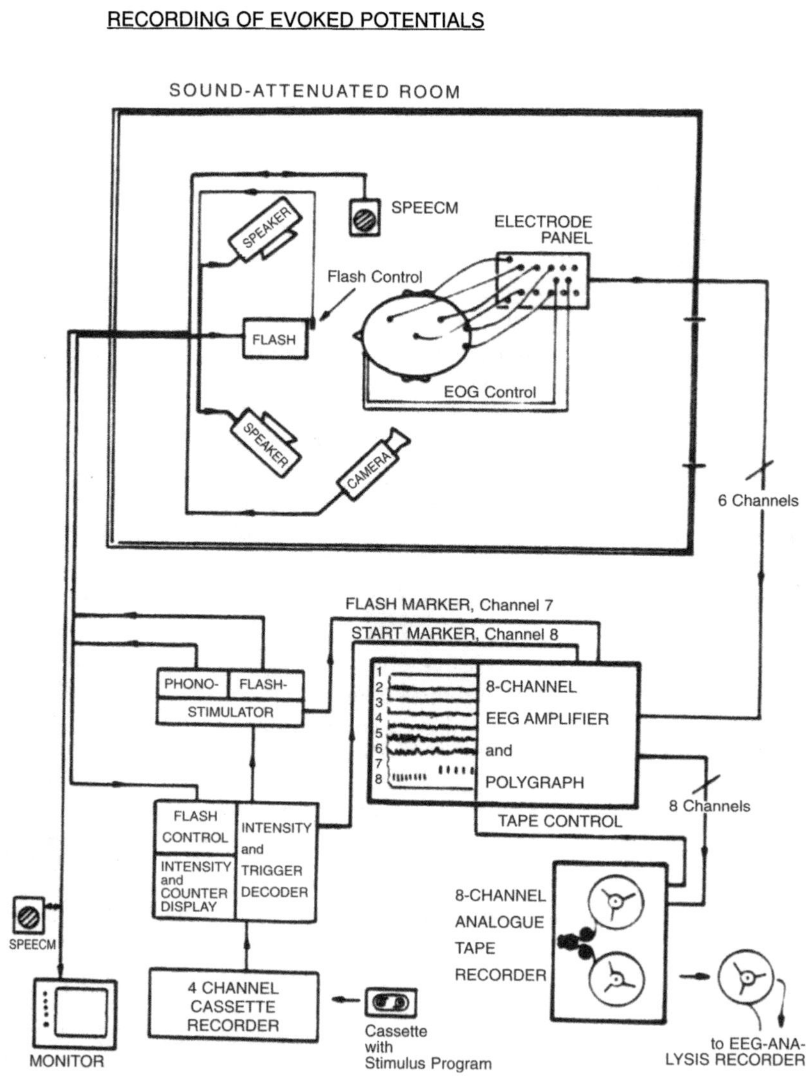

Fig. 5.2. Configuration of instruments for recording of evoked potentials

The following describes a setup that has been used in our own studies on EPs in relation to variants of the normal EEG. The purpose of this study was to determine whether information processing in the brains of carriers of the inherited EEG variants described in Chap. 4 showed any reproducible differences (Vogel et al. 1986). The setup shown in Fig. 5.2 was used. Visual and auditory stimuli were produced by a commerically available stimulator. In distinction to most setups in clinical use, where pattern reversal is used as visual stimulus, light flashes were applied, since the examinations had to be performed with closed eyes; possible disturbance due to eye artifacts were carefully avoided. In each proband, four experiments were performed, each with 255–256 stimuli: two with visual stimuli in fixed inter-stimulus intervals (1.5 s), and a second one with random intervals (1–2 s). Visual stimuli were applied in four intensities to study the augmenting-reducing phenomenon described by Buchsbaum (see, for example, Buchsbaum 1974, 1980; Buchsbaum and Pfefferbaum 1971). Electrodes were positioned according to the 10–20 system; EPs were recorded from the five scalp electrodes shown in Fig. 5.3. For each stimulus, a period of 700 microseconds starting 100 ms before stimulation was digitized of 333 Hz, each period thus being converted into 234 amplitude values for each of the six channels. The amplitudes of the average signals were determined in relation to the zero line of the EEG machine; artifact elimination routines were included. All leads (F_4, C_z, P_4, O_1, O_2) were evaluated separately. For computer evaluation, two methods were used: the period analysis, which permits identification of most of the important peaks described in the literature, and the component analysis for specific identification of the components for which the augmenting-reducing phenomenon was described (Buchsbaum and Pfefferbaum 1971). For details of the delineation of the various peaks against each other and other technical details, see Vogel et al. 1986; Höpp 1983; Fig. 5.4).

Fig. 5.3.

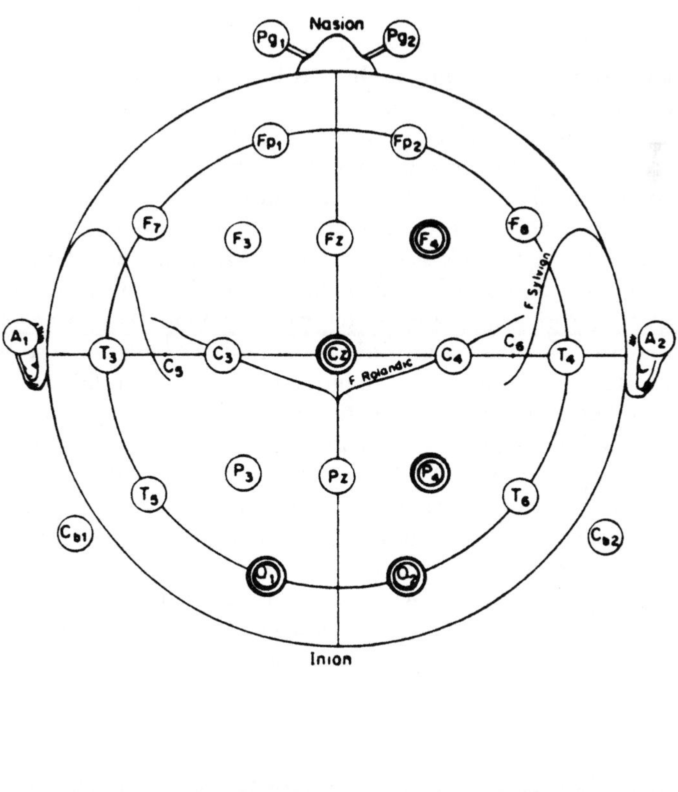

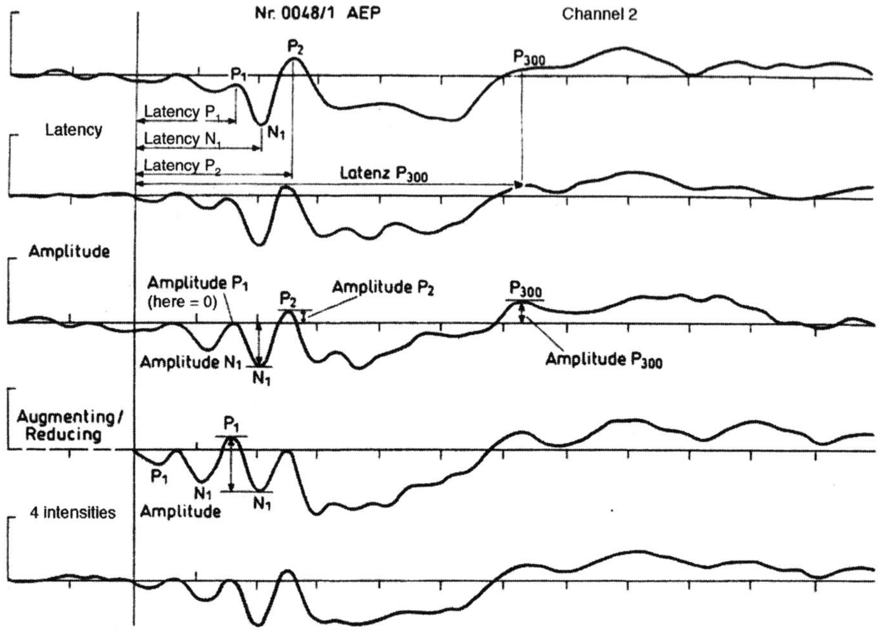

Fig. 5.4. Visually (by light flashes) evoked EEG potentials. Examination with closed eyes; 64 flashes each were given, four levels of intensity, random order. Some characteristic peaks are described; in addition. Peaks used for determining the augmenting-reducing response are indicated. (From Höpp 1983)

In addition to period and component analysis, a new measure for the entire length of oscillation amplitudes has been introduced. Here, we followed, in principle, a suggestion by Hendrickson (1982). However, his "string measure" did not convince us for various reasons. Therefore we developed another measure, the "oscillation," defined as the sum of the absolute values of the differences between subsequent relatively extreme amplitudes of the EP curve plus the amplitudes in the ends of the evaluation interval and the first and last extreme amplitudes (Krüger et al. 1985; Fig. 5.5). We also used a new general measure for latencies – the average latency which was defined as the mean of all latencies of individual peaks. This description gives an example, how evoked potentials may be derived, quantified and evaluated. There are many differences in detail between experimental setups used by different investigators; it cannot be the purpose of this review to describe all of them, but one aspect should be mentioned: The augmenting-reducing reaction described by Buchsbaum and used by his group for characterization of certain types of personalities. With increasing intensity of the stimulus, for example, the light flash, the intensity of reaction also increases in many persons; they were called "augmenters." In others, however, this intensity decreases, at least above a certain level of intensity. These persons are called "reducers." For a possible relationship with personality, see below (Chap. 6). Relationships between properties of EP and the resting EEG are described below in greater detail; here it may be sufficient to note that there are strong individual differences in many properties of EPs.

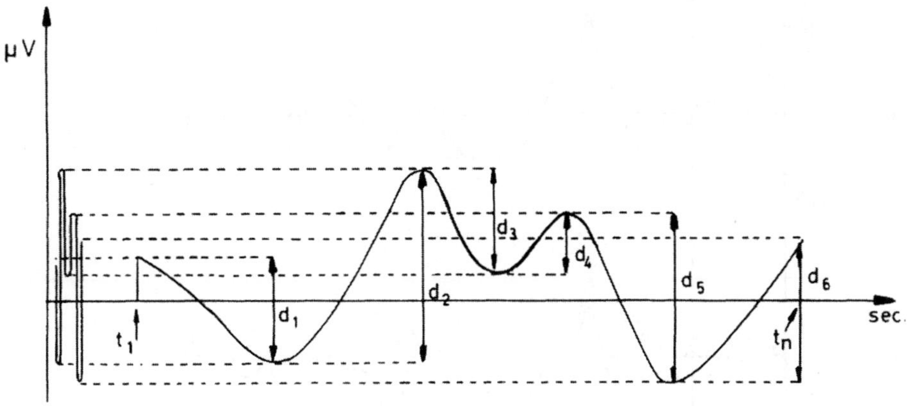

Fig. 5.5. A new over-all measure for amplitudes of evoked potentials ("oscillation S*" within the time interval $t_1 - t_n$). S^*, sum of all intervals $d_1, d_2 \ldots d_n$

5.2 Twin and Family Studies

Evoked potentials show an appreciable interindividual variation while differences between tracings in the same individual tend to be small (see, for example, Dustman and Beck 1963). Therefore it is not surprising that the twin method has been used to examine whether and to what extent this interindividual variation is affected by genetic factors.

The first twin study was reported by Dustman and Beck (1965). The VEPs were studied in 12 MZ pairs (ages between 5 and 17 years), 11 DZ pairs (ages 7–15 years), and, for comparison, 12 pairs of unrelated children matched for age (ages 5–17 years). EPs were recorded from central and occipital regions of the skull (O_1, O_2, C_3, C_4). Flashes were used to elicit the EPs (100 flashes per recording session). Amplitudes were summed and compared for two partially overlapping ranges – 0–250 ms and 0–400 ms. Correlation coefficients of this measure between members of pairs were calculated; they were in MZ twins 0.82 and 0.81 for occipital and 0.74 and 0.69 for central leads; in DZ twins they were 0.58 and 0.54 for occipital and 0.48 and 0.41 for central leads; and in unrelated pairs 0.61 and 0.56 for occipital, and 0.53 and 0.49 for central leads. The order of magnitude of correlations between MZ twins was about the same as that between repeated recordings of the same person. The amplitude measure used for quantification is not sufficient for characterization of EPs; therefore the authors gave figures showing their shape. In MZ twins, they were very similar (Fig. 5.6). The correlations of this amplitude measure in DZ twins, on the other hand, were not higher than the correlations between unrelated age-matched pairs. Other twin studies were reported by Buchsbaum (1974, 1980); they included the augmenting-reducing trait which had been shown before by the Buchsbaum group to be a constant personal trait. Malykh and Ravitch-Scherbo (1986) studied "movement related brain potentials" (MRBP) in 25 pairs of MZ and 25 DZ pairs (age range between 18 and 30). All probands participated in two testings. In the first experiment, the subjects had to push a button approximately every 10–15 s. In the

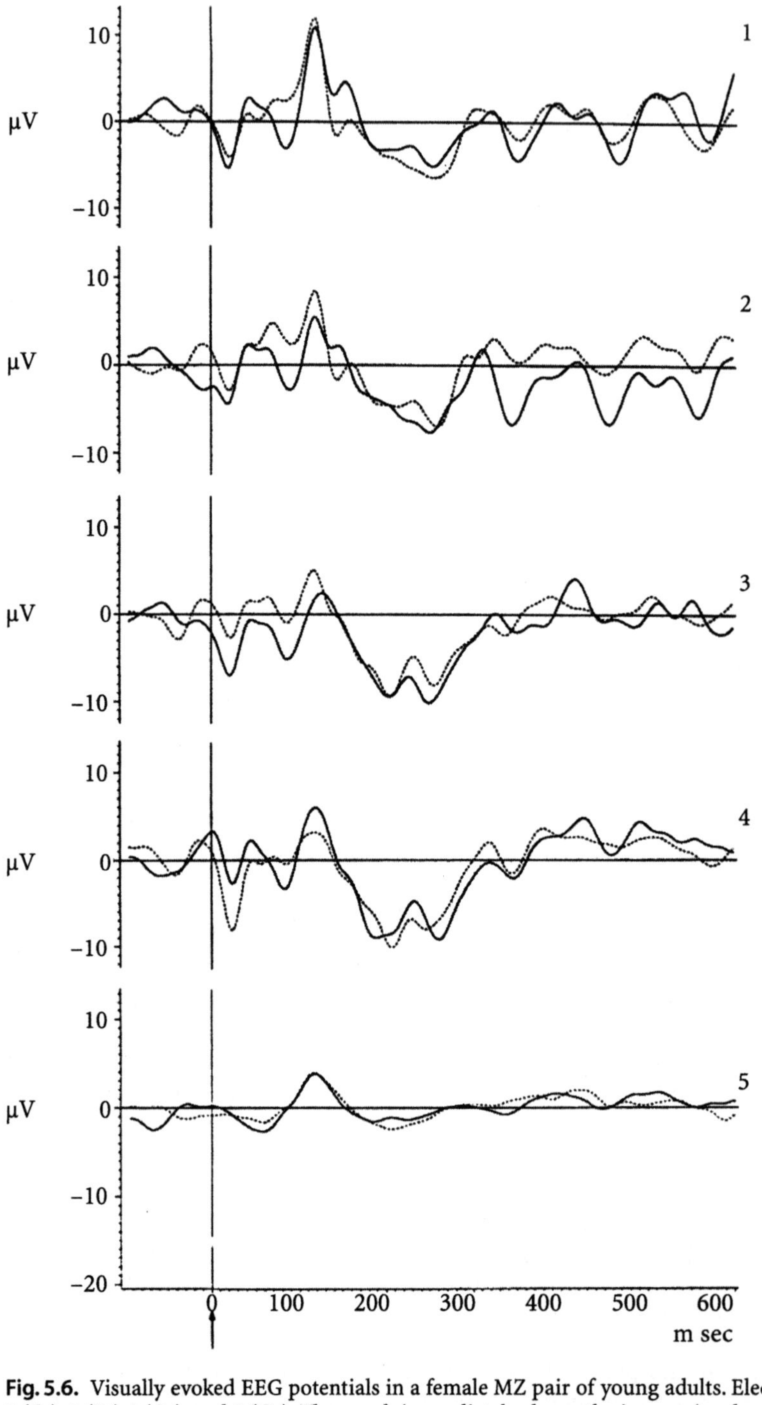

Fig. 5.6. Visually evoked EEG potentials in a female MZ pair of young adults. Electrodes 1 (F_4), 2 (C_z), 3 (P_4) 4 (O_1), and 5 (O_2). The graph immediately shows the impressive degree of similarity (Own observation)

second experiment, probands had to predict the appearance of sounds that occurred with probabilities 0.5 and 1.0. Hence the EPs to be measured included the readiness potential. Intraclass correlation coefficients between MZ twins were not very high but higher than in DZ twins and higher in amplitude measurements than in the time dimension. Cortical EPs after auditory stimulation were studied by Surwillo (1980) in six male MZ pairs (aged 8.11–13.4 years) and in six control pairs of unrelated boys matched for age. Probands were asked to press a button when hearing a click. The cortical potentials were averaged coherently as usual, and peaks were subdivided into exogenous (P_1, N_1, P_2) and endogenous one (N_2, P_3). Latencies of the exogenous components were closely similar in all pairs of subjects. Latencies of the endogenous peaks were significantly more alike in MZ twins than in unrelated subjects. The author concluded that exogenous peaks depend mainly on properties of the stimulus, while endogenous ones are associated "with a person's intention, expectations, and decisions," which largely depend on their individual, genetically affected personalities; therefore their special similarity in MZ twins. Peak amplitudes or other characteristics of the AEP shapes were not considered.

Another twin study has been reported by O'Connor et al. (1994). This study is part of a research program on genetics, and especially the EEG in alcoholism. Therefore we must return to this below (Sect. 7.1). However, to establish a base line, 98 pairs of twins were studied – 59 MZ pairs, among them 33 female pairs and 39 same-sex DZ pairs, among them 22 females (age range: 22–46 years; mean 29.7 years). Base line AEPs were elicited, and an oddball "experiment" was performed; then target and nontarget tones were presented (20% target tones). Subjects were instructed to keep their eyes closed and to press a button in response to the higher-pitched tone. In evaluation of the data, a combination of visual inspection of the AEP curves and measurement of amplitudes and latencies of N_1 and P_3 peaks was used. The N_1 peak as defined as the largest negative deflection between 80 and 180 ms. P_3 peaked within the 250- to 600-ms interval (probably identical with the P300 peak of other authors). For further details, the original should be consulted. For visual evaluation, the maximum of cross-correlations of EPs was used; in addition, a new method for quantifying the difference between EPs by comparing their topographic features was applied. This study had the following results: (a) The amplitude of the target P_3 component was maximal at lead P_z; P_3 amplitudes revealed significant heritabilities ranging from 0.41 to 0.60; analysis of P_3 latencies failed to give any significant differences. (b) Cross-correlation measures revealed significant genetic effect on the shape of the entire ERP response. The topograph method described above proved to be a useful way for describing the individual shape of the EP curve, and was therefore used for describing effects of alcohol on evoked potentials (discussed below).

The twin study reported by Rust (1975) should be mentioned. He studied 20 male MZ and 20 DZ pairs (mean age: 24.2 years). The traits to be evaluated were again AEPs. Heritabilites for amplitudes of the various peaks ranged between 35.17 and 88.53; most of the leads showed very high heritabilities. On the other hand, there was no consistent environmental effect. The results for latencies are less clear; there also seemed to be some environmental effects, in addition to effects of genetic variation. The latter report (Rust 1975) includes some considerations on the short-time individual variation in the EP measurements used. Unfortunately, however, none of these studies, even those using very sophisticated methods of evaluation, contain data on repetition of EPs after a somewhat longer time, for example, some weeks or months. Such studies would help in indicating whether differences between MZ twins indicate a real long-term difference in reagibility of the brain toward stimulation, or indicate only random fluctuations that may occur in the same individual.

In recent years, the P300 component of the auditory EP had found special attention in psychophysiological research as a marker for neural processes related to cognition (Sutton et al. 1965; Pritchard 1981). Twin studies were reported by Polich and Burns (1987) and by Rogers and Deary (1991). In the first study, the EPs in MZ twins were very similar in amplitude and latency in comparison with matched pairs of controls. Striking similarity was also found in the shapes of waves. In the second study by Rogers and Deary (1991), ten adult MZ pairs were compared with 11 DZ pairs regarding latencies and amplitudes. The subjects were advised to count infrequent high-pitched tones given within a series of low-pitch tones. Intraclass correlation coefficients were higher in MZ pairs (latency 0.63; amplitude 0.50) than in DZ pairs (latency 0.50; amplitude 0.35). Both studies indicate "that the neurophysiological mechanisms responsible for P300 generation are themselves highly genetically determined."

The most comprehensive twin studies on the P300 components were reported by the group of Boomsma in Amsterdam (van Beijsterfeldt 1996; van Baal 1997). Their studies on the resting EEG are mentioned above (Sect. 3.7); in that section, the twin samples used were also described. To repeat, the first sample consisted of adolescents; 39 male and 52 female MZ pairs; 36 male and 38 female DZ pairs, and 48 twin pairs of opposite sex. Experimental setup consisted in discrimination and counting of infrequent white figures on black ground among a series of frequently occurring figures. Numerous electrodes, including a reference electrode, were used according to the 10–20 system (for more technical details, see van Beijsterfeldt 1996). Target and nontarget P300 peaks were summed up separately (Fig. 5.7). The P300 peak is especially well visible in the P, P_z and O_1 and O_2 leads. It is developed only weakly in the frontal leads. Quantitative genetic analysis was performed using a relatively sophisticated program designed to break down the genetic variance, shared (common) environmental effects, and specific environmental effects (for details, see the original). This analysis showed no main effect of zygosity, sex or birth order and no significant interactions between them. There was, however, a significant interaction between gender and condition (i.e., reaction to the target vs. the nontarget): For females, the target P300 amplitude was larger than for males, while in males, the nontarget amplitude was higher than in females. The following correlations between cotwins were found: In males MZ correlations were higher than DZ correlations for most leads, both for target and nontargets, pointing to a genetic effect. For females, similar evidence of a genetic effect was found on the P300 amplitude only in central and parietal leads in response to nontargets; MZ correlations were higher than those reported for DZ twins. In response to targets, however, MZ and DZ correlations were the same for most leads; in some instances, DZ correlations were even higher. Following the model used for their genetic statistical analysis, the author concluded that the target P300 amplitude in females may be affected by shared environmental factors. In my opinion, however, it is at least doubtful whether data from a quantitative genetic analysis can be interpreted in such a specific way. In twin pairs of opposite sex (all, of course, dizygotic), very low correlations

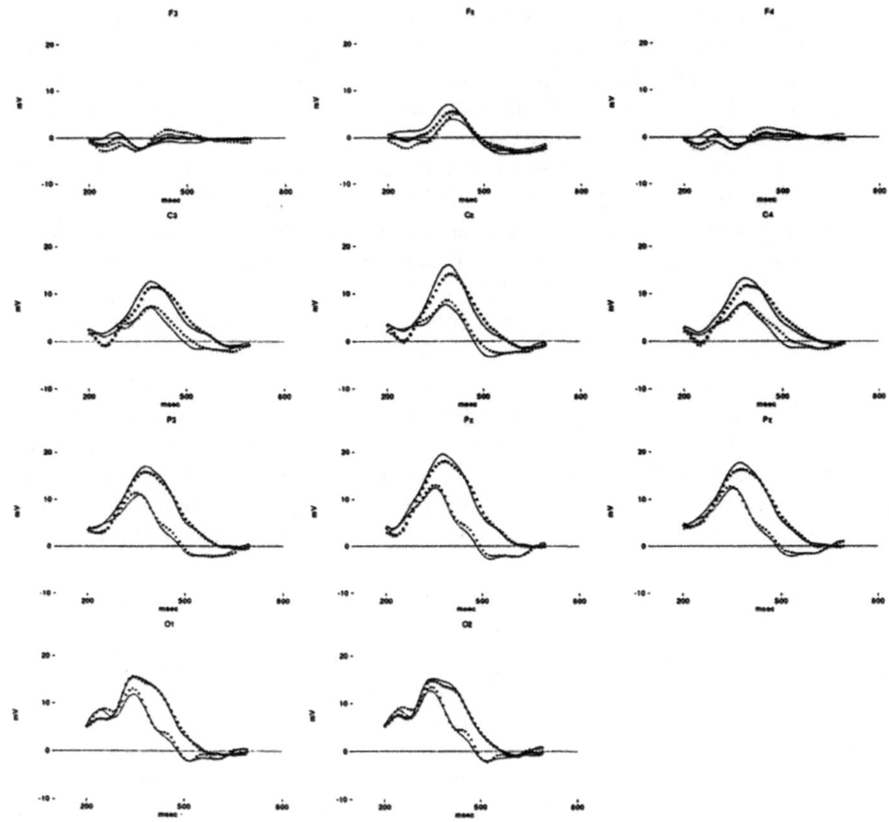

Fig. 5.7. Grand averaged ERPs from the oddball task after the signal is filtered with the Woody filter. For each electrode position the target ERPs of males (··· *line*) and females (— *line*) were given and the nontargets ERPs of males (+++ *line*) and females (-- *line*). The ERP is displayed for the time interval 200–700 after stimulus presentation.(From van Beijsterfeldt)

between cotwins were found. Quantitative evaluation of these amplitude data gave the overall result that the amount of variances explained by genetic factors tends to be somewhat higher than that explained by shared environmental factors. However, in both sexes, a relatively large part of target and nontarget P300 amplitudes had to attributed to nonshared (extraneous) environmental factors. So far, only correlations of amplitudes have been considered; correlations of latencies were generally lower, and no meaningful pattern emerged.

The other study within the same group was performed by van Baal (1997). It was the goal of this study to follow up development during early childhood. Therefore all twin pairs were studied twice; for the first time at the age of about 5 years, and for the second time at the age of almost 7 years. Of the 209 pairs first included in this study, after some dropout had occurred for various reasons, 164 pairs could be studied completely: 33 MZ and 37 DZ males; 33 MZ and 31 DZ females; and 31 DZ pairs of opposite sex. Experimental procedure was the same as that described above for adolescents. The most important result were the following:

- In a large part of the subjects examined, no signals indicating a P300 peak could be discovered in frontal, temporal and occipital locations. Therefore only central (C_3, C_z, C_4) and parietal (P_3, P_z, P_4) leads were evaluated.
- For nontarget amplitudes, MZ correlations were generally higher than DZ correlations mainly for parietal electrodes.
- Twin correlations for nontarget and target latencies were low at age 5; moderate MZ correlations, higher than those in DZ, were found at age 7.
- According to multivariate genetic analysis, heritabilities for P300 amplitudes to targets was low, while it was higher for nontarget P300 at age 5 and age 7.

The latter twin studies, especially those performed on the P300 component differ from those discussed previously before, since they are not performed in the resting proband but require some active participation. It is not surprising that the degree of similarity in MZ twins may be somewhat lower than in experiments in resting twins. This experience appears to accord with results from psychophysical and psychological tests in twins; it would not be too surprising if the effect of genetically determined variation on activities requiring voluntary participation in an experiment would be lower than the genetic effect on variation in aspects of brain physiology that are independent of voluntary action. Especially the studies from the Amsterdam group (van Beijsterfeldt 1996; van Baal 1997) indicate possible ways toward analysis of more specific neuronal mechanisms involved in the P300 formation; for example, possible (although in no way consistent) heritability differences between target and nontarget reactions may indicate such mechanisms, despite the tendencies of these authors to overrate the analytical power of complex multivariate analysis for estimating heritabilities, and the often frustrating scattering of results.

A family study on VEPs was reported by Bulayeva et al. (1993). These authors elicited VEPs by light flashes of two intensities, and by pattern reversal (midfrontal and midoccipital leads). Amplitudes and latencies were measured for the characteristic peaks (Table 5.1). The population studied consisted of families (parents and

Table 5.1. Mean Population Values and Standard Deviations of the Main Components of Visual Evoked Potentials[a] (Bulayeva et al. 1993)

	N60		P100		A(N60–P100)	N70				
	A	L	A	L	A	L	A	L	A(P100–N70)	P240
F1										
M	2.4	66.5	7.0	108.9	9.5	9.1	169.9	15.1	2.6	242.8
SD	2.6	18.7	4.8	28.6	5.5	8.0	44.5	7.0	4.8	68.4
F2										
M	−3.0	61.8	7.5	101.5	10.8	−12.5	168.0	19.1	1.9	246.0
SD	4.2	13.1	6.1	23.1	6.8	8.8	41.4	9.6	7.5	72.3
PREP	N70		P110		A(N70–P110)	N165			A(P110–N165)	P240
M	−1.2	73.5	5.8	111.6	7.1	− 3.81	65.4	8.4	2.2	220.6
SD	1.9	15.0	3.9	20.3	4.5	3.2	32.8	3.8	2.6	47.5

[a] A, amplitude; L, latency; F1, EP to weak intensity light (0.2 J); F2, EP to strong intensity light (1.0 J); PREP, EP to pattern-reversal; M, mean value; SD, standard deviation.

offspring) in a moderately isolated population of Daghestan (northern Caucausus). The most important results were:

- Males and females differed in the amplitude of the N60 component and N60 P100 complex when the flashes were given with lower intensities. There is (again, as in other studies) a consistent tendency toward higher amplitudes in females. Latencies were found to be largely independent of age and sex.
- Familiy studies (50 parent-offspring pairs and 30 sibpairs) gave variances for the additative genetic component (= heritability in the narrow sense) of 22%–88% for amplitudes elicited by flashes; highest heritabilities were found for the amplitude of N60 P100 and P100 N70. Latencies were found to have lower heritabilities (about 30%–40%). For pattern reversal, heritabilities are about the same; these may tend to be slightly higher.

In all these studies, one factor that affects amplitudes and latencies of EPs is not considered: The effect of the resting EEG. This effect is examined in the study discussed below.

5.3 The Effect of the Resting EEG, Especially Hereditary EEG Variants, on Parameters of Evoked Potentials

As shown by the above twin and family studies, there are individual variations in our adult population while EP potentials tend to remain constant in the individual. Genetic determination regarding latencies, amplitudes and shapes of EEG curves and regarding the augmenting-reducing reaction to varying intensities appear to be determined largely by genetic factors as shown by twin studies. So far, such twin studies are not as extensive as for the resting EEG (Chap. 3), but the overall conclusion of a strong genetic effect on normal variation appears to be well-founded. However, these studies did not include an important point of view: The effect of the individual resting EEG on evoked potentials. It was known in principle that such effects do exist (Cigànek 1969, 1975). Our own studies were performed with carriers of the normal hereditary variants described in Chap. 4. The experimental setup has been described in Sect. 5.1. Before the main study was started, a pilot study was performed in 19 adults to test the experimental setup, and the reliability of measurements was tested by repeated examination of the same persons (Höpp 1983). The number of subjects included in the main study can be seen from Table 5.2; there

Table 5.2. Subjects included in the main study

	Monomorphic α-waves (R)	Low-voltage (N)	Fronto-precentral β-groups (BG)	Diffuse β-waves (BD)
Males	32	41	20	31
Females	18	22	25	59
Both sexes together	50	63	45	90

were 248 students altogether; most subjects were between 20 and 25 years old; 124 each were male and female. As expected from the known dependence of the diffuse β EEG on the sex, there were again many more females than males with the EEG with diffuse β waves. The study had the following results:

- As shown by the pilot study (on individuals who had more or less average EEG records) reliability was satisfactory; in VEPs and AEPs, intraindividual variation was lower than interindividual variation.
- Oscillation, the newly developed measure for general amplitude variation, is always higher in VEPs than in AEPs (= auditory EPs).
- There is a clearcut sex difference, oscillations (amplitudes) in females being, on the average, much higher than in males. This sex difference was also apparent among the 19 subjects of the pilot study (12 male, 7 female).
- Within the sexes, there were significant differences between EEG types. Individuals with a low-voltage EEG (N) showed consistently and in both sexes the lowest, subjects with monomorphic α waves (R) the highest oscillations. Probands with frontoprecentral β groups (BG) tended to have the second highest, those with diffuse β waves had the second lowest values. The BG group was the only one without a significant sex difference which could be due to their relatively small number.
- For VEPs the highest oscillations were found in occipital leads (O_1, O_2). AEPs had a maximum in the central lead (C_z). These patterns were found to be consistent for all EEG variants.

In conclusion, there was a consistent oscillation difference between the four EEG variants studied in both sexes.

To obtain an overall impression about the effect of gender and EEG type on the latencies, we calculated and compared the averages of all latencies of all experiments (= average latency; see above, Sect. 5.1). Figures 5.8, 5.9 show the results:

- There is a slight tendency for higher latencies of VEPs in males compared with females, when comparisons are performed within EEG types. The majority of differences, however, is not significant.
- There is a clearcut difference between EEG types in both sexes for VEPs, average latency being largest in type R (= monomorphic α waves). Between the other EEG variants, differences are not so clearcut, but the N type (= low voltage) has a tendency to be the lowest. The difference between R and N is significant in comparison for most leads when sexes are considered together. Differences between EEG types are especially clear in leads C_z and P_4.
- For average AEP latencies, no clearcut sex difference could be observed. The difference between EEG types was in the same direction as for VEPs (R > N).

In addition to the above overall measures, oscillation and average latency, mean values for single peaks were also compared (except the first 70 ms that were not evaluated in this study). As shown by these comparisons, consideration of single peaks revealed that sex differences as well as differences between EEG variants shown by the oscillation measure (for average amplitudes) and by the average latency are fairly consistent for most single peaks. They cannot be traced back to only a few peaks.

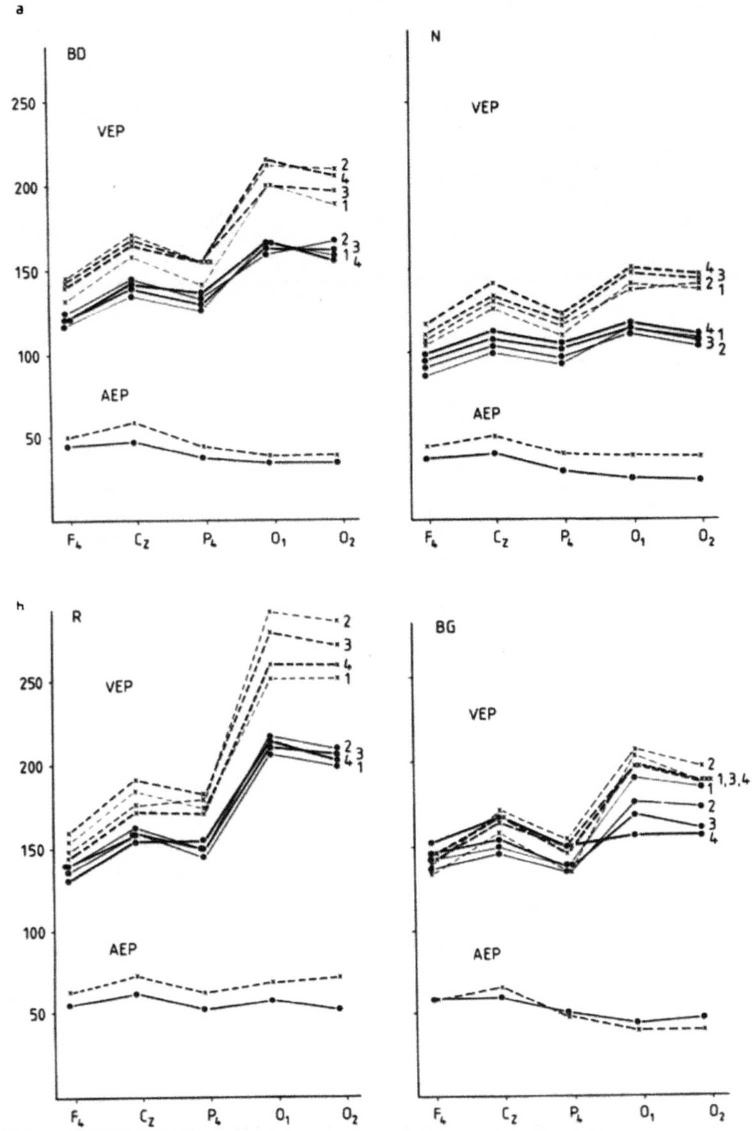

Fig. 5.8. Oscillations for VEPs and AEPs, *R*, monomorphic α waves. *N*, Low voltage EEG; BD diffuse β waves; BG β groups) and the females = --), O_2, see Fig. 2, (1, 2, 3, 4), and for five leads

The last phenomenon to be studied was the augmenting-reducing reaction (Buchsbaum 1974, 1980). As noted, light flashes were applied at four different intensities in (pseudo-) randomized order, and for randomized and regular time intervals. Of the parameters tested, the peaks P_1, N_1, P_2 and the differences P_1N_1, N_2P_2 – the P_1N_1 difference in lead C_z gave the most consistent result in the pilot study: 18 of 19 individuals could be classified either as augmenters (10 males, 2 females) or as reducers (2 males, 4 females). Only one woman gave an inconsistent result. There-

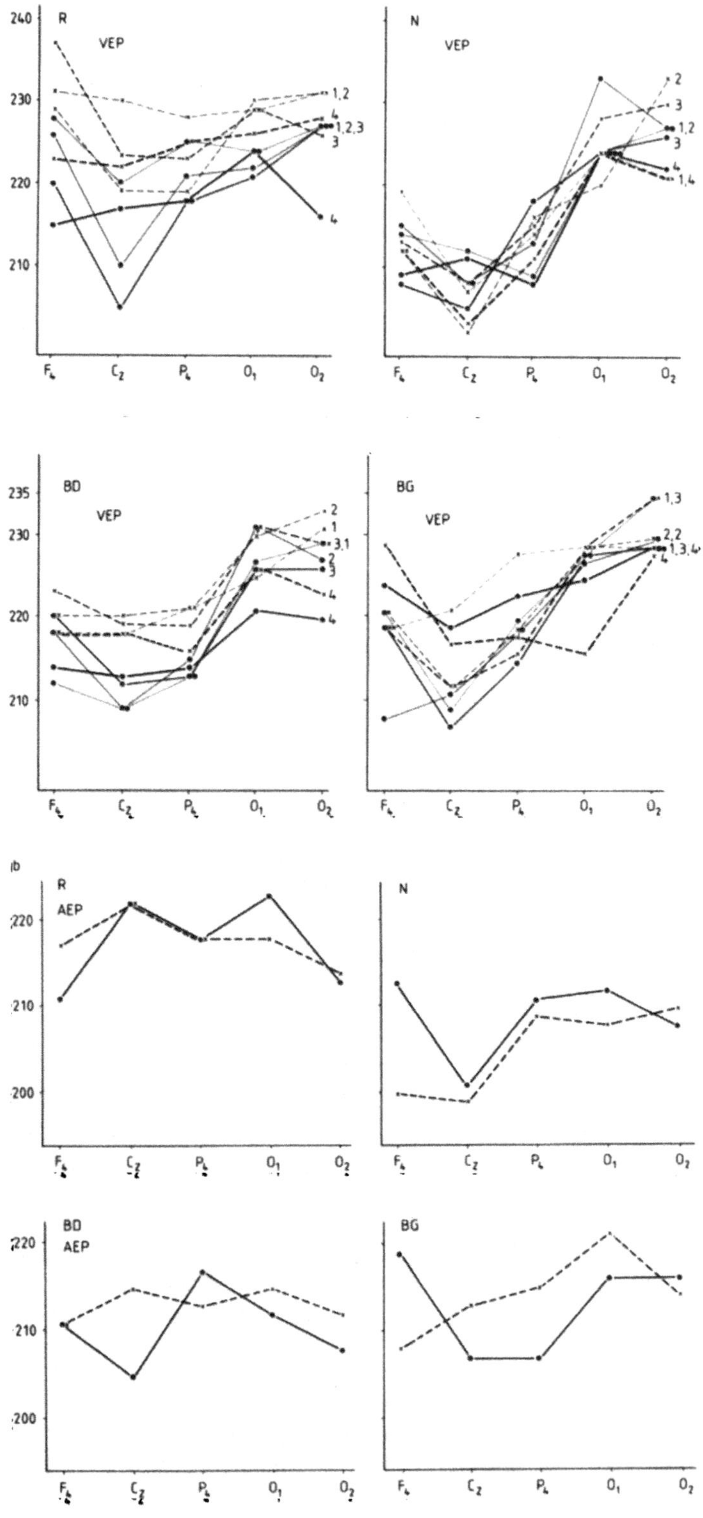

Fig. 5.9. Mean latencies in the four EEG types and the two sexes (*unbroken line*, males; *broken line*, females), the five leads F_4, C_z, P_4, O_1, and O_2, and four light flash intensitites (1, 2, 3, 4,). **a** VEPs. **b** For AEPs

Table 5.3. Distribution of augmenters and reducers according to EEG type (both sexes together)

	R	N	BD	BG	Sum total
Augmenters					
Observed:	34	47	57	34	172
Expected:	35.0	43.0	63.4	30.6	
Reducers					
Observed:	14	12	30	8	64
Expected:	13.0	16.0	23.6	11.4	
Sum total	48	59	87	42	236

$\chi^2 = 5.245$; DF = 3 $p > 0.1$; R = monomorphic α-waves; N = low-voltage EEG; BD = diffuse β-waves; BG = fronto-precentral β-groups

fore the difference P_1N_1 in lead C_z was used to classify probands of the main study. Table 5.3 shows the result. Obviously, there is no visible effect of the EEG variants studied on the augmenting-reducing phenomenon. Among the probands for which classification was possible, 80 males were augmenters and 37 reducers, while among females, 92 augmenters and 27 reducers were found. Hence the difference is in the direction reported by Buchsbaum (more augmenters among women), but the difference is not significant ($\chi^2 = 2.4$). For other references on the augmenting-reducing response and its possible significance see v. Knorring et al. (1978), Perris and v. Knorring (1982).

In conclusion, this study showed strong differences between EEG variants in amplitudes of EPs, and smaller differences in latencies. This result fits well into a hypothesis on neuropsychological differences between carriers of these variants that may lead to corresponding differences in information processing (for details, see Chap. 6). There were some differences in experimental setup between our study and the setup used normally, especially in a clinical setting. For example, we carried out the examinations with closed eyes; and we did not evaluate the first 70 ms after stimulation (we were not interested in these potentials since they are caused by the afferent extracerebral media but not by the brain. For further details on the experimental setup and its possible problems, see Vogel et al. 1986). However, one note of caution is necessary: The possibility has been discussed that some peaks of the EPs may, in part, be summed EEG potentials: α oscillators could be blocked briefly by the stimulus and then, start oscillating synchronously. This effect could be stronger in EEGs with monomorphic α waves than in other EEG types, especially the low-voltage EEG. However, such synchronization would probably be stronger after stimulation with equal than with unequal time intervals. In our study, however, stimulation with unequal time intervals gave consistently higher amplitudes. Moreover, practically no peaks were seen in addition to the known EP peaks, and a lowering of hysteresis from 5% to 0% had almost no effect on the oscillation measure (hysteresis = amplitude change below which the computer does not note this change). Therefore the main amplitude difference is probably caused by true EPs. For the described differences in mean latencies, no other explanation than that given above appears to be possible.

CHAPTER 6

6 The Normal Human EEG as a Research Tool in Human Behavior Genetics

6.1 General Introduction to the Problem

At present, human genetics as a science is developing very fast (see Vogel and Motulsky 1996). An increasing number of genes has been identified, their structure has been elucidated, and their function has been analyzed. Many aspects of general metabolism, many basic functions of the human organism, and mechanisms of interaction with the environment, such as defense against infective agents, have been elucidated. However, the most complex and – despite successful attempts especially in recent years – least understood organ is our brain. On the other hand, feeling tone, behavior, and mental performance are personal properties most specifically human; they are closely connected with our subjective and objective identities as human beings. Therefore the effect of our genetic makeup and its interactions with effects from our environment have been the most interesting and, at the same time, most controversial issues in human genetics research and in the discourse with scientists of other fields, especially with social sciences, and with the general public. It is not incidental that the first serious scientific attempt at investigation of the effect of heredity and genetic variation on a complex personal property addressed human performance: The work by F. Galton (1865) on "Hereditary talent and Character" which was extended some time later into the monograph "Hereditary Genius" (1869). In this work, Galton showed that men who were famous enough for being included with their biographies in biographical handbooks had a very high chance of having close relatives (fathers; brothers; sons) accepted in such handbooks, as well. While Galton assumed that this similarity of performance was largely due to their common hereditary background, many social scientists pointed to inequalities of life chances, and other environmental factors. This problem has not been solved up to the present day as shown by the controversies on books such as H. Jensen's *Educability and Group Differences* (1973) and The Bell Curve (1994) by Herrnstein et al. However, Galton's study has initiated one of the two paradigms by which research in human genetics is guided – the study of measurable traits by quantitative biometric methods (for details, see Vogel and Motulsky 1996; Falconer 1981), and the analysis of genes, their structure and action which was initiated by Mendel (1865), and pushed forward during recent years by the "molecular revolution." The biometric approach for solving the above behavior genetics problems has been used mainly by psychologists interested in human behavior and its genetic determinants but also by psychiatrists trying to disentangle genetic and nongenetic factors involved in the causation of behavioral anomalies and mental diseases. In the cause of all these researches, methods have been diversified becoming more and more sophisticated; in addition to comparing close relatives such as parents, sibs and children, researchers concentrated on MZ and DZ twins reared together and apart and on adopted as compared with biological children. Statistical methods for evaluation and interpretation of data also became more and more sophisticated as shown, for example, by some of the twin data referred to above. However, the results achieved by this approach, while offering some important insights, were, on the whole, not entirely satisfactory. Einstein said: "The significant problems we face cannot be solved at the same level of thinking we were at when we created them."

The new level of thinking required for gaining deeper insights into these problems has been provided, to say in a somewhat oversimplified way, by two developments: The first one was the growth of genetics, the science based on Mendel's paradigm of the gene – from analysis of segregation of phenotypes, and localization of genes to certain chromosomes down to the structure, action, and interaction of genes (see Chap. 1). The second development is that of neurophysiology – analysis of structure and function of that organ which is the main "instrument" of thinking, feeling, and interaction with the world around us – the brain. Even psychology – the science of human behavior that, for a long time, studied many aspects of human behavior, including mental health, intelligence, and performance and individual differences almost without brain physiology – is establishing now closer and closer connections with brain physiology. In their work on "Physiology of psychology" (1987), Bunge and Ardila wrote: "The correct and badly needed synthesis is the merger of all the branches of psychology on the basis of neuroscience, together with developmental and evolutionary biology, and in tandem with social science. This is the correct synthesis because behavior and mentation happen to be biological processes." These two developments – that of human genetics and that of a synthetic psychophysiology – should be combined to achieve deeper insight into the biological mechanisms involved in psychological differences between human beings.

However, there are different ways for achieving this goal: two of these are described: First, it may be possible to achieve it directly, in a "big jump": One could define certain psychological phenotypes and then try to apply the instruments of genetic analysis: Establishing a mode of inheritance and localizing a gene by segregation and linkage analysis, and then, identifying and analyzing this gene and its function. This strategy has been successful in certain anomalies such as some types of mental retardation. In mental disease, such as schizophrenia, a similar approach has been used to identify genes that may contribute to genetic susceptibility in a situation in which not everyone who is genetically predisposed actually becomes affected (as shown by discordance of 50% of MZ twins). Here, study of families showing a pattern suggestive of a dominant mode of inheritance, or of families in relatively small but long-term isolated population groups may help in identifying "main genes" in such predisposition (as an example see Moises et al. 1995).

In addition to such linkage studies with DNA markers whose location in the genome is known, studies on association of certain marker genes with psychologically defined phenotypes may help in identifying and localizing genes affecting such phenotypes (see Vogel and Motulsky 1996). The rationale of such studies is that genetic markers may occur in linkage disequilibrium with genes, various alleles of which may lead to differences in psychological phenotypes. Such linkage disequilibrium may have two reasons: either the time that elapsed to separate by recombination the suspected genes from the tightly linked marker may not have been sufficient for the disequilibrium to disappear, or the marker allele itself affects the phenotype to be studied. In both instances this approach may lead indirectly or directly to one of the responsible genes. In addition to genetic analysis of mental diseases, this approach is also being used in searching for genes involved in the genetic determination of cognitive abilities (intelligence; Plomin et al. 1994). Up to now there has been no convincing success but still, this approach may be successful in the long run.

However, a second, quite different approach could also be tried: There are quite a number of levels in-between the genes, on the one hand, and psychological parameters, on the other. We have come to know, for example, the structure of neurons, groups of neurons, and their interconnections. We know in principle how they communicate with each other chemically, and we have much information about neurotransmitters, their enzymes, and their receptors. We also have a clearcut conception, how certain portions of the brain cooperate, and how information transfer works. One level that has been elucidated especially well is the level of spontaneous electrical activity of the brain – the EEG.

6.2 The EEG and Normal Psychology: General Considerations

As explained in detail in Chaps. 3 and 4, the normal resting EEG shows, in addition to its typical development from infancy and childhood to maturity and old age, relatively strong interindividual variation all over life time; this interindividual variation is determined almost completely by genetic differences as shown by extensive, and repeated studies on twins reared together and apart. This has been confirmed in the course of time by detailed visual inspection of the EEG records and by several methods of both semiquantitative and quantitative measurements and evaluations of increasing complexity. The same is also true for the sleeping EEG and EEG reactions to simple tasks such as eye opening or hyperventilation. Moreover, some normal EEG variants have been identified that can be distinguished clearly from the majority of EEG records; family studies in some of them even suggest a simple, autosomal dominant mode of inheritance. As noted above repeatedly, a simple, monogenic mode of inheritance is a pointer to the genes. Studies on most aspects of physiology normally can be performed over a very short time distance; they give a momentary picture of the function to be examined. To put it somewhat differently, they represent a "state." In genetic analysis, however, we are interested in "traits," i.e., in time – invariant properties of the individual. Most psychological properties of individuals are states; i.e., they tend to vary more or less over time. This is one of the reasons why their genetic analysis is so difficult: The geneticist needs traits. However, the normal resting EEG recorded under carefully maintained standard conditions is a trait, or, at least, it comes very close to a trait. This is true despite the fact that the EEG may vary under the effect of many factors – arousal and fatigue, chemical alterations by narcotics and drugs and many others. However, these factors can be controlled. Therefore the resting EEG offers itself as a promising tool for studying relationships and individual properties that can be determined and measured by psychological methods.

The situation is different with event-related potentials (EPs). They are elicited by exogenous stimuli of various types; it would not be surprising if reaction to such stimuli would depend more on the disposition of the individual at the moment of the experiment than the resting stage. Twin studies on EPs tend to confirm this expectation: There are some strong similarities of EPs in MZ twins but, as a rule, their properties cannot be described as identical. The shapes of EP curves tend to be very similar, and some characteristic peaks show strong similarities, as well, but in general, there were also differences. Unfortunately, studies reported so far do not permit conclusions as to the question whether these differences between MZ cotwins are constant personal properties, or indicate state variations within the same individual. One often neglected factor is the effect of the type of the resting EEG on properties of EPs; as discussed above, a comparative study on carriers of some normal EEG variants has shown that this effect is considerable, suggesting conclusions as to differences in information processing (see below).

In conclusion, looking for associations of EEG patterns, especially the resting EEG, with certain psychological features has a strong prima facie appeal: The EEG undoubtedly represents aspects of brain physiology, and under normal conditions it represents – or comes very close to represent – a trait. Moreover, individual differences in the normal range are genetically determined. The notion that the rhythmic oscillations of groups of neurons indicated by the EEG may, at least in part, represent psychological or psychophysiological processes is not new at all.

Quite the contrary: Hans Berger, the (re-)discoverer of the human EEG (Chap. 2) was a psychiatrist. It was his hope to create an instrument for psychophysiological research (Berger 1932). From Berger to the present day, almost uncountable attempts have been made to find relationships between certain EEG phenomena and normal psychology as well as psychopathology. It is the prevalent feeling among EEG specialists that most of these attempts were not very successful, or even futile. The picture created when one tries to scrutinize relevant literature is confusing. Therefore it is not surprising that some authors have declared all asserted relationships as nonconvincing. For example, Sisson and Ellingson (1955) have stated that "no study has been done conclusively showing a relationship between any feature of the normal adult EEG recorded under standard conditions and any personality trait or variable." During the more than 40 years since that statement was made, a number of studies have been performed which show some fairly convincing results although the field is still open to discussion, and some doubts are still justified. For the design of such studies, a number of conditions must be met:

1. The EEG property to be tested must be as close as ever possible to a "trait" as described above. This condition is fulfilled in neurologically healthy individuals; and in properties, such as α frequency and α index. Presence of the EEG variants described in Chap. 4 is a special advantage since variants have been described clearly, and can be diagnosed by any fairly experienced investigator. In general, adequate methods of EEG measurement and evaluation should be used.
2. For psychological and psychophysiological evaluation, well-established test-methods must be used. If it is the purpose of the study to draw conclusions as to genetic variation in the psychological features examined, it is necessary to examine these tests whether they indicate psychological features that have a genetic basis. It cannot be expected that all carriers of a certain EEG type have a

certain psychological property that is indicated by a test result while persons not carrying the EEG trait are free from it. In view of the well-known complex determination of psychological properties, moderate or even weak associations are to be expected. However, if a psychological test does not show any genetic effect at all, a contribution of a genetically determined neurophysiological property such as an EEG variant cannot be expected. For most standard tests, twin studies are available in the literature. However, reported results may not be entirely reliable for many reasons. Therefore it is advisable to examine the test battery used by adequate studies of a sufficiently large sample of MZ and DZ twins, and to estimate heritabilities for single test items and for the entire tests. Here, adequate statistical methods should be used. Such methods have been described, for example, in Vogel and Motulsky (1996, Appendix 5).

3. Studies on normal psychology and those of pathological conditions should be distinguished clearly; this also applies to the EEG. Christian (1968), in his textbook chapter on the EEG in behavioral anomalies, psychopathy, endogenous psychoses, and neuroses, gave many references, for example, on higher frequencies of abnormal EEG results in children with behavioral disturbances; these data could indicate that many of these children suffer from early brain damage. According to Christian, similar anomalies were often described in psychopaths and criminals, especially those convicted for repeated criminal acts. Such results are important for adequate treatment and, if possible, rehabilitation, but for problems to be discussed here, they are not informative and even misleading without further, more specific information.
4. As considered above, any associations between EEG traits and psychological test results are expected to be weak or, at best, moderate. In order not to be fooled by statistical small-number effects, sample sizes should be adequately high. Moreover, uncontrollable side effects could be avoided by repetition of the entire study using a sample with quite different background. When many tests are applied, and the customary 5% level is used for determining statistical significance, one of 20 tests is expected to give a significant result merely by chance. Such chance effects should be considered when results are interpreted.

6.3 EEG Alpha Activity and Intelligence

Intelligence as measured by the IQ or similar intelligence measures is very suitable for association studies with the EEG since it has been operationalized well, and many studies on heritability are available (Bouchard and McGue 1981). Heritability estimates based on studies of twins reared together and apart are in the order of magnitude between approx.0.5 and approx.0.7, differences depending on selection of twin samples, and, to a surprisingly high degree, on the statistical method of heritability determination (see, for example, Vogel and Motulsky 1996, "Appendix 5"). α frequency and other characteristics of the α rhythm, on the other hand, can be quantified very easily. Therefore it is not surprising that its association with the IQ has been studied quite often. Results were, however, controversial: Mundy-Castle (1958) and Mundy-Castle and Nelson (1960) reported a positive relationship, while in other studies, no significant correlation could be found. W. Vogel and Broverman, in a review, concluded that the available evidence supported the relationship between EEG and test intelligence in individuals with either relatively undeveloped intellectual function such as children or mentally retarded persons. Evidence in the same direction was reported by Gasser et al. (1983), while in normal adults result were ambiguous. Ellingson argued in his review (1966) that the weight of available evidence suggested no relationship between EEG and intelligence in normal adults. In another comprehensive review, Oswald and Roth (1974) noted that most EEG studies of normal adults did not provide evidence of an association between α frequency and psychomotoric intelligence; the few positive findings available suggest a possible relationship with performance rather than verbal IQ. Giannitrapani (1969), on the other hand, reported a significant correlation between IQ and the average EEG frequency (overall frequency bands) and its asymmetry index. However, the sample studied consisted of relatively few (18) adults. In contrast, W. Vogel et al. (1968) did not find any evidence that α frequency is related to general level of intelligence; however, it was correlated with "automatization" cognitive style. The concluded that EEG indices seem to be related to particular cognitive factors, rather than to general mental ability. According to Giannitrapani (1985), on the other hand, there is a significant correlation between dominant α frequency and full-scale IQ and correlation of 13-HZ activity (the upper bound of the α band) with verbal IQ in a sample of normal 11- to 13-year-old children. A relative large series of adults (52 cardiac vascular patients) was reported by Juolasmaa (1986). Although some of the probands were thought to have brain disorders due to impaired cerebral circulation, the mean IQ in this sample was in the normal range. This study found significant correlations between α frequency and intelligence test scores, mainly with verbal and memory subtests. Related aspects of α activity were studied by some other authors. For example, there is evidence that α frequency is associated with memory performance and processing speed. Golubeva (1980), for example, regarded α frequency as one of the indicators of a general CNS activation factor; she found a significant correlation with performance on memory tasks. Lebedev (1990) proposed a theoretical model that allows of an individual limit of short-term memory span from composite electrophysiological indices based on α frequency and the duration of α spindles. Klimesch et al. (1993) reported significant differences in α frequency between poor and good memory test performance which were most pronounced when the probands actually retrieved information from their memories. According to Survillo (1964), α frequency is negatively correlated with decision time in a choice reaction task; he hypothesized that the information capacity of the CNS is a function of EEG period.

In conclusion, the question of whether a frequency is related to test intelligence in normal adults was controversial despite strong indications that such a relationship may exist. Possible reasons for these contradictory results are those discussed in Sect. 6.2: small sample sizes; admixture of patients suffering from brain damage; confounding with age-related effects on EEG and test results; gender-specific effects and differences in methods of EEG evaluation.

We tried to avoid these sources of error in a study of our own (Anokhin and Vogel 1996). The sample of probands included in this study consisted of 101 healthy males (German Air Force personnel) ages 20–45 years (mean 30.6). This sample had been collected for study of possible psychological differences between carriers of hereditary EEG variants (see Sect. 6.4). It also contained, in addition to individuals with these variants, a great number of controls with average EEG. Based on figures found in population studies (Vogel and Fujiya 1969), the sample of 101 to be studied here was composed in a way that it resembled as closely as possible the composition of the general male population in the same age range, excluding, however, the low-voltage records since they showed very little or no α activity (see Sect. 4.3). The average IQ (as assessed by using the Amthauer IST test) surpassed that of the general population, and its range of variation was somewhat restricted (mean IQ = 119.9 ± 9.4). The EEG was recorded in the usual way; eight conventional sites of the 10–20 system were used (F_{p1}, F_{p2}, F_3, F_4, C_3, C_4, O_1, O_2); with reference electrodes to the ipsilateral ear (time constant 0.1 s). For each proband, at least 2 min of records stored on magnetic tape were available. For the purpose of this study, EEG records were digitized at the rate of 128 per second and analyzed by MBN-neurocartography software; an artifact elimination routine was used. The power spectra were divided into 4-s periods and subjected to Fourier spectral analysis. Two parameters, peak frequency (the frequency at which maximum power occurred) and mean frequency (weighted for power) were assessed within the α frequency band (8–13 c/s) at each recording site, and averaged over 30 epochs. For psychological examination, the following mental ability tests were used in addition to the Amthauer Intelligence Structure (IST) test: The Raven Standard Progressive Matrices test, and three primary subtests and two composite subtests of the LPS (Horn 1962).

To reduce the number of variables principle-component factor analyses for α frequency and cognitive ability measures were performed. The first unrotated factors derived from the matrices of intercorrelations among mean and peak α frequencies measured at different recording sites were used as integral measures of mean and peak α frequencies. Similarly, factor analysis was performed for various sets of cognitive performance measures. First, test results were combined to obtain a factor of general abilities (g); then, separate analyses were performed only for subtests based on verbal material, on the one hand, and for those assessing geometrical and spatial abilities. For further details of the analysis, see the original. The main results are shown in Table 6.1: All correlations were positive, but only some of them were significant statistically. Tests indicating verbal abilities showed correlations around 0.35 with both α frequency measures. The correlations with the overall Raven result were somewhat smaller but, for peak α frequency, still significant. For both frontal α frequency measures there was also a significant correlation with the Raven result. According to the experience of some leading psychologists, the "culture fair" Raven test should measure factor g, a general factor of intelligence, especially well. Spatial and arithmetic abilities, on the other hand, showed only small and nonsignificant correlation coefficients with α frequency. A comparison of correlation coefficients showed that the correlations of α frequency measures with verbal ability factors differed significantly from their correlations with "spatial" and "arithmetic" factors.

As noted, a majority of studies published before have failed to show any consistent relationship between measures of α frequency and intelligence, except when mentally backwards or even mentally retarded individuals were included. However, the study of Juolasmaa et al. (1986) which was performed on adult and mentally normal cardiac vascular patients showed a similar result as ours: positive correlations were described between α frequency and intelligence measures, primarily in subtests testing verbal abilities and memory. The correlations described in the

Table 6.1. Correlations between the EEG alpha frequency factors and mental abilities (Anokhin & Vogel 1996)

Factor scores analyzed	*r*	*p*
Mean AF vs. General Abilities	.138	*ns*
Peak AF vs. General Abilities	.162	*ns*
Mean AF vs. Verbal Abilities	.341	<.001
Peak AF vs. Verbal Abilities	.356	<.001
Mean AF vs. Raven's SPM	.190	*ns*
Peak AF vs. Raven's SPM	.266	<.01
Frontal mean AF vs. Raven's SPM	.238	<.05
Frontal peak AF vs. Raven's SPM	.304	<.01
Mean AF vs. Spatial Abilities	.083	*ns*
Peak AF vs. Spatial Abilities	.081	*ns*
Mean AF vs. Arithmetic Abilities	.072	*ns*
Peak AF vs. Arithmetic Abilities	.120	*ns*

Note. Figures in this table represent correlations between the scores on the first unrotated factors derived from intercorrelations with in the following sets of variables. *Mean AF and Peak AF*: mean and peak alpha frequency values, respectively, across all recording sites; *frontal Mean and Peak AF*: the same for frontal areas only (Fp1, Fp2, F3, F4); *General Abilities*: all subtests of the IST and LPS tests and the SPM score; *Verbal Abilities*: verbal subtests of the IST and the LPS; *Spatial Abilities*: spatial and geometric tasks of the IST and the LPS; *Arithmetic Abilities*: multiple correlation of the two arithmetic subtests of the IST with each of the AF factors is presented. For more detail see Methods and Results sections.

above-described studies are, of course, relatively small. Here, however, it must be considered that heritabilities for performance in the tests used in this study are far from 1.0 as shown by twin studies (Sect. 6.4.). Moreover, it should be remembered that the average IQ in this sample is well above the population mean, and the range was reduced accordingly. Here, the correlations found would have been somewhat higher if a really average population sample would have been available for study. There are methods for correcting the bias introduced by a reduction in range (Cohen and Cohen 1983), but we did not use them. There are a number of studies correlating psychological, and especially neurophysiological parameters with mental performance; even the most convincing ones show correlations in the order of magnitude described here for α frequencies. Examples are conduction velocity in a brain pathway (Reed and Jensen 1992); tests for speed of information processing (Vernon and Weese 1993), and others. It should be noted, however, that our attempts at correlating event-related potentials (EPs) with intelligence measures had a negative result (Vogel et al. 1987) in agreement with some, and contrary to alleged positive results reported by other authors. This very controversial topic is discussed in Sect. 6.14.

The study described above also suggests some conclusions regarding possible function of certain areas of the brain for aspects of intellectual performance: Correlation with the Raven test – and also with another measure for logical thinking, the LR score of the LPS test, tend to aggregate in the frontal areas, while verbal scales of the IST and LPS show a more diffuse topographical distribution of significant correlations with the two measures of α frequency. This suggests that (nonverbal) analytical reasoning abilities may be related to frontal areas of the brain. However, differences between correlation coefficients (frontal vs. nonfrontal) are not significant statistically; therefore this observation is preliminary; further studies are needed. This study also suggests a closer relationship of α frequency to more specific rather than to general abilities (g factor). However, the tests used in this study do not seem to be optimal for the assessment of g; they were developed based on Thurstone's primary abilities model; the first unrotated factor found in factor analysis accounted for only 29% of the total variance of individual subtests. Regarding specific abilities, there are distinct and significant differences in the magnitude of correlations with α frequencies: As noted above, there are highly significant correlations with factors of verbal activity but no significant relationships with spatial and arithmetical abilities. This result raises a more general question: Could it be that the importance of factor g is being overrated by some psychologists concerned with cognitive abilities? There is another example not directly connected with EEG research: Complex reaction time, i.e., the time needed to react in different ways to varying stimuli, has been shown to be correlated to performance on the Raven test. Since this test was thought to be a good measure of factor g, it was concluded that factor g is responsible also for performance in the complex reaction task. More detailed analyses using the IST mentioned above show, however, that performance in the complex reaction time test depends much more on specific abilities such as short-time memory. There was even a negative correlation between g loading of IST subtests and their correlation with performance in a complex reaction task (Ruchalla et al. 1985).

What does the result on correlations of α frequency measures mainly with aspects of analytical thinking and verbal intelligence tell us about genetic reasons for individual differences in intelligence? First, it confirms that in such individual differences, genetic mechanisms are involved. α frequency belongs to those properties of the normal EEG individual variation which are determined by genetic differences. This has been shown by extended twin studies in which this problem has been addressed by a variety of methods (Chap. 3). Secondly, it shows that intelligence, or its genetic component, cannot be determined by one gene (or a very small number of them), as asserted occasionally (Weiss 1992). It is certainly a complex human property in which many genes are involved. Even for α frequency there is no indication for a simple mendelian mode of inheritance; there is not even a bimodal distribution of EEG frequencies in families, and in the population. Therefore even that component of intelligence which is represented by the rhythmic activity of groups of neurons visible to us as EEG obviously has a multifactorial genetic basis. Moreover, there are genes involved in individual differences of intelligence that have been "trapped" by a completely different approach. Many autosomal recessive diseases reduce, in addition to other aspects of brain function, intellectual abilities, for example, by causing metabolic anomalies that impair normal function of the neuronal network. A superficial observer could think that these are rare exceptions that should not be included in a description on variation in normal intelligence. However, heterozygotes of these diseases are not rare at all; altogether they comprise an appreciable fraction of our population (Hardy-Weinberg law; see Vogel and Motulsky 1996), and in some of them, such as heterozygotes of phenylketonuria or lipid storage diseases, a sometimes small, but certainly not negligible effect on intelligence has been shown (Vogel 1984). The study on aspects of α frequency in relation to intelligence has been only one step in the stepwise elucidation of the genetic basis of intelligence. However, it permits insight into the complex functional network determining mental performance and its variations from an interesting angle. It may be possible in the future to combine comparative studies of individuals with various types of α activity, as have been analyzed here, with EEG studies to localize special types of mental performance in special areas of the brain by quantitative analysis of the EEG at rest and during performance of special tasks (Liberson; Giannitrapani; see Giannitrapani 1985). At the moment, it may be premature to speculate on a possible relationship.

6.4 Variants of the Normal EEG and Personality: Concepts and Data

Intelligence is only a part – although an important part – of the psychological makeup of a person. Other aspects are quite as important; their examination is discussed below in the context of our own studies. Many of these are characterized as "personality" or "performance." According to Herrmann (1972) personality is considered as a construct that can be defined and characterized from empirical data. Such data have been subdivided into L data (from the life history of the proband); Q data (derived from self-rating of the proband; today the most widespread way of collecting such self-rating data is the personality questionnaire, but psychological exploration also provides Q data); and T data (evaluation of a personality by others). Sensory and motoric performance can be measured by special devices for psychophysiological studies, such as fusion of flicker light, tachistoscopy, reaction time to simple or complex stimuli; or coordination of both hands. All these methods have been used for characterization and comparison of carriers of hereditary EEG variants (Vogel et al. 1979a,b). They are described in somewhat greater detail below; before we proceed to these studies of our own, however, another study is described that may be regarded as a kind of forerunner of our studies (Schmettau 1969, 1970). This author examined a series of 118 male students in the age group between 19 and 32 years. All of then were healthy and there was no indication for any neurological anomalies. The EEGs were studied using a program of time-domain analysis of reference leads from O_1. The following main quantitative measures were used: Mean and standard deviation of α waves, α index, kind and number of β waves and β index and number of ϑ waves (amplitude above 50 μV). In addition, the EEGs were classified by visual inspection into the following categories: Pure α EEG, mixed α EEG, β EEG, "flat" EEG (20% of all records; therefore this category must have contained, in addition to the low-voltage EEG according to our definition (Sect. 4.3) many EEGs with relatively low α waves), irregular EEGs, and irregular EEG types with paroxysmal wave groups. For assessment of personality, a number of personality questionnaires was used: Eysenck's MMQ and MPI; the German version of the MMPI, including a number of additional scales (Hathaway et al. 1963); Cattells's 16 PF-test (Cattell et al. 1970) and a few German tests. For quantifying performance, a number of psychophysiological tests were used such as complex reaction time; tachistoscopy with numbers and figures; coordination of right and left hand; and, in addition, a test for quantifying speed and precision of work (d 2-test; Brickenkamp 1962; for details see below). There were many positive and negative correlations, and those between EEG variables and test results were low. However, taken together, they indicated a clearcut pattern. Analyzing this complex pattern of intercorrelations between EEG variables and test results, the author was able to establish two dimensions of EEG activity which she characterized as "dynamics" and "speed." The first dimension comprises high α index, high α and ϑ amplitudes, and very little variability of α activity. The "countertype" of this EEG type, with emphasis on "speed," is the "flat" EEG often combined with irregular α activity and β activity. Correlations with the psychological test results gave the following picture for individuals showing a high degree of "dynamics": The common feature of these individuals was an autochthonous activity. They show spontaneous energy; there are "sthenic" (this expression is used in the original) and, on the other hand, stable and well-controlled. There is a tendency to independence in thinking and acting. As to performance tests, they are good in tests requiring strong motive power, but not so good in tasks requiring sensitivity. There was no clearcut relation to the level of intellectual performance, but the battery of tests used did not comprise any of the customary intelligence tests. Individuals showing a "flat" EEG – in the definition of the author – are in many aspects the "countertype" of the first group. Their dynamics is much lower. Instead of tension and critical restraint, they show a relaxed attitude, an even temper, and appear to be rather carefree. In performance tests, they are not so good in tests requiring much motive power; they are often fast but frequency of errors tends to be higher.

The results of this study which has been described here in an abbreviated and, probably oversimplified, way suggest a certain association of aspects of the EEG record with dimensions of personality. The author did not mention in her report that the EEG characteristics analyzed in her studies have a strong genetic basis as shown by extensive twin studies (Chap. 3). Therefore she did not realize that her investigation has been a pioneering study in human behavior genetics. Her main results were confirmed in a study of our own that is now described (Vogel et al. 1979a,b,c). It was the main difference between the investigations described here and those of Schmettau (1969, 1970) that we did not study an unselected population sample, but samples of individuals with defined EEG variants that had been studied before genetically by family investigations (Chap. 4). Hence the genetic basis of these variants has been clarified before our studies on the behavior started. Two normal samples were examined: one of them consisted of EEGs collected in the Institute of Air Medicine of the German Air Force (Fürstenfeldbruck). In Germany, all applicants for service in the flying units of the Air Force, marine and army, who have passed a psychological test program must undergo a thorough medical checkup, which includes a routine EEG. Therefore EEG records from many thousands of healthy man were available, from which the variants to be included in this study could be collected. After having obtained agreement to these examinations from the military authorities, we first informed the commanding officers and, then, the prospective probands to obtain their agreement. All examinations were then performed at the places of service. Only in some instances, when the probands had already left the Air Force, they were examined in human genetics departments of Heidelberg and Düsseldorf.

The test result of this sample has already been published before (Vogel et al. 1979b). Later, however, we had a chance for studying a second, and quite different, sample. It consisted of 248 students of the University of Heidelberg. A great number of students have been asked through the university authorities to cooperate in this program; about 20% of those asked did actually cooperate. In all of them, a resting EEG with reference leads was taken; those who showed one of the EEG variants in which we were interested, were asked to be available for study on visually and auditory evoked potentials (Vogel et al. 1986; see also Sect. 5.3) and, in addition, for a comprehensive psychological test program. While the Air Force sample only consisted of males, both sexes were represented in the student's sample. The reasons for reexamining the problem in a second sample with exactly the same test methods was first that heritability of most of the test methods used was relatively low, and the sample size was necessarily limited. Therefore it was possible that we were fooled, in part, by statistical errors. Secondly, a sample of males wanting to serve, and, generally indeed serving, in the Air Force is certainly not an unbiased population sample; conclusions drawn from such a biased sample need to be checked by reexamination in another, and if possible quite different, sample. Here, we tried to follow the rule set up by Sir John Eccles; it is always preferable to disprove one's own hypotheses oneself instead of having them disproved by others (the data from the student's sample have been analyzed statistically by A. Anokhin; he followed the same procedure that we had used in analysis of the first series). The following tests were used:

- Formal intelligence: The *Intelligenz-Strukturtest* (IST), Amthauer 1955. This standard intelligence group test is widely used in German-speaking countries. It contains 9 subtests with altogether 176 items. Abilities to be tested are: Practical knowledge; abstract thinking (2 subtests); arithmetic abilities (2 subtests); geometric and spatial abilities (2 subtests); and short-time memory. From another group test, the LPS (Horn 1962), 9 of the 14 subtests were used. In addition, Raven's standard progressive matrices (Raven 1960) were applied.
- Concentration; attention to detail: Here, we used the *Aufmerksamkeits-Belastungstest* (attentiveness-burdening test) of Brickenkamp (1962). The test consisted of 14 lines with d's and p's combined with one, two or three commas; the letter d had to be crossed out if, and only if, two commas were added. Speed and precision are scored. The *Konzentrations-Belastungstest* (KLT) of Düker comprises simple arithmetic tasks; speed and accuracy were evaluated.
- Personality: The MMPI (Minnesota Multiphasic Personality Inventory), see Hathaway 1967, was used in its German version (Hathaway et al. 1963), it consists of 566 statements; the proband states whether he considers them true or false. Four scores have been designed to test whether the proband answers the questions honestly; 10 scales test the personal attitudes: Hypochondria (Hd), depression (D), hysteria (Hy), psychopathy (Pp), masculine-feminine interests (Mf), paranoia (Pa), psychasthenia (Pt), schizothymia (Sc), mania (Ma), introversion, extroversion (Si). In addition to these standard scales, other scales can be constructed; in this study, we only used standard scales. The second personality questionnaire used was a German adaptation of the 16 PF (Cattell et al. 1969). In this test, the proband has the choice between three statements for each item. The profile to be constructed from the single answers consists of 15 first-order and 4 second-order factors; these second-order factors are the following:
  - Factor I: low anxiety vs. high anxiety
  - Factor II: introversion vs. extroversion
  - Factor III: tender-minded emotionality vs. alert poise

  - Factor IV: subduedness vs. independence.
  - In addition, a test for readiness to take risks (RSK) was used (Schubert). It consisted of 25 questions.
- Performance tests: In addition, some sensory and motor abilities were tested using a number of machines: Flicker fusion; tachistoscopy with ten pictures showing colored objects, and with numbers, reaction time to simple and combined stimuli; coordination of both hands; "pursuit rotor," requiring to follow with a pencil a small rotary light on a screen; and tapping (hitting one or two metal plates with a pencil).

Before the main study began, we not only tested and optimized the course of examination in a pilot study with a small number of men with the same background and under the same conditions. We also estimated heritabilities of abilities assessed by the tests used by a twin study of limited size. As considered above, the EEG variants included in these studies are determined entirely by genes. Therefore they cannot possibly determine a higher proportion of the variance of the test result than is determined by their entire genetic variance. This proportion will probably be lower since, in addition to genetic factors expressed in the EEG, other sources of genetic variation are expected to affect the psychological phenotype. In fact, for most of the tests used in our studies, or at least for similar ones, twin studies were available in the literature; we regarded it safer to examine at least a small twin sample of our own (a few years later a very comprehensive twin sample was offered to the present author for studying aspects of the EEG in relation to psychological test results. The tests had been performed in a different language. A heritability study of test results in MZ and DZ twins did not reveal any appreciable heritabilies; therefore it would have been meaningless to study association with genetically determined EEG traits).

The twin series to be studied consisted of 52 pairs, 26 MZ and 26 DZ – healthy adult males between ages 18 and 34 years, mean age 23.3 (MZ) and 23.8 (DZ). The same twins were also used by Propping (1977) in his alcohol studies and by Stassen et al. in cooperation with Propping. The tests were performed in the same way as in the study on soldiers. Heritabilities, i.e., the share of genetic variance on the phenotypic variance of a quantitatively varying trait, may be estimated from twin data in various ways. This is not the place to discuss critically these approaches, and their advantages and disadvantages. The problem has been discussed in detail in "Appendix 5" of Vogel and Motulsky (1996). Suffice it to say that an ideally unbiased estimate is impossible.

Heritability (in the broad sense) is defined as follows: $h^2 = V_G/V_P$. Here V_G is the genotypic variance and V_P is the phenotypic variance. If covariance and interaction are neglected, V_P may be defined as: $V_P = V_G + V_E + V_M$. V_E is the environmental variance and V_M the variance due to measurement errors (or due to the intraindividual variability of the measurement; in psychological tests, this is equivalent to the well-known fact that test-retest reliabilities are <1). Three estimates of h^2 from twin data are possible: the first one ($h_1{}^2$) is based on comparison between MZ and DZ twins: $[h^1{}_2 = V_P(D_Z) - V_P(MZ)]/[V_P(DZ) - V_M)$. Here $V_P(DZ)$ and $V_P(MZ)$ are the variances within DZ and MZ pairs, respectively. This estimate contains systematic errors. On the one hand, DZ twins have a part of their genetic variance in common since they are genetically normal sibs. On the other hand, as with MZ twins, they share part of the same environment. Therefore a second estimate (h^2_2) was proposed, in which the DZ twin pairs are replaced by control pairs that can easily be matched by age and sex from unrelated individuals within the twin series. h^2_2 is biased in direction of overestimating h^2 since MZ twins not only share their genes but a part of their environment as well. As a third possibility, h^2 may also be estimated by comparing the intraclass correlation coefficients: $h^3_2 = 2\ (r_P, MZ - r_P, DZ)$. This estimate is also biased since it assumes that r_G, DZ = 1/2 and there is neither dominance nor epistasis (for details, see Vogel and Motulsky (1996). Evaluating the twin sample described above, all three estimates were used; a new estimate of V_M was not tried; and V_M was not considered in h^2 estimation. Reliabilities of the tests used tend to have an order of magnitude of approx. 0.8 (and sometimes higher).

Heritabilities for all tests have been published (Vogel et al. 1979a). Table 6.2 gives a small selection. Heritabilities for items of personality questionnaires varied much more between the various items; as shown by relatively large standard deviations, this was caused in part by the relatively small sample size of this twin series (a few h^2 values were even negative). However, in general, heritabilities tended to be lower than in those reported in the literature. This suggests another tentative conclusion: Not only heritability of such questionnaire results may not be ideal for the purpose

Table 6.2. Selected heritability estimates for intelligence and performance tests from 26 adult MZ and 26 DZ pairs and for selected items from personality tests

Test	h^2_1	h^2_2	h^2_3
Intelligence and performance tests:			
IST	0.353	0.883	0.084
LPS (selected items)	0.399	0.839	0.196
Raven:	0.174	0.561	0.350
Speed and precision:			
d2 – GZ	0.473	0.708	0.112
F	−0.736	0.300	0.609
GZ – F	0.621	0.807	0.349
KLT – No. of tasks solved	0.473	0.858	0.411
Tachistoscopy Numbers:	0.503	0.529	0.061
Pictures:	0.909	0.854	0.890
Pursuit rotor:			
No. of errors/min, 10 rotations/min	0.622	0.696	0.738
No of errors/min, 20 rotations/min	0.675	0.667	1.212
MMPI:			
D (Depression)	0.435	0.333	0.095
MA (Mania)	−0.075	0.368	−0.101
SC (Schizothymia)	0.205	0.349	−0.262
SI (Introversion-Extraversion)	0.526	0.400	0.927
16 PF:			
Q1 (Conservatism vs. Radicalism)	0.207	0.347	−0.016
Q2 (Group adherence vs. Selfsufficiency)	−0.222	−0.029	0.358
Q3 (Group integration vs. Self-concept control)	−0.009	0.325	0.255
Q4 (Low ergic tension vs. High ergic tension)	0.031	0.250	−0.514

Table 6.3. Samples available

	EEG variant: Air force sample	Student ♂	Student ♀	Student ♂+♀
N (Low voltage)	47	38	24	62
NG (Low voltage borderline)	14	–	–	7
BO (Occip. beta waves)	13	–	–	8
R (Monomorphic alpha waves)	45	32	18	50
BG (Frontoprecentral beta groups)	25	22	27	49
BD (Diffuse beta waves)	65	27	59	86
KO (Controls)	79	–	–	–

of this study – even their validity, i.e., their ability for tapping relevant aspects of the "true" personality is not as good as it should be. On the other hand, more basic properties such as working speed or ability to identify tachistoscopically offered pictures and numbers, reaction time and even aspects of "intelligence" appeared to give clearer results. And a fairly clean relationship between IQ and α frequencies, especially in frontal and precentral leads has, indeed, been shown (see Sect. 6.3). In conclusion, not too much can be expected from the main study.

Table 6.3–6.16 show the results of the main studies. Table 6.3 contains the samples available. For the single tests, small deviations from these figures occurred since very few results were not available for evaluation. These deviations are not contained in the tables; we did our best to keep the samples as complete as possible. For a few tests, such as the KLT test and the pursuit rotor, data are available only for the Air Force sample, or evaluations proved not to be readily comparable. Therefore they have not been included in the present report.

Statistical analysis was carried out in two steps separately for the Air Force and the student sample: (a) Heterogeneity between EEG groups was tested by analysis of variance, and (b) differences between single EEG groups were tested for significance by the T test. This method of analysis is well suited for offering hints about the direction of possible between-group differences. However, it also has some disadvantages: when applied to test scores, it requires many statistical comparisons, some of which would be expected to be significant even if there were no differences between the groups. Deciding which of these deviation may be biologically meaningful requires additional considerations. This inevitably introduced as element of subjectivity. Moreover, considering test scores separately neglects their interrelations. Data reduction by factor analysis or by any other methods, on the other hand, may tend to obscure important hints. We decided to follow the above path, comparing, in addition, the results from the Air Force sample, which was exclusively male, with that from the student sample. In addition to an analysis of the two sexes together in the student sample, we also tabulated the results for the two sexes and for four categories (N, R, BG, BD) for which sufficient data were available, separately. We are aware of the fact that these samples do not represent unbiased population samples – not even of populations of the same age group. The two samples share two biases: (a) Their intelligence level is well above the population average. The means are higher and the ranges are more restricted. (b) Major deviations in the personality field and in neurological diseases with EEG anomalies such as types of epilepsy are rarer than in an average population. This leads to extreme rarity, if not absence, of special EEG results. On the other hand, the two samples are sufficiently different in origin and composition to allow recognition of possible generalities. However, we refrained from carrying out further statistical analyses after pooling of the two samples. In the following, the results of various analyses are reported in condensed form; for those readers who want to go into details, more detailed analyses have been reported before for the Air Force sample (Vogel et al. 1979b).

6.5
Variation in the Normal EEG: Performance and Personality: Results

The following compares the results of our two studies (Air Force personal and students), between the two sexes within our student sample and between our studies and those of Schmettau. In the student sample various EEG variants were unequally represented in males and females ($\chi_3^2 = 17.82$; $p = 0.0005$). Both variants of β activity (BD, BG) show higher incidences in females, while the variants of the α rhythm (N and R) are more frequent in males. The age effect is small; BG is the "youngest" EEG variant, while R and N are the "oldest" ones ($P_{hd} = 0.02$). However, the differences are small, and probably are without biological significance. In the Air Force sample (Vogel 1979b), the group showing diffuse β waves (BD) was the oldest one. This could be explained easily by the well-known fact (Sect. 2.6) that the prevalence of EEGs with diffuse β waves increases with advancing age. This increase was not shown in the student sample, but both mean ages and age ranges were lower in this sample than among our Air Force probands. Here we discuss the results for single groups of tests.

Cognitive Abilities

Here we compare the result of the intelligence tests (Tables 6.4–6.8). IST test: No scale of this test showed significant heterogeneity in either of the two samples; heterogeneity, however, was revealed in male and female subsamples. A similar, statistically negative result has been reported for the Air Force sample; marginally significant heterogeneities were found for three tests when three computed categories (R + KO; N + NG; BG + BD + BO) were compared. The two groups achieving best had been N (114.87) and BO (114.85) in the Air Force sample; in the student sample, groups R (114.3) and BO (113.7) scored best.

For selected items of the LPS test (Tables 6.7) the Air Force sample has shown a number of significant heterogeneities (8 and 9, space; 7–10, technical skills; 11, 12, and 12 + 12, guessing; 14, recognition). The student sample did not reveal any significant heterogeneities. The groups achieving best in this sample were R (in four subtests), BO and BG (in three subtests each), while in the Air Force sample, group BG had been the best group in 7 categories; BO, N and the controls (KO) rated best in one category each. The Raven test had shown significant heterogeneity ($p = 0.0005$) in the Air Force sample, with BO showing the highest and BG the second highest score. In the student sample, there were no significant differences between EEG groups; in fact, results were very similar ($P_{het} = 0.8131$). The best group was BG, the worst one was N. The two sexes scored very similarly.

Table 6.4. Mean values, F values, and corresponding P values for the IST test (old: Air force sample, new: Student sample)

		SE x̄	WA x̄	AN x̄	GE x̄	RA x̄	ZR x̄	FA x̄	Wü x̄	ME x̄	Total x̄
N	Old	113.21	113,28	110.34	111.40	110.19	111.30	111.79	112.19	108.32	114.87
	New ♂	110.7	109.9	112.3	110.2	111.7	110.8	108.2	107.9	108.7	113.7
	New ♀	109.7	111.4	108.5	110.2	103.3	103.0	103.3	104.7	109.7	109.8
	New ♂+♀	110.3	110.4	110.8	110.0	108.2	107.6	106.0	106.4	109.3	112.0
NG	Old	114.07	115.60	108.87	112.20	111.87	108.53	107.93	110.00	102.67	113.40
	New ♂+♀	107.6	113.1	111.4	114.1	108.3	108.6	103.4	109.1	108.7	113.0
BO	Old	110.46	110.62	112.92	112.92	113.92	106.69	111.77	109.08	110.23	114.85
	New ♂+♀	112.6	115.6	110.5	108.0	112.1	110.7	110.1	99.8	112.5	113.7
R	Old	109.93	112.67	110.85	108.85	112.20	108.61	110.76	108.78	109.70	113.39
	New ♂	111.5	115.2	113.4	110.7	110.2	110.9	109.4	107.7	111.1	115.0
	New ♀	111.5	111.5	108.9	110.8	105.0	112.5	105.8	107.1	112.9	113.2
	New ♂+♀	111.5	113.9	111.5	110.8	108.1	111.8	107.7	107.4	111.9	114.3
BG	Old	110.20	116.92	115.56	109.08	110.08	111.60	110.36	111.16	107.92	114.36
	New ♂	111.2	113.0	112.9	110.1	111.5	112.1	106.8	109.5	109.3	114.5
	New ♀	108.4	112.7	107.7	109.5	102.5	107.6	101.6	101.0	109.4	109.4
	New ♂+♀	109.7	112.9	110.0	109.8	106.5	109.6	104.0	104.8	109.4	111.7
BD	Old	115.55	112.71	108.60	109.37	107.92	105.60	110.03	107.35	108.91	111.83
	New ♂	111.9	112.2	113.6	112.7	111.1	108.5	108.4	106.2	108.5	114.2
	New ♀	110.1	111.8	110.7	111.6	106.4	109.6	106.1	104.5	113.8	113.1
	New ♂+♀	110.7	111.9	111.6	111.9	107.9	109.2	106.8	105.0	112.2	113.4
KO	Old	111.65	112.78	110.87	109.91	108.97	108.76	111.70	107.68	108.42	113.30
Overall mean		111.55	112,74	110.32	110.04	110.00	108.49	110.88	109.00	108.45	113.41

Concentration: Attention to Detail

The test used in both samples has been the *Aufmerksamkeits-Belastungstest* (attentative-burdening test; Brickenkamp 1962). This test consists of 14 rows with the letter d, which is accompanied by one, to or three commas. All d's with two commas must be crossed out. Speed (number of d's crossed out per unit time) and percentage of errors were evaluated (Table 6.9). No significant heterogeneities between EEG groups were discovered either in the Air Force or in the student samples. However, in both samples, the same EEG groups had the first three rank places for speed; in the Air Force sample, their rank order was BO > BG > R, and in the student sample, it was R > BO > BG. For technical reasons, errors were given as a proportion for the Air Force samples, and in absolute numbers for the student samples. There is no significant heterogeneity between EEG groups within any of these samples. R which held a second position regarding low frequency of errors in the Air Force sample, held the third rank in the student sample.

Table 6.5. Statistical comparison, IST test

		SE	WA	AN	GE	RA	ZR	FA	WÜ	ME	Total
Hetero-geneity	Old sample	–	–	–	–	–	–	–	–	–	–
	New sample	–	–	–	–	–	–	–	–	–	–
Rank	Old sample	NG > N > KO BD > BO > BG > R	BG > NG > N KO > BD > R > BO	BO > BG > KO R > N > NG > BD	BO > NG > N KO > BD > BG > R	BO > R > NG BG > N > KO > BD	N > BG > KO R > NG > BD > BD	N > BO > KO > NG	N > BG > NG BO > R > KO	BO > R > BD KO > N > BG > NG	N > BO > BG NG > R > KO > BD
	New Sample	BO > R > BD > N > BG > NG	BO > R > NG > BG > BD > N	BD > R > NG > N > BO > BG	NG > BD > R > N > BG > BO	BO > NG > N > R > BD > BG	R > BO > BG > BD > NG > N	BO > R > BD > N > BG > NG	NG > R > N > BD > BG > BO	BO > BD > R > BG > N > NG	R > BO > BD > NG > N > BG

Table 6.6. Mean for the LPS test

		3 (Sequence of figures) $\bar{x}$	6 (Verbal fluency) $\bar{x}$	7 (Space) $\bar{x}$	8 (Space) $\bar{x}$	9 (Space) $\bar{x}$	10 (Space) $\bar{x}$	7–10 (Technical skills) $\bar{x}$	11 (Guessing) $\bar{x}$	12 (Guessing) $\bar{x}$	11+12 $\bar{x}$	14 (Recognition) $\bar{x}$
N	Old	29.60	38.34	26.68	32.96	30.15	30.89	120.68	24.57	29.87	54.87	24.40
	New ♂	31.0	45.1	27.0	33.0	28.9	31.3	120.2	26.1	30.3	56.4	26.9
	New ♀	29.7	45.2	25.2	33.1	29.2	29.1	116.6	26.2	31.0	57.1	27.5
	♂ + ♀	30.6	45.2	26.3	33.0	29.1	30.6	119.4	26.2	30.6	56.8	27.1
NG	Old	28.27	38.20	24.33	27.20	29.47	28.33	109.33	23.60	30.93	54.53	22.93
	♂ + ♀	30.1	45.3	25.6	35.4	28.0	34.0	123.0	27.1	31.6	58.7	27.6
BO	Old	30.23	35.08	27.53	28.46	29.38	30.08	116.23	27.15	30.53	57.69	25.92
	♂ + ♀	33.8	51.9	25.6	30.3	29.3	30.8	115.9	24.0	31.1	55.1	30.4
R	Old	30.09	37.39	25.70	31.57	30.46	29.17	117.33	26.33	29.96	56.26	24.74
	New ♂	31.9	43.7	26.2	34.8	30.6	31.2	122.8	27.0	32.4	59.5	25.6
	New ♀	31.6	43.1	29.1	34.6	28.8	31.9	124.4	26.2	32.1	58.3	27.7
	♂ + ♀	31.5	43.5	27.5	34.6	29.6	32.1	123.8	26.6	32.5	59.1	26.7
BG	Old	31.28	36.40	25.64	33.88	30.16	31.28	120.96	27.16	31.76	58.92	26.84
	New ♂	30.4	44.0	25.8	34.0	28.2	31.4	119.5	26.2	32.6	58.8	24.6
	New ♀	31.4	46.0	26.7	33.3	28.8	29.4	118.2	24.9	31.0	55.9	27.1
	♂ + ♀	30.9	45.1	26.3	33.7	28.6	30.3	118.8	25.5	31.7	57.2	26.0
BD	Old	28.26	35.71	24.73	26.60	27.34	27.00	105.66	25.25	28.38	53.78	23.12
	New ♂	31.9	41.4	25.8	34.9	30.8	33.5	125.0	26.3	31.7	58.0	26.1
	New ♀	31.7	48.6	25.4	34.4	29.2	31.6	120.6	26.2	31.6	57.8	26.8
	♂ + ♀	31.8	46.2	25.6	34.5	29.7	32.3	122.1	26.3	31.6	57.9	26.6
KO	Old	29.75	37.42	26.30	32.05	30.62	29.51	118.50	27.90	30.29	58.13	25.14
Overall mean:	Old	29.52	37.03	25.81	30.64	29.63	29.23	115.43	26.20	29.91	56.19	24.57
	New											

Table 6.7. Statistical comparison, LPS items

	3	6	7	8	9	10	7–10	11	12	11+12	14
Heterogeneity											
Old sample:		–	–	P = 0,003	P = 0,003	–	P = 0,002	P = 0,001	P = 0,025	P = 0,010	P = 0,009
New sample:		–	–	–	–	–	–	–	–	–	–
Rank											
Old:	BG > BO > R > KO N > NG > BD	N > NG > KO > R > BG > BD > BO	BO > N > KO > R > BG > BD > NG	BG > N > KO > R > BO > nG > BD	KO > R > BG > N > NG > BD > BD	BG > N > BO > KO R > NG > BD	BG > N > KO > R > BO > NG > BD	KO > BG > BO > > R > BD	BG > NG > BO > KO > R > N > BD	BG > KO > BO R > N > NG > BD	BG > BO > KO > R > N > BD > NG
New:	BO > BD > R > BG > N > NG	BO > BD > N = NG > BG > R	R > N = BG > NG=BD=BO	NG > R > BD > BG > N > BO	BD > R > BO > N > BG > NG	NG > BD > R > BO > N > BG	R > NG > BD > N > BG > BO	NG > R > BD > N > BG > BO	R > BG > NG = BD > BO > N	R > NG > BD > BG > N > BO	BO > NG > N > > R > BD > BG

Table 6.8. Raven test (Old = Air force sample; New = Student's sample)

EEG variant		mean	n
N	Old	53.04	47
	New ♂	55.7	41
	New ♀	53.5	20
	♂ + ♀	54.8	61
NG	Old	52.64	14
	New ♂		
	New ♀		
	♂ + ♀	55.6	7
BO	Old	55.38	13
	New ♂		
	New ♀		
	♂ + ♀	55.0	8
R	Old	55.55	45
	New ♂	55.3	30
	New ♀	54.6	20
	♂ + ♀	54.9	50
BG	Old	54.24	25
	New ♂	55.6	22
	New ♀	55.7	27
	♂ + ♀	55.7	49
BD	Old	50.89	65
	New ♂	56.0	28
	New ♀	55.3	58
	♂ + ♀	55.5	86
KO	Old		79
	New ♂		
	New ♀		
	♂ + ♀		

Heterogeneity	Rank
p = 0.005	BO > BG > R > KO > N > NG > BD
–	BG > NG > BD > BO > R > N

Motoric Performance

Tapping test (Tables 6.10, 6.11): for tapping. i.e., hitting of a metal plate with a metal slate-pencil, the following parameters were measured: total number of hits on one plate when the proband is asked to hit as fast as possible, time during which the pencil does not touch the plate in this experiment, total number of hits on two plates, times during which the pencil does not touch these plates, total number of hits when the proband chooses the most comfortable tapping speed, and time during which the pencil does not touch the plate in this experiment. When the Air

Table 6.9. D2 test

EEG variant		GZ (Sum total)	Errors	Heterogeneity, sum total
N	Old	458.45	3.586%	
	New ♂	497.2	19.9%	
	New ♀	498.7	18.3%	
	♂ + ♀	500.1	20.4%	
NG	Old	445.13	2.628%	Rank; sum total BO > BG > R > KO > N > BD > NG Heterogeneity sum total: No heterogeneity
New	♂ + ♀	477.5	16.3%	R > BO > BG > N > BD > NG
BO	Old	491.00	3.636%	Heterogeneity, errors
New	♂ + ♀	526.0	18.4%	Old and new samples: No heterogeneity
R	Old	480.96	2.912%	Rank; errors (Low values are good)
	New ♂	516.2	20.2%	NG > R > KO > NO > BO > BD > BG
	New ♀	542.6	20.3%	BD > NG > R > BO > BG > N
	♂ + ♀	535.8	18.0%	
BG	Old	487.28	4.745%	
	New ♂	508.8	18.5%	
	New ♀	509.2	20.8%	
	♂ + ♀	511.8	20.0%	
BD	Old	455.43	4.179%	
	New ♂	478.8	13.9%	
	New ♀	505.5	14.2%	
	♂ + ♀	497.7	13.9%	
KO	Old	477.46	3.320%	

Force sample was evaluated, there was significant heterogeneity for one parameter: off-time at preferred speed. Moreover, there were a number of significant 1 : 1 differences: In tapping on one plate at maximum speed, the R group was lower than the controls (KO) and lower than group N. In off-time at the preferred speed experiment, group N was lower than group R. In the student sample, there were no significant heterogeneities. The ranks also differed from those found in the Air Force sample: While in the Air Force sample, BO held the highest rank in maximum speed at the one-plate experiment, its rank was lowest among the students. R was lower than N in all three tests in the student group and in two of the three tests in the Air Force sample.

Coordination of the two hands (Table 6.12): Speed, number of deviations from the small track along with the pin must be directed, and time that the pin was outside the track were measured. In the Air Force sample, analysis of variance for number of errors rendered significant heterogeneity ($p = 0.035$). In the student group,

Table 6.10. Tapping speed (Old = Air force sample; New = Students)

EEG variant		One plate: Maximum speed	Two plates: Maximum speed	One plate: Preferred speed
N	Old	202.85	152.06	152.55
	New ♂	207.3	158.1	127.3
	New ♀	199.5	147.6	113.3
	♂ + ♀	202.9	153.5	124.4
NG	Old	204.93	153.43	139.86
	New ♂ + ♀	208.2	157.2	104.2
BO	Old	211.08	151.62	136.85
	New ♂ + ♀	191.9	152.8	117.7
R	Old	196.04	152.62	142.20
	New ♂	206.5	151.7	124.2
	New ♀	187.6	148.8	122.6
	♂ + ♀	198.6	150.3	122.1
BG	Old	197.40	151.28	144.84
		196.7	151.6	116.9
		190.3	146.0	114.8
	New ♂ + ♀	193.1	148.3	116.0
BD	Old	203.83	150.86	141.86
		204.0	160.0	131.1
		195.2	147.6	118.8
	New ♂ + ♀	198.7	152.4	123.1
KO	Old	203.47	152.51	141.49
	New ♂ + ♀			

Table 6.11. Evaluation, tapping speed

One plate, maximum speed: Heterogeneity	Rank	Two plates, maximum speed: Heterogeneity	Rank	One plate, preferred speed: Heterogeneity	Rank
Old	BO > NG > BD > KO > N > BG > R	-	NG > R > KO > N > BO > BG > BD	-	N > BG > R > BD > KO > NG > BO
New	NG > N > BD > R > BG > BO	-	NG > N > BO > BD > R > BG	-	N > BD > R > BO > BG > NG

no significant heterogeneity was found. Among the Air Force sample, R needed the longest time; in the student sample, this group needed the shortest time. The lowest number of errors was found in both series by group BO, followed, again in both series, by R.

Table 6.12. Two-hand coordination

	EEG variant	Time needed	No. of errors
Old	N	111.19	17.68
New ♂		138.5	23.2
New ♀		180.5	29.1
♂ + ♀		155.6	25.6
Old	NG	122.07	18.79
♂ + ♀		147.7	34.7
Old	BO	105.77	12.39
♂ + ♀		188.6	21.6
Old	R	127.67	15.93
New ♂		128.7	22.4
New ♀		163.5	26.8
♂ + ♀		143.4	24.3
Old	BG	119.36	17.00
New ♂		174.6	24.7
New ♀		186.2	32.4
♂ + ♀		180.3	29.0
Old	BD	102.41	20.23
New ♂		155.6	25.1
New ♀		180.5	28.9
♂ + ♀		172.9	28.0
Old	KO	113.29	16.24
No hetero-geneity	time (low values = good) ERRORS p = 0.034 (low values we good)		
Rank (Old)	BD > BO > N > KO > BG > NG > R R > NG > N > BD > BG > BO		
(New)	BO > R > KO > BG > N > NG > BD BO > R N > BD > BG > NG		

Sensoric Performance

Reaction time (Tables 6.13, 6.14): The parameter tested was the time needed to react to stimuli offered at random time intervals. Each experiment consisted of three parts: first, a red light was offered, then a sound and finally a mixture of lights and sounds. Accuracy of reactions was checked by counting the total number of reactions in all experiments; it was only rarely higher than the number of stimuli. Hence all probands understood the design of the experiment; in very few instances, probands reacted without stimulus. In the Air Force sample, there were significant heterogeneities for the reaction time ($p = 0.00087$) and for the range of reaction ($p = 0.028$) in the experiment with red light. The reaction time on sound did not

Table 6.13. Reactions time; medians and ranges (Old = Air force sample; New = Student's sample

EEG variant:		Red light Median	Range	Noise Median	Range	Mixture Median	Range
N	Old	20.96	4.40	28.27	4.62	56.27	19.14
	New ♂	23.43	5.61	28.57	5.30	62.34	19.45
	New ♀	21.47	4.50	25.89	6.43	59.24	20.91
	♂ + ♀	22.27	5.09	26.83	6.08	60.86	20.41
NG	Old	26.50	6.46	29.54	6.71	55.36	19.71
	♂ + ♀	20.75	5.00	27.25	5.75	56.08	17.33
BO	Old	22.69	6.31	29.27	4.69	58.03	20.15
	♂ + ♀	24.00	4.13	31.19	4.80	66.63	20.19
R	Old	23.54	6.12	28.81	6.59	55.24	19.67
	New ♂	22.74	4.71	29.61	4.92	58.58	19.87
	New ♀	21.10	4.09	27.90	5.72	55.13	18.67
	♂ + ♀	21.79	4.22	28.70	5.44	55.93	18.86
BG	Old	21.72	4.68	27.52	5.08	55.66	19.00
	New ♂	23.50	5.83	27.21	5.90	61.69	20.58
	New ♀	21.26	4.16	24.95	4.66	60.41	21.02
	♂ + ♀	22.59	5.10	26.44	5.40	61.23	20.92
BD	Old	23.58	5.60	29.35	5.37	57.24	21.15
	New ♂	22.68	4.70	27.37	5.68	60.45	20.25
	New ♀	21.78	4.40	26.78	6.67	59.24	18.62
	♂ + ♀	22.34	4.50	26.68	6.10	58.94	19.69
KO	Old	22.22	4.91	28.90	4.94	55.16	18.99

show any heterogeneity in the Air Force sample, but there was heterogeneity regarding range in the student sample ($p = 0.00067$). The ranks differed in the two samples.

Personality Questionnaires

Two personality questionnaires were used, the MMPI (Minnesota Multiphasic Personality Inventory) and the 16-PF (16 Personality Factor test; Cattell). Table 6.15 shows the MMPI data. There is only one significant heterogeneity in the Air Force sample; in the Mf (male-female) score. In a number of scores, the student sample differs strongly from the Air Force sample: This applies especially to the Hd (hypochondria), Hy (hysteria) and Pp (psychopathy) scores, but for the Pt (psychastenia) and Sc (schizothymia) scores as well. In all these items, the students score much higher than the Air Force personnel. This hold true despite the fact that in the Air Force sample, but not in the student sample, the K correction was added to the results. The students also show higher values on the Mf (male-female) scale; their interests and attitudes are much more in the direction regarded by the test constructors as

Table 6.14. Evaluation, reaction time (low values are good)

Red light Median Het.	Rank	Range Het.	Rank	Noise Median Het.	Rank	Range Het.	Rank	Mixture Median Het.	Rank	Range Het.	Rank
Old: P = 0.0087	N > BG > KO > BO > R > BD > NG	P = 0.028	N > BG > KO > BD R > BO > NG	-	BG > N > R > KO > BO > BD	-	N > BO > KO > BG > BD > R	-	KO > R > NG > BG > N > BD	-	KO > BG > N > R > NG > BO > BD
New:	NG > R > N > BD > BG > BO	-	BO > R > BD > NG > N > BG	P = 0.0069	BG > BD > N > NG > R > BO	-	BO > BG > R > NG > N > BD		R > NG > BD > N > BG > BO		NG > R > BD > BO > N > BG

Table 6.15. MMPI scores (Old, Air force sample, with K correction; New, Student's sample, without K correction)

EEG		L	F	K	Hd	D	HY	Pp	Mf	Pa	Pt	Sc	Ma	Si
N	Old	4.57	5.43	15.72	11.66	19.62	19.15	21.85	22.68	8.87	23.77	24.81	18.77	25.28
	♂	4.5	7.5	16.2	13.0	22.7	23.5	24.6	28.5	10.7	28.5	28.5	19.9	29.6
	♀	4.6	7.0	15.1	17.6	24.4	26.0	22.8	38.5	11.1	28.6	28.0	20.1	29.1
New	♂+♀	4.5	7.3	15.8	14.7	23.2	24.4	23.9	–	10.8	28.5	28.2	19.8	29.5
NG	Old	4.27	5.47	16.33	11.80	21.27	20.07	22.87	26.33	9.60	24.73	25.80	20.80	25.40
New	♂+♀	42.9	7.3	16.0	11.4	20.3	20.0	24.6	–	8.0	25.7	25.6	19.3	29.6
BO	Old	4.38	5.54	14.92	11.46	21.08	19.00	21.85	24.69	8.69	23.15	24.46	18.77	27.23
New	♂+♀	4.5	7.0	15.1	14.4	27.4	24.9	23.9	–	11.8	31.8	30.1	17.9	34.1
R	Old	4.24	6.30	14.87	12.22	20.67	19.43	21.89	25.13	8.76	24.13	25.39	20.70	26.26
	♂	4.2	9.1	15.9	12.5	21.4	21.8	24.6	27.5	9.7	27.2	29.5	21.0	28.8
	♀	4.0	6.8	15.0	15.3	24.4	23.0	24.9	37.5	10.2	30.3	30.4	20.3	34.9
New	♂+♀	4.1	8.2	15.6	13.7	22.7	22.5	24.8	–	10.0	28.6	30.2	20.9	31.3
BG	Old	5.12	6.04	15.44	11.32	20.28	19.52	20.84	23.40	8.96	23.28	23.36	18.48	23.52
	♂	4.1	7.5	14.4	11.9	21.7	21.7	23.5	27.2	9.2	25.7	26.5	18.9	30.9
	♀	5.0	6.8	15.1	14.0	24.8	25.1	23.7	37.5	11.0	28.5	28.4	20.0	32.2
New	♂+♀	4.6	7.1	14.7	13.0	23.3	23.5	23.6	–	10.2	27.2	27.5	19.5	31.5
BD	Old	5.22	5.71	15.95	12.54	20.88	19.85	22.28	23.66	8.75	24.17	24.42	19.85	24.66
	♂	3.8	7.7	15.6	12.6	21.4	21.5	23.8	27.7	10.0	27.4	27.3	20.4	29.7
	♀	4.1	7.8	15.5	14.3	24.3	23.4	23.9	37.8	10.7	28.9	29.7	19.9	32.3
New	♂+♀	3.8	7.9	15.2	14.1	23.4	22.9	23.8	–	10.6	28.7	29.1	20.1	31.3
	Old	4.30	6.42	15.91	11.97	21.27	19.59	22.86	23.92	8.71	25.49	25.91	19.87	27.41
	Het.	–	–	–	–	–	–	–	P = 0.007	–	–	–	–	–
		–	–	–	–	–	–	–	(P = 0.0004)	–	–	–	–	–
Rank	Old	BD>BG>N >BO>KO>NG>R	KO>R>BG> BD>BO>NG	NG>BD>KO>N >BG>BO>R	BD>R>KO NG>N>BO>BG	NG=KO>BO>BD >BG>R>N	NG>BD>KO>BG >R>N>BO	NG>KO>BD >R>N=BO>BG	NG>R>BO>KO >BD>BG>N	NG>BG>N >R>BD>KO>BO	KO>NG>BD >R>N>BG>BO	KO>NG>R>N >BO>BD>BG	NG>R>KO>BD >BG>N=BO	KO>BO>R>NG >N>BD>BG
	New	BG>N=BO >R>BD>NG	R>BD>N= NG>BG>BO	NG>N>R >BD>BO>BG	N>BO>BD >R>BG>NG	BO>BD>BG >N>R>NG	BO>N>BG >BD>R>NG	R>NG>N=BO >BD>BG	♂=N>BD>R>BG ♀=N>BD>R=BG	BO>N>BD >BG>R>NG	BO>BD>R >N>BG>NG	R>BO>BD >N>BG>NG	R>BD>N >BG>NG>BO	BO>BG>R=BD >NG>N

Table 6.16. 16-PF values; Old = Air force sample; New = Student sample

EEG		A	B	C	E	F	G	H	I	L	M
N	Old	5.212	7.458	6.125	6.368	6.056	5.532	5.889	5.671	5.002	5.467
	♂	4.353	6.774	4.445	5.563	5.582	3.915	4.432	6.496	5.141	6.830
	New ♀	4.680	6.050	4.019	6.062	5.513	4.760	4.057	6.740	6.211	7.430
	♂+♀	4.472	6.510	4.290	5.745	5.558	4.224	4.295	6.585	5.532	7.049
NG	Old	5.777	7.400	6.112	6.089	5.713	5.890	6.139	7.202	4.264	5.235
	New ♂+♀	3.903	7.556	5.244	5.839	3.893	3.140	3.819	6.486	7.209	6.669
BO	Old	4.637	6.692	6.371	7.377	4.968	4.806	5.346	6.811	5.517	6.398
	New ♂+♀	4.240	7.065	3.506	4.029	4.164	4.170	3.600	5.834	6.030	6.958
R	Old	5.287	7.076	5.947	6.254	5.508	5.331	5.747	5.510	5.466	5.705
	♂	3.849	7.276	4.941	6.136	5.259	3.714	4.604	7.302	5.366	6.384
	New ♀	3.092	6.600	2.893	5.962	3.987	4.415	2.546	5.903	6.636	7.695
	♂+♀	3.540	7.000	4.105	6.064	4.740	4.000	3.764	6.731	5.884	6.919
BG	Old	5.493	7.238	6.330	6.227	7.017	5.707	6.592	5.158	5.241	5.162
	♂	3.791	6.537	5.007	6.169	5.319	3.301	4.184	6.890	6.020	6.615
	New ♀	4.054	7.429	3.913	5.871	4.852	4.163	3.458	6.632	5.680	7.482
	♂+♀	3.928	7.002	4.436	6.013	5.073	3.751	3.805	6.755	5.843	7.067
BD	Old	5.047	6.660	5.832	6.158	5.840	5.407	6.121	5.539	5.423	5.826
	♂	4.129	7.302	4.808	6.830	5.828	3.423	4.444	7.212	5.320	6.998
	New ♀	3.706	7.180	3.791	5.604	4.374	4.077	3.415	6.573	6.597	7.234
	♂+♀	3.842	7.219	4.117	5.997	4.841	3.867	3.745	6.778	6.187	7.158
KO	Old	5.022	7.095	5.998	6.204	5.635	4.594	5.292	6.291	5.373	5.565
Het.:		–	–	–	–	–	P = 0.035	–	0.006	–	–
		–	–	–	–	–	–	–	–	–	–
Rank:		NG>BG>R>N >BD>KO>BO N>BO>BG>NG >BD>R	N>NG>BG>KO >R>BO>BD NG>BD>BO>BG >R>N	BO>BG>N>NG >R>KO>BD NG>BG>N>BD >R>BO	BO>N>R>BG KO>BD>NG R>BG>BD>NG >N>BO	BG>N>BD>NG >KO>R>BO N>BO>R>BD >BO>NG	NG>BG>N>BD >R>BO>KO N>NG>BG>R >BG>NG	BG>NG>BD>N >R>BO>KO N>NG>BG>R >BD>BO	NG BO>KO>N>BD >R>BG BD>BG>R>N >NG>BO	BO>R>BO>KO >BG>N>NG NG>BD>BO>R >BG>N	BO>BD>R>KO >N>NG>BG BD>BG>N>BO >R>NG

Table 6.16. 16 PF values; II

EEG		N	O	Q_1	R_2	R_3	R_4	R I	R II	R III	R IV
N	Old	5.240	4.613	5.458	5.479	4.934	5.311	6.082	4.944	6.420	6.051
	♂	3.776	6.445	4.962	6.250	4.460	6.976	4.970	6.624	6.526	5.788
	New ♀	4.126	7.362	5.540	6.755	3.531	8.210	4.853	7.667	4.703	6.643
	♂+♀	3.903	6.780	5.173	6.434	4.121	7.427	4.928	7.005	5.861	6.100
NG	Old	5.068	4.932	4.443	5.028	5.159	5.487	6.090	5.101	5.224	5.254
	New ♂+♀	2.474	6.749	5.644	7.020	4.420	7.781	4.114	7.076	6.463	6.734
BO	Old	6.075	5.179	5.945	5.034	5.337	6.295	5.589	5.450	5.825	6.578
	New ♂+♀	2.658	7.713	6.336	6.771	4.150	7.086	3.861	7.459	3.500	6.091
R	Old	5.294	5.165	5.092	6.419	4.769	5.864	5.619	5.435	6.298	6.146
	♂	3.511	6.350	5.068	6.390	4.477	7.102	4.929	6.558	6.531	6.121
	New ♀	4.155	8.244	4.346	6.884	3.485	8.325	3.419	8.414	4.441	6.259
	♂+♀	3.774	7.123	4.773	6.592	4.072	7.602	4.313	7.316	5.678	6.177
BG	Old	6.251	4.661	4.271	5.643	4.603	5.563	6.639	5.101	6.717	5.657
	♂	3.588	5.519	5.056	6.854	4.700	7.076	4.745	6.348	6.739	6.572
	New ♀	3.637	6.477	4.786	6.559	3.981	7.197	4.224	7.007	4.155	6.580
	♂+♀	3.613	6.019	4.915	6.700	4.325	7.140	4.473	6.692	5.391	6.576
BD	Old	5.681	5.451	5.225	5.716	4.771	5.683	5.899	5.455	6.344	5.934
	♂	3.491	6.145	5.238	6.312	4.285	7.573	5.317	6.696	6.805	6.575
	New ♀	3.709	7.006	4.802	7.026	3.725	7.773	3.888	7.525	4.521	6.484
	♂+♀	3.639	6.730	4.942	6.797	3.905	7.709	4.347	7.259	5.254	6.513
KO	Old	5.507	5.289	5.291	5.984	4.671	5.971	5.463	5.544	6.040	5.971
Het.		–	–	–	–	–	–	–	–	–	–
		–	–	–	–	–	–	–	–	–	–
Rank	Old	BG>BO>BD>KO >R>N>NG	BO>KO>BO>BD >NG>BG>N	BO>N>KO>BD >R>NG>BG	R>KO>BD>BG >N>BO>NG	BO>NG>N>BD >R>KO>BG	BO>KO>R>BD >BG>NG>N	BG>NG>N>BD >R>BO>KO	KO>BD>BO>R >BG=NG>N	BG>N BD>R >KO>BO>NG	BO>R>NG>KO>BD >BG>NG
	New	N>R>BD>BG >BO>NG	BO>R>N>NG >BD>BG	BO>NG>N>BD >BG>R	NG>BD>BO>BG >R>N	NG>BG>BO>N >R>BD	NG>BD>R>N >BG>BO	N>BG>BD>R >NG>BO	BO>R>BD>NG >N>BG	NG>N>R>BG >BD>BO	NG>BG>BD >R>N>BO

"female," which includes arts, etc. These differences between soldiers, on the one hand, most of them professional and keeping more or less elevated ranks in the Air Force, and university students are not surprising. However, they may tend to obscure communalities in EEG category-specific differences. One such communality is obvious: Among both samples – Air Force personnel and students – and students of both sexes – group R holds a high rank in the Ma (hypomania) score. In students of both sexes, it is the highest, in the Air Force sample it is the second-highest rank. There were only two heterogeneities of the 16-PF test in the Air Force sample, and no ones in the student sample (Table 6.16). However, there was an interesting sex difference in this sample, and a number of pair-wise differences between special EEG variants: Moreover, R and N variants show opposite extreme values for five scales; the difference between them is significant ($p < 0.05$). In the female sub-sample, N has the highest scores on scales A, B, F, H, I and Q_1; for these scales, R had the lowest score. N also shows a minimum score on B, and R has a maximum score on O. This allows personality "syndromes" to be defined for N and R (see below). For groups NG and BO, no separate analysis in relation to gender was performed in the student sample; numbers of probands were too small.

6.6 An Attempt at Characterization of EEG Variants Based on Test Results

The following attempts to characterize the average psychological profiles of the various EEG variants. This is made difficult by a number of problems, however:

a) Heritability of test scores is not very high, and in some instances even low (and not significant statistically) as shown by our studies on an – admittedly small – sample of young adult twins (Vogel 1979 a; see also Sect. 6.4).
b) The two samples studied by ourselves, the Air Force and the student samples, are "biased" in partially different ways: Both samples show an elevated mean intelligence and, probably, also aspects of sensory and motor performance and, accordingly, a restricted range of measured intelligence. While there were definite differences between the two samples regarding some personality characteristics, they overlap in other aspects of personality: Both are biased in the direction of "normalcy." The questionnaires used had been constructed in part for characterization of the individuals showing deviant behaviors, especially mental anomalies and diseases, but also certain types of neuroses and, in general, failures of social adaptation and success in life. Such individuals were, at least, unusually rare in both samples. This led to a restriction of test scores also in evaluation of personality questionnaires and therefore to diminishing of possible group differences.
c) The third series to be included in our evaluation, the series studied by Schmettau (1969, 1970), started with a series of probands showing "normal" EEGs but not with defined EEG variants. Therefore results should be compared taking into account critically this major difference. Obviously, this creates difficulties of interpretation; it may also have certain advantages.

Psychological Characterization of EEG Variants

The low-voltage EEG (N) and low-voltage borderline EEG (NG). It has been described in Sect. 4.3. Its most characteristic feature is the almost complete absence of α waves. Both β and ϑ waves may be present.

Based on the Air Force sample, this EEG variant was characterized as follows (Vogel 1979b): "This group had relatively high intelligence scores, except in guessing ability in the LPS test. Spatial orientation was especially good. Their MMPI scores were average or low, indicating a conspicuous degree of "normality." In the 16 Pf test and in tests requiring concentration, the N group tended to average values. Among the sensorimotor results, their short reaction time to color and sounds stands out. In motor skills and tapping, the group showed average or good values." The student sample showed some differences to this description. For example, the N group had somewhat lower values in the general intelligence test (IST); for almost all subtests, performance was within the lower half. In the LPS items, the N group showed average to below-average values. In the Raven test, it had the lowest rank of all groups within the student sample; in the Air Force sample, it had held position 5 (of 7). As to all reaction time items, the group had average values. The group was especially fast this time for tapping speed; in preferred speed it was the fastest one in the Air Force and student samples. In two-hand coordination, it showed average values in both series as regards time needed as well as errors; regarding number of errors, group N was worse in both samples (Air Force and students) than group R. Regarding working speed (D2 test), the N group scored average, but it was the most error-prone group; as noted above, results of personality questionnaires were quite different within the student sample than in the Air Force sample. Here, the N group scored highest of all groups in Hd (hypochondria), second highest in Hy and Pa, and lowest in Si. It also had the highest Mf scores in both sexes, pointing to interests in the direction of those regarded by the test constructors as "female." The high Hd and Hy scores seemed to indicate a higher degree of psychosomatic complaints. We examined this point of view in greater detail by reexamining the greater portion of our student sample with a questionnaire designed specifically for studying bodily complaints (Freiburger *Beschwerdeliste*, FBL). This test comprises 78 items testing subjective feelings on health; emotional reactivity; and condition of certain organic areas such as heart, stomach and intestines; pain; skin anomalies; and others (for details, see Förg 1984). The subsample studied with this questionnaire consisted of 187 subjects (Table 6.17). The result can be summarized very briefly: There was no significant differences between EEG groups; not even a tendency could be discovered.

Table 6.17. Subsample studied by the "Freiburger Beschwerdeliste"

	R	N	BD	BG	Total
♂	23	33	24	11	91
♀	16	17	52	11	96
♂ + ♀	39	50	76	22	–

As regards the 16 PF-scores, group N had the highest score of the student sample in A ("outgoing, easygoing, participating") and in N ("astute, polished, socially aware") and the lowest values in L ("trusting, accepting conditions") and Q2 ("group dependent, a 'joiner' and sound follower"). It kept the second-lowest ranks in QII ("adjustment" vs. anxiety) and QIV ("subduedness" vs. independence; the descriptions in the 16 PF handbook).

When one tries to compare the results of the student sample with those of the Air Force sample, and to give a more general characterization of the N group, the following characteristics stand out:

The N group does not show any characteristics in the traditional intelligence range. Average intelligence was somewhat higher in the Air Force sample, especially in comparison with the R group, but there were no special strengths or weaknesses. Working speed was average but this group was slightly more error-prone than others. In concordance with the Air Force sample, it showed a certain tendency for high speed, this time not expressed by reaction time but by a preferred high speed of tapping. In the personality field, the high Hd and Hy scores should be mentioned again. These suggest a higher susceptibility for psychosomatic complaints in members of the student sample, but not in the Air Force sample. This difference may well be due to the stronger group dependency and the more outgoing (= extrovert) temperament of the members of this group. A low tendency for hypochondric complaints certainly belongs to the conventional self-image of the professional soldier but not to the self-image of the university student (especially in the humanities). Therefore more group-dependent persons tend to follow the group image of their group. In three personality characteristics, the N group is distinguished most clearly from other groups, especially the R group.

This group is now described in greater detail. Based on the Air Force sample, it has been described as follows: "This group showed average performance in the majority of intelligence scores; short time memory and practical calculation were especially good. In the MMPI, the clinical scores were average or above average. Average scores were also seen in the 16-PF. In concentration tests, ... the group performed with average speed but above-average precision. Motor skills and tapping were average." This description is not very characteristic; therefore the characterization by Schmettau of one of her two psychological syndromes should be added; her study was described above, in the beginning of Sect. 6.4. She did not start with special EEG variants but with a series of young men representing the entire variety of normal EEGs. By studying of correlations between EEG characteristics such as α index, α amplitude and others, she was able to identify a syndrome comprising the following aspects: "Personality traits associated with this syndrome" (comprising high α index and high α amplitude) "were found to be distinguished by activity and tension, affective excitability, frustration tolerance and readiness to dysphoric reactions. ... (These individuals) tend to be active and tense, inclined to experiment rather than to go along with tradition, self-sufficient, critical and self-opinionated, sober, pessimistic, emotionally easily upset and annoyed, low in frustration tolerance, dominated by a drive for achievement and sometimes by a strong sense of duty. Typically, these subjects are never really at ease. There is a faint tendency to introversion." We should remember that this characterization is not confined to the EEG type with monomorphic α waves (the R type) but it certainly comprises this type.

The two above descriptions above are now compared with the test data for the R type from the student sample (Tables 6.5–6.16). In the IST tests, students of both sexes together had the highest total score; they had excellent results in all fields. In the Air Force sample, the N group had scored highest. In the LPS test, R probands were especially good in items measuring technical skills. Here, the R probands of the Air Force sample had shown average results. In the Raven, R scored average in both samples, but was better than the N group in both. In the D2 (concentration-burdening) test, the R group scored highest of all groups in the student sample in speed; it had been the third one (of seven) in the Air Force sample. In both samples it scored higher than the N group. Regarding number of errors (low error rate regarded as good), the R group scored better than the N group in both samples; in ranking, it was within the first three in both samples. As to motor tests, the R group that had been low in the Air Force sample, was now the fastest in working speed – faster this time than the N group. With its low number of errors, it was excellent in both samples; in both of them only the relatively small BO group scored better (the BO group is discussed separately; see below). As regards tapping speed (Tables 6.10, 6.11), the R group held average positions; in all three experiments, it was lower than the N group in the student sample. Regarding reaction time, the R group showed better scores in the student than in the Air Force sample. In five of six tests, it scored higher than the N group, and in five of six subtests, it was among the first three groups.

The most interesting results were found in the personality questionnaires. The R group scored highest in the Ma (hypomania) score; this applied to both sexes. In the Air Force sample, it had been the second in this score. It was also highest in the student sample for the Sc (schizotymia) score where it has held the third position in the Air Force sample, and it was among the first three for Si (introversion-extraversion) in both samples. In all three scores, and in both samples, it was higher than the N group. The N group, on the other hand, was higher in the Hd (hypochondria), the D (depression), the Hy (hysteria) and the Pa (paranoia) scores. It was the highest in the Mf scores in both sexes. Here, the R group scored much lower. The results of the MMPI are supplemented by the 16-PF results as follows: R has the lowest score in subtest A ("reserved, detached, critical, aloof-stiff") – quite in contrast to group N (see above). In B (intelligence), both groups scores low – a surprising result in view of their performance in intelligence tests. In C, group R scores as the second- lowest ("emotionally less stable"; lower ego strength). In E, it scored the highest, much higher than N ("assertive, aggressive, competitive"; dominance). In F and G, this group held average values in both samples; in both subtests it was lower than that of N. In H, its position was lower in both samples than that of N. In score M, group R is again lower than N; it tends toward "practical, down-to-earth," while N is more "imaginative, bohemian absent-minded." In the Air Force sample, this relationship between R and N was reversed. In category N (artlessness vs. shrewdness"), there was no consistent difference between groups N and R. It is interesting that in category Q1, R in both samples tended more toward conservative, respecting "traditional ideas" while N tended more to "experimenting, liberal, free-thinking." As to Q2, group R tended more toward "self-sufficient, resourceful, prefers own decisions" while N tended to be "group-dependent; a 'joiner' and sound follower." In Q3, N has a slightly higher value than R in both series, this would mean that N individuals would have a "higher strength of self-sentiment" while R persons tend more toward "low self-sentiment integration." Scale Q4 is more interesting; here, R tends more toward "high ergic tension," while N shows "low ergic tension (relaxed, tranquil)." Again, this difference was found in both series.

More interesting than these "first stratum factors" are the "second stratum factors" that were calculated by the test-constructors from intercorrelations of the "first-stratum factors" described above. QI ("invia vs. exvia") coincides with the classical concept pair introversion vs. extraversion. Here, N shows higher scores in both series. N individuals are on the average more extravert than R persons. In QII ("adjustment vs. anxiety"), the R group has higher scores than the N group in both samples; they are more "anxious" and less well "adjusted." In Q III, the term "contertia" (tough pause) is thought by the Cattell school to indicate high "cortical alertness." The opposite term ("pathemia"; low score) characterizes persons who "show a tendency to feel rather than think." In QIV ("subduedness vs. independence"), R individuals in both samples tend more toward "independence" while N persons show a stronger tendency for "subduedness."

It could be criticized that most if not all these comparisons are based on non-significant group differences. However, this is unavoidable since all psychological differences between EEG groups are found to be small for reasons explained above (only moderate heritability test scores; probably contribution also of other genetic factors that do not affect the EEG). It is all the more interesting, however, that there were significant pairwise differences especially in the female subsample of students. Here, R and N variants show opposite extreme values for five scales – with significant differences ($p < 0.05$). Therefore it is possible, on the basis only of the 16- PF test to give a personality characteristic for these two variants in females, while in males significant findings are insufficient for such generalization. Here, results from the Schmettau data as well as from our Air Force sample must be used additionally. In the subsample of female students, N has highest scores on scales A, B, F, H, I and Q1; for these scales, R had the lowest scores. Also, N has minimum score on B, and R has a maximum score on O. Based on the 16-PF data alone, the carriers of the N variant can be characterized as cyclothymic, easygoing, happy-go-lucky, carefree, spontaneous, tender-minded and group-dependent. Carriers of the R variant, on the other side, can be described as schizothymic, reserved, cool, critical, sober, prudent, serious, introspective, tough-minded, self-reliant, realistic, conservative, tending to oppose and postpone changes. These personality features of carriers of these two EEG variants form rather consistent syndromes which are opposite to each other. In the Air Force sample, we were also looking for some characteristics of personality that were apparent from life histories (L data). While other aspects failed to give any objective and controllable evidence, there was one characteristic difference: Among the R group, very few persons were involved in flying accidents as compared with N probands who had been involved in flying accidents more frequently than all other EEG groups. This also points to the high degree of work precision of the R group. However, this group had been involved more often than the N probands in car accidents (Vogel et al. 1979b, c). Obviously, involvement in car accidents depends on personal properties different from those increasing the risk for flying accidents; this results fits with the self-assured and, sometimes, ebullient attitude of R probands. Below we discuss whether and to what extent the conclusion regarding these two syndromes can be generalized and how our data from the Air Force sample and the Schmettau results can be used either to corroborate or to modify and, possibly to complement these conclusions.

Before we proceed to conclusions, however, the other variants must be discussed. Here, another variant of α activity, the EEG with occipital fast α variants (BO) are discussed first. As noted above, this variant is relatively rare (0.6% among German young males; 0.42% among male Japanese; Vogel and Fujiya 1969). Its mode of inheritance is autosomal dominant (Vogel 1966). Relatively few probands could therefore be studied (13 in the Air Force sample, 18 in the student sample). Therefore results should be regarded with restraint, since sampling errors are expected to be still more important than in the other EEG types. Our description that was based on the Air Force sample went as follows (Vogel 1979b): "The BO group performed very well in the IST test and especially in the abstract thinking (IST, LPS, Raven). Their MMPI scores tended to be low, albeit not quite as low as the N group scores. They also tended to extreme scores in the 16 PF. Results of the D2 and KLT tests were not consistent. Reaction times were average. The group stands out for excellent performance in motor skills. ..." The eight probands from the student sample scored excellently again in the IST intelligence test, they were the best ones in five of nine subtests, and scored second in the total test. They also scored best in three of nine single LPS subtests. In the Raven, however, they only have rank 4 (of 6). In the D2 test, they held the second rank in working speed (the first rank in the Air Force sample). In working precision (number of errors) they only had average positions in both samples. In two-hand coordination they were relatively slow this time, but again were the best in coordination. In tapping speed, their performance was average to low. There were no outstanding results for reaction time in both samples or in MMPI scores, possibly except for a certain tendency for introversion or shyness (= high Si score in both samples, low H and I scores in the 16-PF). The other 16-PF subtests, and especially the second-stratum factors, show noncharacteristic results that are often contradictory between the two samples. This may, but does not necessarily, mean that this EEG variant does not affect personality at all; it could also be caused by the small sample sizes. Studies of much larger samples would be necessary to establish reliable personality and performance profiles for individuals showing this EEG variant. However, one result stands out: The excellent performance of BO individuals in intelligence tests. As explained in Sect. 6.3, there is a positive correlation between frequency of α waves and performance in intelligence tests. Individuals showing the BO variant, on the other hand, have by far the highest α frequencies; as explained before, the occipital waves which are in the β range (approx.14–16 c/s) are to be regarded functionally as α waves. Therefore their high intelligence test scores fit well into the observation that high α frequency is one of the factors affecting intellectual performance.

The next group to be discussed is the group of individuals showing a diffuse distribution of β waves in their EEG (BD). As explained in Sect. 4.8, diffuse β activity increases with advancing age in both sexes and is more common in females than in males, especially in older age groups. Both twin and family studies have shown a strong genetic effect but no hint for a monogenic mode of inheritance. Moreover, this EEG variant (or group of EEG variants) is generally more common than the other variants discussed in this chapter; therefore the number of this BD group is highest in both samples – the Air Force and the student sample. In our first report (Vogel 1979a), this group was characterized as follows: "In most of the intelligence tests, this group scored the lowest. Their low LPS scores were partially due to the fact that raw scores were evaluated (the BD group had the highest average age). ...

However, the IST scores are standardized for age, and here too their average result was low, both overall and for spatial and arithmetic abilities. This did not seem to be caused by their having unstable personalities: Most of their MMPI scores were average. Also remarkable was their relatively high percentage of errors in the two concentration tests. ... Reaction time for red light, sound and the mixture was relatively long. This may partly be due to their higher mean age. On the average, they scores too low in tests for motor skills. ..." For this EEG type, the results of the student sample were quite different. This difference was caused in part – but not completely – by the fact that females were more common in this group than males (59 vs. 27). In the entire IST test and in most of its subtests, the BD group now held an average position. There was no conspicuous sex effect. The same was true for the LPS subtests – except for item 6 (verbal fluency), where BD females scored much better than BD males but this is not surprising. The group as a whole also kept a middle position in the Raven; here, the sex difference was very low. A middle position was found for tapping speed, as well (Tables 6.10, 6.11); here, males were slightly faster in both maximum and preferred speed, but this applied for individuals of all EEG variant groups. In the D2 test which tests for concentration, speed and working precision, the BD group again scored low in speed; here, females were much faster than males. In precision (number of errors), this group as a whole scored higher this time than all other EEG groups; it had shown the second worst result in the Air Force sample. The low present errors rate was not caused by a preponderance of females; this rate was almost equal in both sexes. In two-hand coordination, this group now held an average position; this time, in contrast to the Air Force sample, is was not especially error-prone. As to reaction time, it now kept average positions; in the Air Force sample, its position tended to be lower. Here, too, there was no conspicuous sex difference. Their MMPI results were also inconspicuous; small sex differences generally correspond to sex differences in the entire student sample. The inconspicuous personality profile was also documented by the more or less average scores in the second-stratum scores of the 16-PF. Whether the highest rank of BD in the I factor ("tender-minded, sensitive") is of any importance will have to be determined by later studies. In conclusion, the description given for the BD group, which was based on the Air Force sample, cannot be corroborated by the student sample. This difference is not, or at least not predominantly, caused by the fact that, in the student sample, the majority of BD individuals consisted of females. On the other hand, the difference in age distribution of the two samples – the students were much younger than the Air Force probands, and especially those of the Air Force BD sample – may have a strong effect on these different results; it even may be the decisive factor.

The next EEG variants to be considered are those characterized by clearcut groups of β waves that are concentrated in, but not confined to frontoprecentral leads (BG). This trait occurs in a small percentage of the normal population (Vogel and Fujiya 1969), and as a rule it has a simple autosomal-dominant mode of inheritance (Sect. 4.8). Our earlier description of psychological test results went as follows: "The BG group showed excellent results in space perception and guessing abilities. MMPI scores were especially low, the lowest of all EEG categories. Hence this group is especially 'normal' and has a low tendency to neurotic disturbances. Results of concentration tests... were generally very good; reaction times low; and motor skills good to average." Student sample: In the total IST test, the BG group scored average, but it was good in subtests scoring abstract thinking (AN). Average results were also achieved in the LPS items; especially good abilities in space perception were not confirmed. In the Raven, however, the BG group held the first rank this time; it had held the second rank in the Air Force sample. Together with the good result in AN and GE scores of the IST this points to a good ability for abstract thinking. In tapping, the group scores average to low in both series. Average scores were also seen in two-hand coordination and in reaction time. A noncharacteristic pattern was also seen in MMPI scores – in both samples. The same applies for the 16-PF scores. The entire pattern of test results in the BG group is not very different from that of the control (KO) group in the Air Force sample. This is not too surprising, since both groups, BG and KO comprise almost the entire range of α wave patterns, except for only the two extreme variants – monomorphic α waves R, and the low voltage EEG (N), on the other. These results suggest that the a pattern is important for psycho-physiological correlations while presence or absence of frontoprecentral β waves may have little or no effect.

The last group to be discussed are the "borderline" cases of the low-voltage EEG. As shown by family studies, this group appears to be a mixture of persons belonging to the true low-voltage group and those having more or less regular α activity with low amplitude (Reinke 1966; and sometimes many β waves). Based on the (small) Air Force sample, this group has been described before (Vogel 1979b) as follows: "This group differed conspicuously from the N group. The average intelligence score showed slight weaknesses in abstract thinking (IST, LPS and Raven), in short-time memory, and in motor skills and tapping. On the other hand, they were the highest in 8 of 10 "clinical" MMPI scores. This indicates a relatively strong tendency to neurotic complaints. ... In the D2 tests, they were relatively slow.... Reaction time to red light and sound was poor, as were motor skills. ..." In the student sample, only seven probands were classified as belonging to this group; therefore all results should be regarded with great caution. There is no such strong difference any more to probands showing a typical low-voltage EEG (N), largely because their test pattern in the student sample differs from that in the Air Force sample, mainly due to higher values in "clinical" MMMPI scores such as Hd, Hy, or Pa. In the total IST test, the NG group showed an average result – slightly better even than the N probands. In LPS items, especially those testing spatial ability; they were this time especially good and they score higher than the N group in the Raven. In the D2 test, this group was the lowest one in both samples but had a low error rate in both. In maximum tapping speed, they were high in both samples, but their preferred speed was low, also in both samples. In two-hand coordination, this group showed a relatively high speed in the student sample as compared with a lower speed in the Air Force group but error rate was high in both samples. In reaction time, the NG group of students showed excellent results in reaction to light and to mixture; contrary to the Air Force sample and its low scores. In the MMPI, the group scored lower than the N group in Hd, D, Hy, Pa, Pt, Sc and Ma; it was high in the Pp score. Hence the tendency is opposite to that found in the Air Force sample. A similar tendency is found regarding the 16 PF-items. Here, NG probands appear, in comparison with N probands more reserved (A), more intelligent (B), emotionally more stable (C), more "serious and sober" (F), but have a weaker "super-ego strength"(G), are more suspicious (L) and more practical (M). They are more forthright (N), more self-sufficient (Q2) and more controlled (Q3). As to second-stratum factors, they appear to be more introverted (QI) and more independent (QIV). In conclusion, the student NG probands differ strongly from the NG probands of the Air Force sample; their negative characteristics appear not to be present (weaknesses in performance; high scores in aspects of personality). They still differ from the N group, especially in personality scores but, this time, in the opposite direction: now, they look more stable, self-sufficient and also "healthier." This contradiction is discussed in the context of possible neurophysiological mechanisms.

6.7 "Cognitive Styles" and EEG Variants

So far, results of studies have been discussed, in which a variety of psychological standard methods were used for comparative characterization of EEG variants. These studies have led to the hypothesis that such EEG variants lead to differences in information processing within the brain. One method to test this hypothesis by a neurophysiological method is the study of evoked (event-related) potentials (Sect. 5.3). Another method which may permit to test it by using a psychological concept and psychological methods is the study of "cognitive styles." The central concept in definition of the cognitive style is the "conceptual tempo" or "the consistent tendency to respond slowly or rapidly when confronted with a problem-solving situation that had uncertainty" (Kagan et al. 1963, 1964). Here, the contrast of "reflexivity" vs, "impulsivity" (R/I) appears to be most important. It has been operationalized, for example, by tests in which that element which corresponds closely to a given model must be selected from a number of pictures. Such an examination was performed on students showing the above-described EEG variants by Walter (1982). Her sample consisted of most of the students that have participated in the EEG and test studies. Table 6.18 shows composition of the sample. We cannot go into details of the results; suffice it to say that the concept of "cognitive styles" tests for its examination and correlation of test results with those of some other tests, for example, those designed to examine introversion-extraversion, neuroticism, and others, were studied in great detail. The results regarding EEG variants are summarized by the author in Table 6.19.

Table 6.18. Number and sexes of EEG variants included in the study of cognitive styles (Walter 1980)

EEG variant	n (♂)	n(♀)	n (♂ + ♀)
N	33	13	46
NG	5	1	6
BO	0	4	4
R	25	20	45
BG	14	12	26
BD	45	45	90
Sum total	122	95	217

Table 6.19. Cognitive styles and classification of EEG variants

Strategies of test solution	
Reflecting	Impulsive
Steady	Variable
Analyzing	Perceptive
Cognitive	Intuitive
EEG variants	
♂ Monomorphic α waves R	Low-voltage (and low-voltage borderline) EEG (N + NG)
♀ Low-voltage and low voltage borderline EEG (N + NG)	EEG with diffuse β waves (BD) and EEG with frontoprecentral β groups

Most differences between EEG variants, however, were nonsignificant; therefore these are, again, tendencies. However, they show a certain correspondence with those found with more conventional tests, especially the MMPI and 16-PF, in the same student sample (see above). They correspond especially well with the observation that the student BD group (diffuse β waves) differs substantially from the BD group in the Air Force sample. These findings are included in the discussion on possible neurophysiological mechanisms of psychological differences between EEG variants.

6.8 Possible Neurophysiological Mechanisms

These psychological studies call for an interpretation in terms of neurophysiology. For such an interpretation, however, not only these results should be used, but also the results of comparative studies on visually and auditory evoked potentials described in Sect. 5.3. They should be interpreted in terms of present theoretical concepts on the formation of EEG patterns. These concepts have been described, for example, in various chapters of the standard textbook of Niedermeyer and Lopes da Silva (1993) and in a paper of our own (Vogel and Schalt 1979c). Here only a short outline is given (for more comprehensive reviews, see for example, Andersen and Andersson 1968, 1974; Creutzfeldt 1971; Creutzfeldt and Houchin 1974; Steriade et al. 1990). Three levels must be considered: The EEG waves are produced by a "battery" in the cerebral cortex; their "pacemakers" are found in the thalamus; and the EEG is modified by input from lower-level brain structures, especially the ascending reticular activating system (ARAS) and the limbic system

First to the battery: According to one leading hypothesis (see Creutzfeldt 1971), EEG waves are summarized excitatory postsynaptic potentials (EPSPs) of cortical pyramidal neurons. To produce voltage fluctuations that become visible as EEG waves groups of neurons must fire in unison. Secondly: To make them fire in an ordered way, an ordering principle – a kind of pacemaker – is necessary. According to many experimental results, this pacemaker – or, better, these pacemakers – are located in the thalamus, especially in the intralaminal nuclei. At present, it looks as if the thalamus may contain numerous facultative pacemaker regions that can affect activity in corresponding cortical areas (for many more details, see Speckmann and Elger 1993). The third brain structure important for synchronization of neuronal discharges and therefore for the EEG waves is the ARAS as shown first in animal experiments by studies on the *cerveau isolé* and *encéphale isolé* preparations, and analyzed in greater detail in the classical work of Moruzzi and Magoun (1949 and subsequent studies). The tonus of the ARAS is affected by input from the periphery, but also from a variety of cerebral structures. This tonic activity may depend on this input, but it may also be to a certain degree autonomous (Schlag 1974). It is certainly an oversimplified statement, but it is useful as a first approximation to the truth, to say that an increased level of "tonic arousal" tends to lead to desynchronization of EEG waves.

According to more recent animal experiments, "a small territory of the mesopontine junction between the levels of collicular midpontine transsections, contains the neurons involved in the ascending activation of the thalamus and the cortex" (Speckmann and Elger 1993; here, many references). Two groups of nuclei containing cholinergic neurons have been identified by immunohistochemical studies (see Steriade and McCarley 1990). These and other studies suggest an important rule of cholinergic neurons in creation of EEG potentials, and it changes, for example, in wakefulness and sleep. In recent years, cholinergic neurons and, especially, acetylcholine receptors have become elements of junction between experimental neurophysiology and molecular genetics starting from analysis of special types of genetically determined epilepsies (Steinlein et al. 1994; see also Chap. 1). However, elucidation of molecular mechanisms of neuronal discharges at the single-cell level does not explain the ways of cooperation between cells, nuclei, and brain areas. For explaining of the "emergence" of new properties of such systems, new approaches from systems theory may be useful (Haken 1996; Haken and Haken-Krell 1997).

The third brain structure which has a strong effect on brain wave patterns, in addition to thalamus and ARAS, is the limbic system with its significance for emotionality. This cannot be the place for discussing the complex functions of this system, and its effect on brain function at many levels. Suffice it to say that it induces slower waves (especially in the ϑ range) in the EEG.

6.9 A Possible Function of EEG Waves, Especially Alpha Waves

Many speculations have been proposed on the physiological function of the rhythmic patterns of neuronal activity recognized as EEG. (See also Vogel and Schalt 1979.) G. Walter (1963), for example, developed the hypothesis that the α rhythm acts as a scanning device for memory patterns which are stored somehow in the brain. In his opinion, α oscillations are seen as long as the brain has not identified a certain pattern. As soon as some specific pattern has been spotted, for example, a visual impression after opening of the eyes, or an imagined picture, the oscillations disappear and are replaced by less-well synchronized EEG waves. Walter and his coworkers recognized the interindividual differences of EEG patterns and corresponding psychophysical reactions and tried to account for them in a highly preliminary typology.

Another, fairly elaborate hypothesis, was proposed by Andersen and Andersson (1968, 1974): "It is tempting to propose that the rhythmic thalamic activity is necessary to produce a sufficiently effective impact by the afferent volleys of the cortical system. A single stimulus to the cortex or to certain thalamic nuclei is not sufficient to produce a perceived reaction. ... However, even when a single receptor is activated, the ensuing response is received. ... It may be conjectured that a single afferent volley from a receptor is transformed to a train of impulses of about 10 c/s by the thalamic recurrent inhibitory mechanism. Such a train may have far greater effect on the cortical synapses than the single excitation. ... In this context, it is important to note the greatly increased efficiency of the transmission across many synapses when repetitive stimulation is used instead of a single stimulus."

An increase in EPSPs with increasing number of stimuli has been observed in various experimental systems. The hypothesis of Walter (1963) and Andersen and Andersson (1968) are not mutually exclusive; they could be regarded as describing the functions of α waves at two different levels. For example, the Walter hypothesis accounts for the α blocking after (sensory and other) stimulations, an aspect not covered by the Andersen and Andersson hypothesis, which attempts to explain the events at the neuronal level. For the latter hypothesis, experiments are important that showed that the efficiency of propagation of artificial electric stimulations of thalamic structures to the corresponding areas in the cerebral cortex varies with the phase of the (experimental) thalamic spindle rhythm (assumed to be homologous to the human α rhythm) in which the stimuli are administered. According to these authors, this favors the view that the neurons involved in the thalamic spindle rhythm are identical with those utilized for the orthodromic volleys after peripheral stimulation.

According to this concept, α waves could be involved in selective amplification of incoming stimuli. These stimuli could originate either in the outside world, or in other parts of the brain itself.

6.10 Earlier Attempts at Connecting Neurophysiological Mechanisms with Aspects of Personality

Such attempts have been described before in detail (Vogel and Schalt 1979); in the following, this description can be repeated only in brief outline. According to Eysenck (1964, 1967 1970) interindividual variability of personalities may be described using two dimensions that are orthogonal to each other: introversion vs. extraversion, and neuroticism vs. stability. At the neurophysiological level, both dimensions are characterized by a number of parameters, among them the EEG. For example, Eysenck generalized the somewhat contradictory evidence from the literature by stating that "introverted neurotics tend to have fast EEG activity." This statement has not been confirmed in our studies. According to Eysenck, introversion corresponds to a high level of activation (arousal) in the ARAS; neuroticism corresponds to high activity in the "visceral brain" (limbic system). He made a strong point that these basic and physiologically defined personality dimensions are largely genetically determined. However, he founded this argument on classic biometric twin and family studies of a very general type, and not on specific studies on genetics of EEG phenomena. His generalizations were therefore premature and not sufficiently well based on empirical evidence. To avoid differences that may be caused by incongruencies between the personality questionnaires used in our studies and those used by Eysenck, the student sample was also investigated using the Eysenck questionnaires (MPI neuroticism; MPI extraversion; Walter 1982). However, the results were similar to those achieved with the other questionnaires; group R tended to be slightly more introverted and group N had a higher neuroticism score.

The personality model of Claridge (1967; Claridge et al. 1973) was developed as a modification of Eysenck's typology. In his system, the two underlying dimensions "high tonic arousal vs. low tonic arousal," and orthogonal to them "extraversion vs. introversion" are superimposed by two other dimensions, "hysteria vs. dysthymia" and, orthogonal to it, "active psychosis vs. retarded psychosis." Combination of dimensions at these two levels leads to various personality types. This system comes closer to the neurophysiological evidence: The lower level of "tonic arousal" may be homologized with the ARAS (and, in addition, the limbic system), while the higher level, also called "arousal modulation," corresponds to the function of the thalamus (or, to put it less simple, to the thalamocortical feedback circle). Unfortunately, Claridge reduced information from the EEG so much that, apart from the α rhythm, no additional information was utilized.

6.11 Results of Our Psychological Studies in the Light of Neurophysiological Evidence

The EEG with Monomorphic α Waves

This EEG variant shows regular α waves, often with high amplitudes, over the whole cortex. This cortical activity is triggered by a group of interrelated pacemakers in the thalamus. The function of α activity may be to modulate and amplify selectively stimuli coming from lower levels of the brain so that the cortex can recognize them better. It could therefore be predicted that brains with especially regular and widespread α activity would be especially efficient for this function. Such individuals would be especially good modulators and amplifiers. They should process relevant information very efficiently and transform it into well-controlled activity without being overly confused by irrelevant information.

This prediction can be compared with the actual results of the three studies: the Schmettau study (1969, 1970), the Air Force sample and the student sample. All three studies agree in the average personality picture they show: Probands tend to be intelligent, precise, reliable and forceful in their personality profiles. Certain aspects of information processing within the brain can be studied, for example, by examining summarized evoked (=event related) potentials (Chap. 5, especially Sect. 5.3). A comparative study on probands with various EEG variants (they were the same individuals who were studied psychologically in our student sample) showed strong differences between EEG variants in amplitudes of the responses to visual and auditory stimulation (VEPs and AEPs); probands with monomorphic α waves (the R group) showed the highest responses (Vogel et al. 1986). This points to a strong reaction (= high amplification?) of stimuli: Differences in average EP latencies, on the other hand, were much smaller. Here, probands of the R type showed slightly higher latencies than those having the low-voltage EEG. In our Air

Force sample, this corresponded to a certain tendency toward slowness in tests requiring quick reactions and fast action. In the student sample, this picture was less clear; R individuals could also be fast in some experiments. However, the entire picture of strong, forceful, active personalities with good intelligence and high reliability remains valid throughout all three studies.

The Low-Voltage EEG

From the EEG point of view, the low-voltage EEG (N) is the countertype of the R variant. Consequently, one would expect a low degree of modulation and amplification of stimuli. It is not as easy to predict specific personality characteristics for the N as for the R variant. On the one hand, the reduced amplification would be expected to lead to lower intensity of the stimuli admitted to the cortex. On the other hand, it is possible that favorable or unfavorable stimuli, for example, from the ARAS or the limbic system, are less efficiently screened and may therefore cause more modifications – disturbances or "positive" changes. For this group, the empirical results showed strong differences between the Air Force and the student sample; our student sample was more similar to the description of the low-voltage pole by Schmettau (1969, 1970). Here, it is important to know that Schmettau's probands were students as well. In all three series, the N group showed lower self-sufficiency, lower psychic energy as expressed by the lower Ma (hypomania) score in the MMPI, and, generally a somewhat higher degree of extraversion and, especially, group dependence than the R group. In the Air Force sample, this let the probands appear inconspicuous and especially "normal" – with a low Mf (male-female interest) score. In the student group, the Mf value of male probands was, on the contrary, high and that of the female N probands was low – both results pointing to a direction of interest in the "female" direction (arts, literature etc.). As noted above, the difference between the two samples could be caused by the group-dependence of this EEG class; they may tend to internalize especially easily values of their own social group.

Formal intelligence seems not to be impaired by the lack of α activity. This results does not favor hypotheses, especially that of Walter (see above) according to which the α rhythm is a screening mechanism for recognition of memory pictures. According to the hypothesis of Andersen and Andesson (1968), the α rhythm not only amplifies but also modifies afferent volleys, helping to screen out unfavorable stimuli. Considering this, one would expect in some probands an increased tendency to be unduly irritated even by average or only slightly above average levels of tonic arousal in the ARAS or other untoward stimuli. In the Air Force sample, this expectation was not fulfilled; rather, the "average" N probands showed a relaxed and "normal" attitude. The "irritable" group was represented rather by the small group of probands with borderline EEG (NG) which consists of two subgroups – true dominantly inherited low-voltage EEGs and the tail of the non-low-voltage, more average EEG. The student sample gave a different picture of the N group: Contrary to the Air Force sample, these probands, in addition to their high (or in females low) Mf scores, also showed high Hd (hypochondria) and Hy (hysteria) scores. Both scores suggest a high degree of irritation by minor bodily complaints of various kinds. As discussed above, a look for concrete, and more specific signs of impairment by diseases or subjective disturbances in the same sample failed to show positive results (Förg 1984). As discussed in the description of EEG variants (Chap. 4), females show on the average, a higher level of β waves pointing to a higher degree of tonic arousal. Therefore it is not surprising that the fraction of "typical" low-voltage EEGs with dominant inheritance is hidden in the borderline (NG) group and even in the group of EEGs with "diffuse" α waves, which is be discussed below.

The EEG with Diffuse β Waves

The amount of β waves is higher in females than in males (see for example, Vogel and Götze 1962; Friedl and Vogel 1979). Considering the experimental results discussed above, the most likely neurophysiological mechanism is a relatively high level of tonic arousal in the ARAS leading to disturbances of an α activity of low or medium strength. Hence the expected personality correlates would be hypersensitivity and low resistance to stress. Probands with this EEG variant would be expected to avoid excitation, if at all possible. This is exactly Schmettau's (1969) description of individuals with high β index.

Our Air Force sample BD (diffuse β waves) showed inconspicuous scores in personality questionnaires. Hence there was no direct evidence of the hypersensitivity and psychastheny expected when the tonic arousal level was increased. More indirect evidence, however, seemed to be obvious: The probands showed high error percentages in the concentration tests in spite of relatively low working speed (for example, D2). These tests are generally experienced as stressful. Hence poor performance is related to low stress resistance. Moreover, the BD Air Force probands achieved relatively low scores in the intelligence test scales designed to test spatial orientation. As discussed in Sect. 6.6, this was not confirmed in the student sample; neither in males nor in females there was a special weakness in space perception. In the D2 test, the BD group scores low in speed, with faster performance in females. However, this time, their percentage of error was lower than that of all other EEG groups in both sexes. Hence the conclusion drawn from the data in our Air Force sample that individuals showing diffuse β waves (BD) suffer from disturbance of the α system by having a weakness in their space performance, for example, by disturbance of an α mechanism according to Walter's hypothesis, is not corroborated by the new set of data. Likewise, the possibility that the well-known difference in space perception between the sexes (lower ability in females) could be, at least in part, due to more frequent disturbance of this α mechanism cannot be held up any more. (By the way, our student sample showed a small tendency in direction of this sex difference – subtests FA and WÜ in the IST and subtests 7–10 in the LPS – for the other EEG groups as well – except for the R group, in which females were better than males in LPS categories 7–10).

In properties of visually and auditory evoked potentials, the BD group scores between the R and N groups in average amplitudes and in latencies.

The difference in the entire outcome of test results between the BD Air Force and the student sample of the same EEG type is difficult to explain. In view of the fact that number of individuals examined was relatively high in both samples (65 in the Air Force sample; 90 of the students), it would probably be too easy to assume a chance effect due to small numbers. The age difference between the two samples may provide a partial explanation. Within the Air Force sample, BD probands were, on the average, older than carriers of all other EEG variants. This was not the case in the student sample.

The EEG with occipital fast α variants has been discussed before; probably its relatively high performance in intelligence and performance tests is related directly with the high frequency of α-like waves which may link to especially specific and fast amplification of incoming stimuli. However, whatever the precise interpretation, it may be the same as for the general correlation between intelligence scores and α frequency that is supported by numerous data (Anokhin and Vogel 1996; see Sect. 6.3).

The EEG with frontoprecentral β group (BG): Contrary to the α rhythm, there seems to be little if any experimental evidence that could explain at least tentatively the neurophysiological mechanism of the frontoprecentrally accentuated, often spindlelike β waves. These β groups are completely compatible with an undisturbed, normal α rhythm with occipital location; occasionally, they can even be observed in combination with a low-voltage (N) EEG. Moreover, there were no indications for any psychological peculiarities of this group either in the Air Force or in the student sample. A possible hint for elucidating the physiological origin of this EEG group is the observation that similar spindles are often produced by a variety of drugs, such as barbiturates (Sect. 2.9; see for example, Wauquier 1993; Bauer 1993). However, it would be premature, to formulate a more specific hypothesis.

6.12 Critical Evaluation on the Results About EEG Characteristics and Normal Psychology: What Can Be Regarded as Confirmed, What Is Likely, and What Is Hypothetical and Could Be Clarified by Further Research?

Table 6.20 summarizes the results from the psychological studies in two samples of individuals showing various inherited EEG variants. They are compared with the results of a study by Schmettau (1969, 1970); older reports were discussed critically not only in this publication, but by Vogel and Schalt (1979) as well. These discussions cannot be repeated here in great detail. Suffice it to say that in most of these reports, psychological studies were not performed on samples of sufficient size, and using adequate methods. In most of them, the EEG criteria used were not defined sufficiently well. Therefore the contradictory results are not surprising. The studies reported here are be discussed critically below. The following questions are asked:

- Which results can be regarded as well-established, which ones can only be regarded as hints for planning of new studies?
- What can be said about the hypotheses on psychological differences between individuals showing different EEG variants, and their attempted explanations in term of brain function?
- What could be done to pursue the line of research suggested here further? How could the developed concepts be refined, and the experimental approaches be improved? Can the process made in recent years in molecular genetics be utilized to gain deeper insight into aspects of brain physiology in relation to behavior and mental performance?

Table 6.20. Somewhat oversimplified characteristics of EEG variants

Low-voltage EEG (N):
Performance: Average intelligence; average working precision;
higher than average working speed.
Personality: Often extravert; "outgoing; easygoing; participating".
Dependent on attitudes and preferences of the group to which the proband belongs.
Not very self-sufficient and energetic. Neurophysiological explanation: Below-average selection and amplification of stimuli.

EEG with monomorphic alpha waves (R):
Performance: Average intelligence with emphasis on technical skills; slightly above-average working precision; average to slightly below-average working speed.
Personality: Often a tendency to self-sufficiency and even introversion; strong energy and "sthenic" attitude; high internal tension. Individuals with this EEG variant tend toward marriage partners with similar EEG types (= assortative mating).
Neurophysiological interpretation: Strong selection and amplification of stimuli.

EEG with fast alpha variants (BO):
Above-average intelligence, working speed, and coordination; no characteristic personality scores.
Neurophysiological interpretation:
Fast (and precise) selection and amplification of stimuli.

EEG with diffuse beta waves (BD):
This group – the largest one of all – does not provide a consistent picture. While older males with this variant showed below-average performance in tests requiring intelligence and various aspects of performance, this was not the case in the (younger) student's sample.
BD EEGs are more common in females than in males; in females, they point to a more varied response. –
Personality: An inconspicuous profile.
Neurophysiological interpretation:
Sometimes (in males?) selection and amplification of stimuli disturbed by influences from the ARAS. – In younger persons – and, especially, in females – a higher level of tonic arousal may have a more positive effect.
EEG with fronto-precentral groups of beta waves:
For this variant, no characteristic psychological features emerged.
Neurophysiological interpretation: These beta waves appear to be independent of cortico-thalamic mechanisms of selection and amplification of stimuli influencing performance and personality.

- In which way may the concepts developed here be helpful in understanding abnormal behavior – from mild abnormality, for example, in neurosis, to behavioral anomalies such as alcoholism (and, possibly, other types of addiction), and to outright mental diseases such as affective disorders or schizophrenia?

We begin with the first question: Which of these results can be regarded as well-established? This is primary the positive correlation between α frequency and intelligence (Sect. 6.3). It has been found in a number of different studies and should now be accepted. It is another question how this result could be integrated into a more comprehensive concept on the biological foundations of intelligent behavior and performance. A second result which is not quite as well-established, but still looks quite reliable is the personality profile of individuals showing an EEG with monomorphic α waves (our R type), or, in more general terms, a regular α pattern not only in occipital and, often, central leads, but over precentral brain areas, as well. This profile is obvious in results from personality tests: the "sthenic" attitude of the carriers of this variant is supported by their good intelligence and reliable performance. Unfortunately, our attempts at establishing a basis for their personality profile at a more basic level (sensory and motor abilities; precision of working etc.) gave interesting single results but did not lead to an unequivocal answer. The results on visually and auditory evoked potentials (high amplitudes, slightly longer latencies) could be regarded as such an answer, but there still remains a lingering doubt whether this result could be feigned, at least in part, by partial blocking of α oscillators and subsequent synchronization of α waves. In the field of basic mechanisms, much work is still to be carried out.

The personality profile of the "countertype," the low-voltage EEG, appears to be less well-established. Description of this group as "group oriented" fits the results from all three samples; there are always low introversion scores (=high extraversion). The conspicuous difference between our Air Force and student samples in the Hd, Hy and Mf scores can be explained by their identification with different group standards. The low values of second-stratum factors QII and QIV in the 16-PF (adjustment; subduedness) support this view. Low working precision especially in the student sample (D2 test; high error rate) may indicate weak thalamic amplification.

Information of the third major group – EEGs with diffuse β waves – is contradictory; here, results from the Air Force and the student sample contradict each other. The characterization in our earlier report (Vogel and Schalt 1979) "tense, disturbed, spatial orientation, susceptible to stress" cannot be held up any more as a general rule. It certainly does not apply to our student sample.

The group BG (frontoprecentral β wave groups), on the other hand, has been inconspicuous in both samples; our conclusion that probands of this group fail to show any conspicuous and group-specific psychological peculiarities has been confirmed.

For a geneticist accustomed to precise methods and unequivocal results, working with psychological concepts and methods is sometimes similar to looking through a pane made from frosted glass: very interesting and important structures seem to emerge but their boundaries appear to be somewhat hazy.

6.13 Psychological Observations on Carriers of the 4–5 c/s Rhythm

This EEG variant has been described in Sect. 4.6. It is rare (approx. 0.1%) but concordant in MZ twins and was seen in several members of some families. In Sect. 4.6, psychological abnormalities observed in probands belonging to this group were reported. Many of these individuals (not all of them) showed a "retarded psychological development with infantile behavior and disturbances in human contacts and ability for social interactions." These psychological abnormalities were found predominantly in male probands. In view of present-day neurophysiological concepts, especially the well-known significance of the limbic system for emotionality; this variant could be caused by an abnormally disturbing influence of the limbic system to the thalamocortical circuit. This EEG variant is especially common in younger adults but may also be seen in old persons. It may, but must not disappear, and be replaced by inconspicuous α activity, some time during adult age, as shown, for example, by long-time observation of an MZ twin pair (Heintel et al. 1986). Both this and the fact that superficially similar EEG patterns are observed among normal children may justify the somewhat nonspecific description of a "maturation anomaly."

6.14 EEG and Normal Psychological Development in Childhood

In Sect. 2.5, the development of the EEG during childhood and youth was described. We stressed the high variation in EEG patterns commonly regarded as indicating brain maturation, for example, the development of α frequency, percentage of sub-α waves, persistence as a measure of regularity of occipital α waves, and coordination of phases between left-hand and right-hand occipital waves. Since MZ twins continue to be absolutely concordant during childhood (Chap. 3), the speed of "EEG maturation" and its characteristic phases are determined genetically. Here, the question arises whether EEG maturation is associated with psychological maturation. If such an association could be shown, this would be an important indication for a genetically determined aspect of psychological maturation with possible consequences for educational strategies.

A pilot study on this problem was reported by Vogel et al. (1982). The twin sample consisted of 110 MZ and 98 DZ pairs in the age group between 5 and about 30 years, most twins were between 10 and 20 years old. The methods used during the EEG studies were described by Vogel (1958; see Sect. 3.3). In addition to the above EEG parameters, a number of psychological tests were performed: The Rohrschachtest, the "Wartegg-Zeichentest" and the "Baum-Test" (tree test) of Koch (1976). Correlations with genetically determined EEG parameters, and especially those indicating a common genetic component, can be expected only if the test results reveal genetic variation, i.e., if test scores are more similar in MZ than in DZ twins. This was the case only for the Baum-Test; therefore result from the other tests were eliminated from further analysis. The Baum-Test consists of two parts. (Figs. 6.1, 6.2)

First, the proband must draw a tree. Then, s(he) is asked to write a short essay on the tree. The degree of immaturity was assessed by standard criteria; it is graded from "very immature" (20 points) to "very mature" (0 points). Figure 6.1a,b shows a very immature (score 13) and a very mature (score 2) tree. The essays were classified into three categories: Advanced for age; normal for age; and backwards. Classification was performed by a teacher with more than 30 years teaching experience, who did not know the twin sample. The means of immaturity indices are seen in Fig. 6.2. A significant rank correlation ($r = -0.157$; $p < 0.05$) was found between mean α frequency in occpital leads and the immaturity index in the Baum-Test. The teacher's essay rating gave a positive rank correlation with α frequency as well. The other EEG measures, especially sub-alpha percentage in frontoprecentral and occipital leads, failed to give any relationship with psychological maturation. This result fits excellently into the evidence discussed above (Sect. 6.3) that there is a positive correlation between α frequency and intelligence in adults.

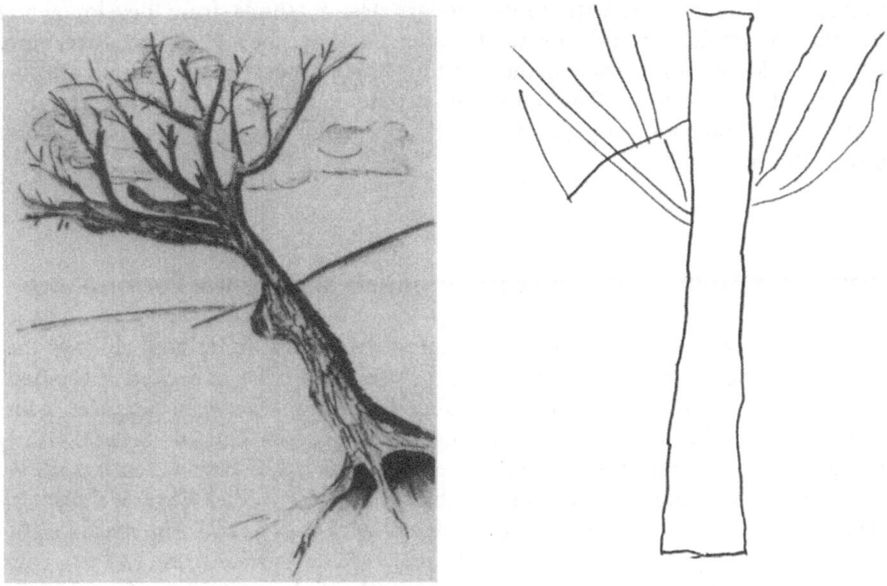

Fig. 6.1. Examples of two drawings at different stages of maturity. **a** Male, 17 years, very mature (score 2). **b** Female, 6 years, very immature (score 13)

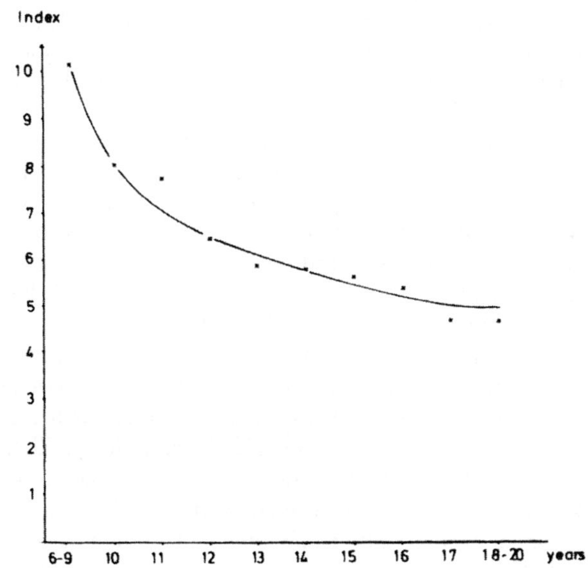

Fig. 6.2. Means of Baumtest scores (immaturity indices) in relation to age

Still, it should be regarded as preliminary – and the entire study should be classified as pilot study – since the data have been collected many years ago, in the 1950s, when suitable methods for computerized EEG evaluation were not yet available, and the psychological methods used must be regarded as outdated. A repetition of this study with a new twin series, and with methods of computerized EEG evaluation and, mainly, with more modern test methods from developmental psychology would certainly be worthwhile: Possibly, they could produce more detailed evidence for answering the question which aspects of maturation are correlated with α frequency. The notion of "psychological maturation" is certainly a very general one; modern psychology may offer much more specific concepts and test methods.

6.15 Visual and Auditory Evoked EEG Potentials and Mental Performance

Another attempt at discovering basic neurophysiological functional abilities that may contribute to "intelligence" has been the study of aspects of evoked EEG potentials, and especially, the attempt at finding correlations between latencies, complexity and amplitudes of EPs and intelligence test results. Ertl and Schafer (1969) described strong correlations between latencies of visually evoked potentials (VEPs; see Chap. 5) and intelligence scores. Subjects of their studies were 573 primary school students (grades 2–8; probable range of ages 8–14 years). The negative correlations between IQ grades (Wechsler, Primary Mental Abilities Test, and Otis) and latencies of VEPs were in the order of magnitude of about −0.30 to −0.35 for later VEP peaks (about 200–250 ms) and smaller but still significant for earlier peaks.

This study elicited comprehensive examinations of the Eysenck school (Eysenck 1982; A. E. Hendrickson 1982; D. E. Hendrickson 1982) as well as of many other research works (for references, see Callaway 1973, 1975). The discussion was lifted to a theoretically more ambitious level when Eysenck, together with the Hendricksons, developed a theory according to which more or less intelligent behavior depends on "a probability R, that a given message encoded in a series of pulse trains will arrive at its destination in the identical form in which it was encoded while 1-R presents the probability of an error occurring during transmission." According to the Hendricksons, this probability can be assessed by measuring the complexity of average evoked EEG potentials. A number of additional studies in which in the relationships between EPs and measures of intelligence was examined are discussed in the following; their results were contradictory. We begin with a study of our own (Vogel et al. 1987) (Tables 6.21, 6.22).

The Hendricksons have measured the complexity of EPs by a "string measure," i.e., by measuring the length of the EP curve up to a certain time (for example, 600 ms) after simulation. The longer this "string," the more complex the shape of the EP curve. In the study to be described here, the "oscillation," a measure proposed by Krüger and Vogel (1985) and described in Chap. 5 was used instead. However, all correlations were also performed using the original string measure; the results deviated only trivially; 236 university students (118 males, 118 females) were included in this study. Their age distribution was described in Chap. 5; suffice it to say that most of them were in their (early) twenties. The methods used for evaluation of EPs were also described in Chap. 5. In addition to the above "oscillation," latency was measured by another new measure, the "average latency": Moreover, the three main peaks of the late EPs were evaluated separately. The IQ was determined using the IST test, a German standard group test; some items of the LPS (*Leistungs-Prüfsystem,* Horn) and the standard Raven. The *Aufmerksamkeits-Belastungstest*

(Brickenkamp 1962) was also used (for details of these tests, see Sect. 6.4). In addition to the student sample, 24 inpatients from an institution for the mentally retarded (8 females, 16 males; age range 15–29) were examined. All were mildly or moderately mentally retarded; individuals, in which retardation could be traced back to a major cause (for example, severe brain damage during birth or trisomy 21) were excluded from this study. They were compared with 19 normal individuals (13 males, 6 females in the same age range; mostly students or employees of the institute).

Details of VEP and AEP studies have been reported in Chap. 5; suffice it to say that EEGs were recorded in a sound-attenuated chamber and with closed eyes to keep unplanned, external stimuli at a minimum. Four different intensity levels were used for VEPs to test the "augmenting-reducing" phenomena (see Chap. 8). As in earlier studies from other authors, recordings from the C_z electrode of the international 10–20 system were used for comparing parameters of VEPs and AEPs with the test results. Results have been published in great detail (Vogel et al. 1987). To summarize them in one sentence: There was not even a hint of any possible relationship between IQ and degree of attention, on the one hand, and any of the EP parameters tested, on the other. In Tables 6.21 and 6.22, the main results for oscillation and for mean latencies are repeated. When the peaks used for measuring the augmenting-reducing response (Chap. 5) were evaluated separately, the results were also negative. Moreover, a comparison of mentally retarded individuals with normal controls of the same age had an absolutely negative result. What is the reason for such a discrepancy in the results?

To clarify this question, we compared our experimental setup with that of the Hendrickson group (Hendrickson 1982; Blinkhorn and Hendrickson 1982; Haier, et al. 1983) in every detail (Vogel et al. 1987). This comparison is not repeated here. There were three main differences:

- Their studies were performed mainly in children and adolescents, while we used adults in our studies. There may be differences in brain maturation – even in youngsters of the same ages – that may be reflected in differences of EPs. In this connection, we should remember that in the first study, that of Ertl and Schafer (1969), the probands were also children.
- As noted above, our studies were performed in a sound-attenuated chamber, and we tried to avoid additional stimuli. In case such additional – and more or less regularly repeated – stimulation is not avoided, this may lead to additional smaller peaks that enhance the "string" measure.
- As shown in Chap. 5, the resting EEG has a strong effect on the shape of the EPs, especially their amplitudes. And the string measure is an amplitude measure. However, in none of the studies discussed so far, except in our own, have aspects of the resting EEG even been mentioned. It is a strange result of compartmentalization of science along borders determined by competence in research methods that, for a long time, scientists using the resting EEG as their medium and those working with evoked potentials did not even recognize the other group's result. This has changed only recently, when EPs have been found to be useful in medical diagnostics.

Table 6.21. Product-moment correlations between visually and auditory EEG potential (VEP and AEP) "oscillations" and intelligence test scores; all EEG groups together (118 males, 118 females)

Evoked potential oscilla-tion	Lead	Inten-sity level	IST combined score (I.Q.)	LPS subtests			d2				Standard Raven
				3	7–10	11 + 12	Gz	F	Gz-F	SB	
VEP	Cz	1	−0.063	0.042	0.031	0.075	0.028	0.022	0.022	−0.095	−0.026
		2	−0.087	0.038	0.015	0.045	0.046	0.038	0.036	−0.057	−0.037
		3	−0.037	0.118	0.022	0.071	0.088	−0.020	0.095	−0.078	−0.005
		4	−0.016	0.059	0.010	0.050	0.089	−0.018	0.096	−0.016	−0.026
AEP	Cz		0.035	0.110	0.019	−0.000	−0.006	−0.038	0.005	0.021	0.068

Table 6.22. Product-moment correlations between visually and auditory EEG potential (VEP and AEP) "mean latencies" and intelligence test scores; all EEG groups together (118 males, 118 females)

Evoked potential mean latency	Lead	Inten-sity level	IST combined score (I.Q.)	LPS subtests			d2				Standard Raven
				3	7–10	11 + 12	Gz	F	Gz-F	SB	
VEP	Cz	1	0.093	−0.030	−0.000	0.049	−0.041	−0.031	−0.033	−0.096	0.046
		2	−0.081	−0.020	−0.102	−0.034	−0.067	−0.017	−0.063	−0.193[a]	−0.055
		3	0.036	−0.058	0.059	−0.014	0.070	0.023	0.065	−0.004	−0.021
		4	0.041	−0.057	−0.073	−0.025	0.011	−0.052	0.026	−0.034	−0.021
AEP	Cz		−0.035	−0.062	0.043	−0.041	−0.097	−0.047	−0.085	0.028	0.034

[a] Significant at the 1% level

Point one – studies in children and adolescents with positive, in adults with negative results – should be considered very seriously if correlations in younger persons would always have positive results. However, this is not the case at all. For example, the studies of Engel and Henderson (1973) which were performed at school age, had a negative result. The same is true for the probands examined by Pietz (1984). However, it is possible that the above studies did not tap the correct portion of the EP, or did not use the appropriate experimental setup. Polich et al. (1983) found positive correlations between digit span – a trait strongly correlated with intellectual performance – and late EP peaks (P300) during mental activity. Reed and Jensen (1992) reported on "conduction velocity in a brain nerve pathway of normal adults" that was correlated with intelligence; they measured a specific EP peak. In P300 experiments – and in similar experimental setups – the proband is usually not passive, but is asked to perform a certain task or to react in a certain way to a stimulus or set of stimuli; a judgment is need for their proper recognition. Obviously, this is not required in a simple VEP or AEP experiment. Therefore it would not be surprising, if experiments of the first kind would reveal an association between speed of performance and intellectual level; discussing these results in any greater detail would go beyond the scope of this review. However, such results suggest the possibility that subjects studied, for example, by the Hendricksons, may have been busy in observing other things in addition to the experimentally applied stimulation and that the more intelligent subjects indulged in more such diversions than the less intelligent ones; traces of such additional stimuli would not be removed by the averaging process if they would occur in a regularly repeated way. In this connection, it may be important that the probands in the studies of Hendrickson and Haier were studied with open eyes, while our probands and also the probands in the Pietz (1984) study, the results of which were also negative, were examined with closed eyes.

There are numerous studies on EPs in subjects who have suffered some traumatic impact to their brains and on patients with a variety of brain and mental diseases. Discussion of such studies and their results would go beyond the scope of this review.

CHAPTER 7

7 EEG Variation in Psychologically Borderline Conditions such as Alcoholism, Anxiety Disorders, and Certain Neurotic States, Psychiatric Disorders

7.1 Alcoholism and the Resting EEG

Alcoholism is defined as a dependence on alcohol which leads to social deterioration. Alcoholism depends strongly on the environment. In a society in which alcohol-containing drinks are not available, no one can become an alcoholic. However, there are individual differences in alcohol susceptibility, and the possible genetic basis of such differences can be studied (Propping 1989, 1992). According to a review of 27 different studies (Cotton 1979), almost one third of all alcoholics had at least one affected parent, in most cases the father. Twin and adoption studies confirm the effect of genetic factors. Specific genetic mechanisms were identified at two levels – alcohol metabolism and reaction of the brain to alcohol as measured by the EEG. Alcohol degradation occurs in two main steps, requiring two enzymes: In a first step alcohol is oxidized to become acetaldehyde; this requires the enzyme alcoholdehydrogenase (ADH). This enzyme has genetic variants that do not appear to affect susceptibility to alcoholism. The second step – oxidation from acetaldehyde to acetic acid – is determined by the enzyme acetaldehyde dehydrogenase (ALDH). A variant of this enzyme with reduced activity is common among Orientals. Leading to accumulation of acetaldehyde after alcohol intake, it causes symptoms such as sweating, heart trouble and nausea. Discouraging drinking, this enzyme variant tends to protect persons from alcohol addiction (see Vogel and Motulsky 1996).

After some animal experiments (cat; rat) had suggested alcohol effects on EEG parameters of the cerebral cortex and the ARAS, Propping (1977) performed a twin study. He examined 52 healthy young males (26 MZ, 26 DZ). This twin sample has been described in Sect. 3.7 and Sect. 6.4. On the first day of their examination, the twins underwent a psychological test program (Sect. 6.4). On the second day, the twins came to the institute in the fasting state after having slept sufficiently during the preceding night. Then, the alcohol experiment was performed. First, the resting EEG was recorded. Then, the probands got a light, standard breakfast. Immediately thereafter, they took a dose of 1.2 ml/kg ethanol as a 30% solution in orange juice. The EEG was recorded 60, 120, 180 and 240 min after the start of drinking; at the same time interval, a series of psychophysiological experiments was repeated. Venous blood samples for determination of blood alcohol were taken seven times (Kopun and Propping 1977); these are not discussed here in any detail. The EEGs were recorded and analyzed as usual; for computerized evaluation, a program for time-domain analysis was used (Sect. 3.7).

Figures 7.1–7.5 show the means of the main results of the alcohol experiment: On the average, alcohol produces a better synchronization of the EEG, i.e., the amount of α and ϑ waves and the amplitudes for all frequency classes increase, while the β activity is diminished. This result corresponds with some earlier reports (for references, see Propping 1977). The mean frequency decreases significantly by about 1 c/s; this effect persists during nearly the whole experiment. Figure 7.1 shows the alcohol effect in an MZ pair with average α activity, while Fig. 7.2 shows a pair with very good and regular spontaneous α activity. In both instances, a clearcut increase especially in α amplitude is obvious. Figure 7.3, on the other hand, shows a true low-voltage EEG (Sect. 4.3). This EEG remains virtually unchanged after alcohol intake. EEG similarities between MZ twins were compared with repeated experiments in the same individuals. These twins proved to be as similar as these intraindividual repetitions. The results may be summarized as follows:

- The EEG of MZ twins, especially the α activation, remain (at least) as similar in MZ twins, as in the normal resting state. In DZ twins, on the other hand, the EEG differences that were present in the resting EEG become still more pronounced during the experiment.
- While most EEGs react by increasing their α activity, low-voltage EEGs may be resistant to α activation. However, this observation cannot be readily generalized; in another proband with a "flat" EEG – partner in a DZ pair – alcohol led to α activation.
- While β activity measured in average, α wave dominated EEGs normally decreases after alcohol intake, it is increased in some instances. Figure 7.4 shows a DZ pair; in one of the twins, β activation in the shape of frontoprecentral β groups can be seen. Similar changes were observed in one partner of another DZ pair and, concordant, in an MZ pair.
- These differences in EEG reaction are not caused by differences in alcohol absorption and elimination (Kopun and Propping 1977); they are caused by a different reaction of the brain.

In conclusion, the EEG usually shows a clearcut alcohol effect. Type and extent of this effect is genetically determined. In the majority of instances, it consists in α activation; it is especially strong in persons having a relatively irregular spontaneous α activity. However, increase in β waves may also occur. These effects are not caused by differences in alcohol metabolism but by genetic variation within the brain. This conclusion, however, is valid only for persons having the active ALDH (allele ALDH2–1, see above). Many Asians have the less active enzyme variety; in these subjects, EEG reaction strongly depends on the enzyme variety present; those having the less active (Asian) variety (ALDH $2 \times 2/2 \times 2$ genotype) show a much weaker EEG reaction (less of slow α activity) in the falling-phase of their blood alcohol curves (90–150 min, after alcohol intake; Wall et al. 1993).

Another twin study was reported by Sorbel et al. (1996). They used about the same experimental setup as Propping (1977) but a lower alcohol dose (0.35 g/kg in males and 0.325 g/kg in females), while Propping had used 1.2 ml/kg. Their twin sample consisted of 53 MZ and 38 DZ pairs, aged 30.0 ± 7.0 years. In distinction to the Propping sample, this sample also contained female twins. Resting EEGs were recorded, following standard techniques, before and about 35 min after alcohol

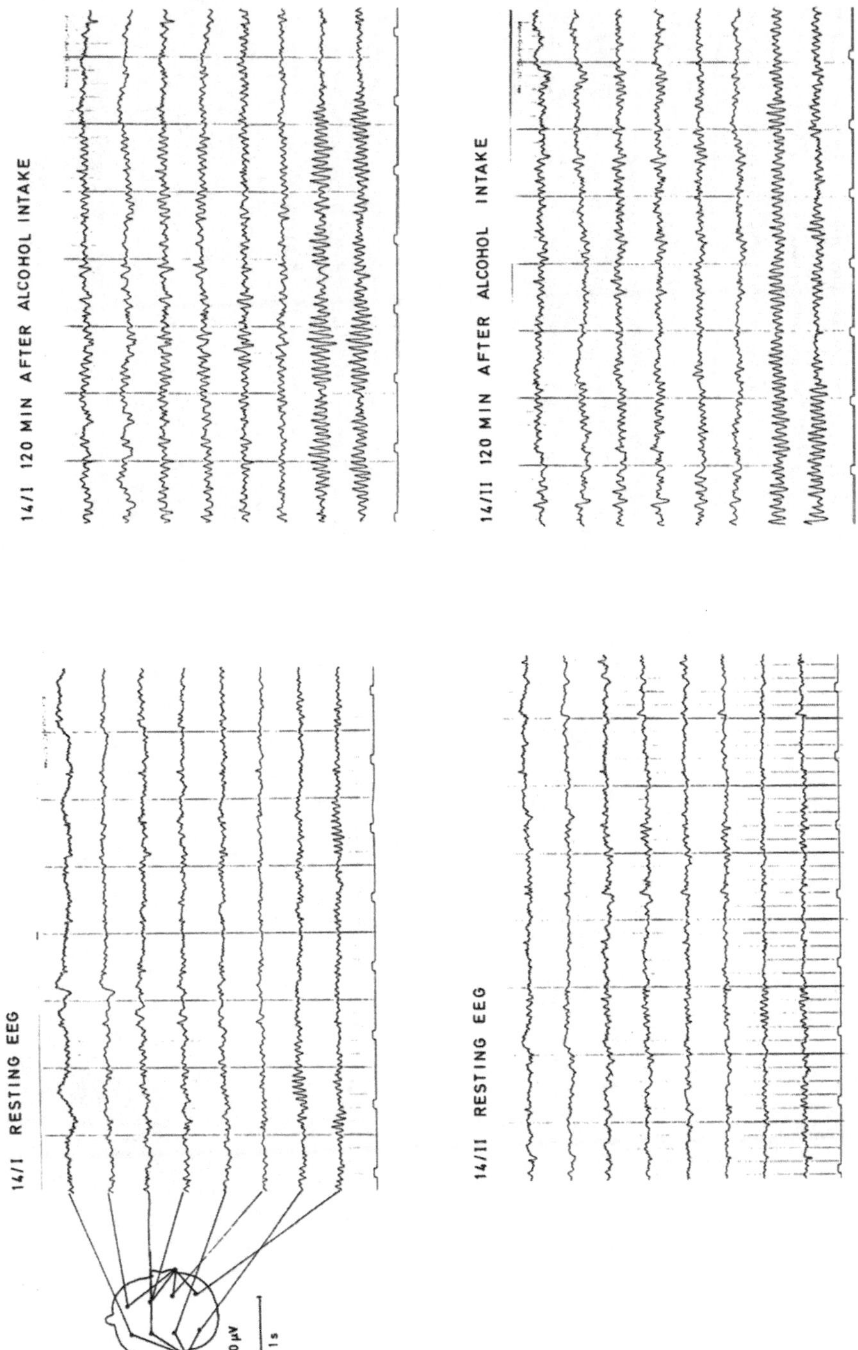

Fig. 7.1. Effect of alcohol on an average α EEG in an MZ twin pair

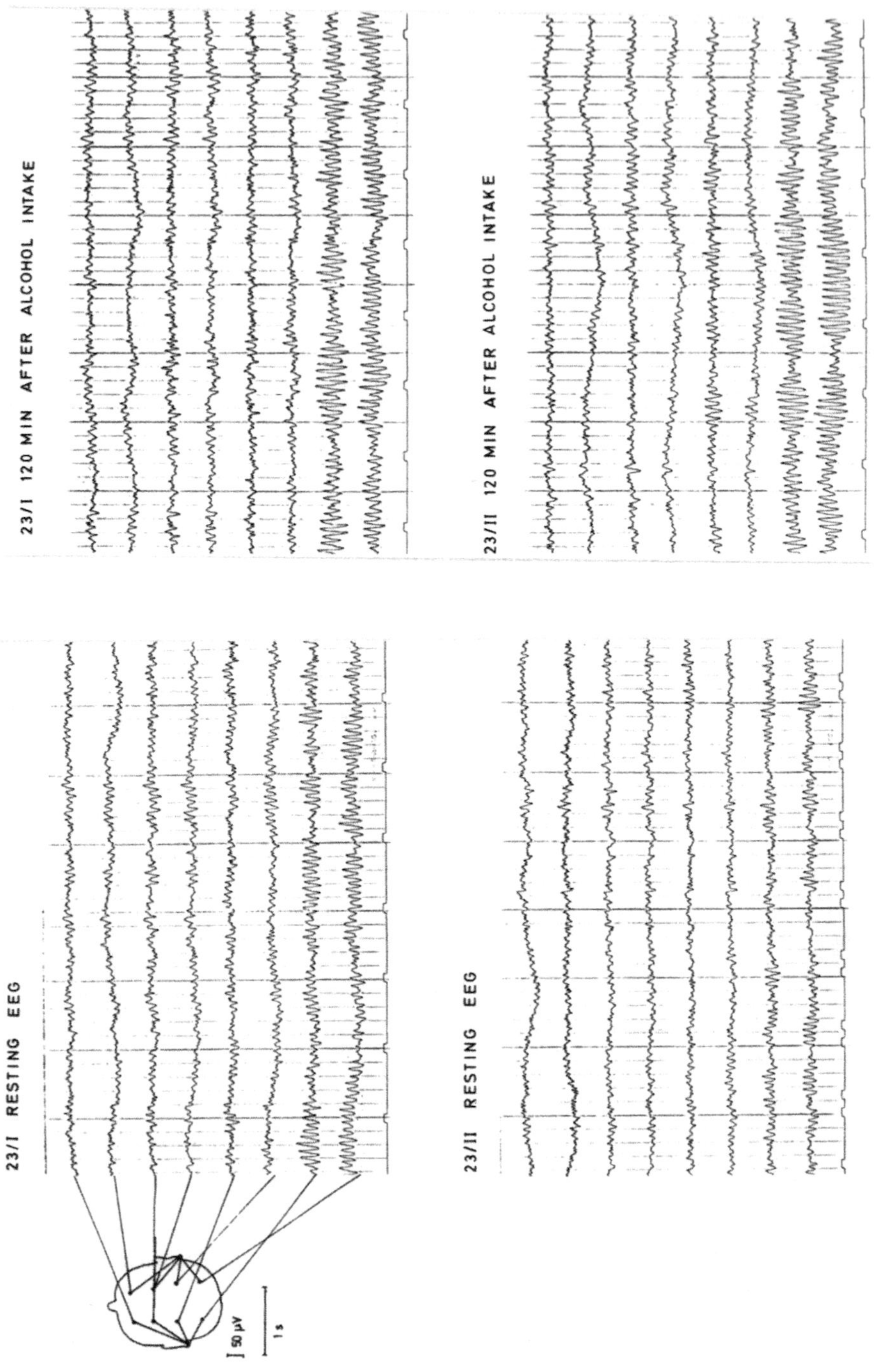

Fig. 7.2. Effect of alcohol on an EEG with good α production in an MZ twin pair

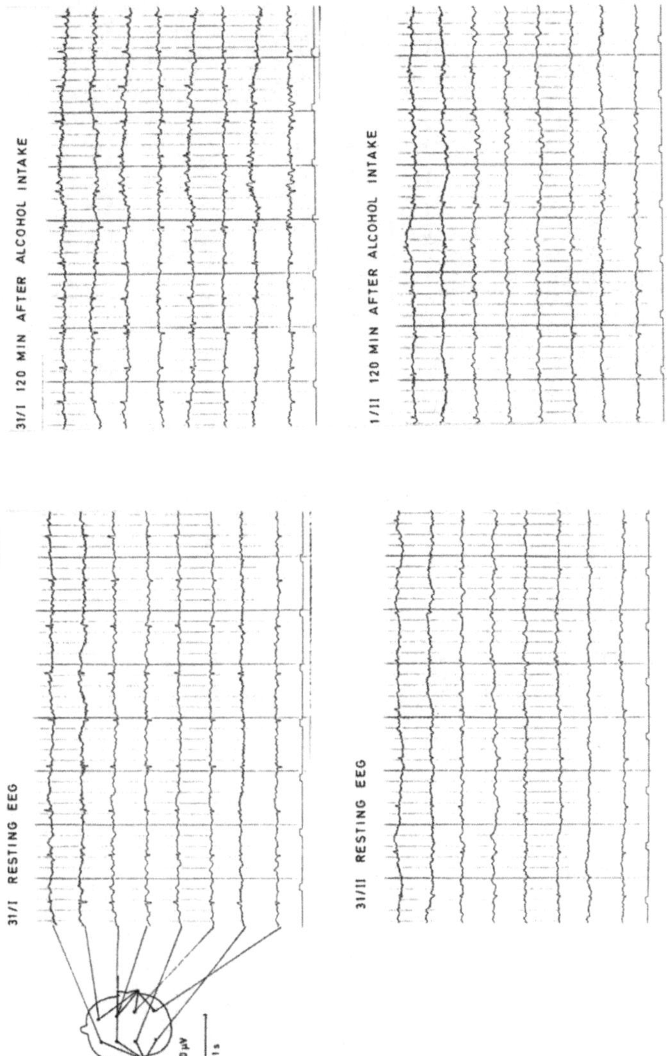

Fig. 7.3. Low-voltage EEG (with ECG spikes) in an MZ twin pair which is nearly resistant to alcohol

ingestion. Seventeen leads were used in each individual; computerized evaluation following the rules given by Christian et al. (1996) was performed. There was an increase in band power over all frequency bands except for the δ band. Obviously, this increase corresponded to the enhancement of α activity, especially α amplitudes, observed by Propping. An increase in β bands was observed as well which may be compared with the β activities observed by Propping. For power spectral intensity, heritabilities were estimated before and after the alcohol load; in addition, within-twin pair differences were computed. There was a significant increase in heritability for all frequency bands, except, again, for the δ bands. HenceProppings result that EEGs of MZ twins become more similar after alcohol intake and heritability increases, has been confirmed with a slightly different method.

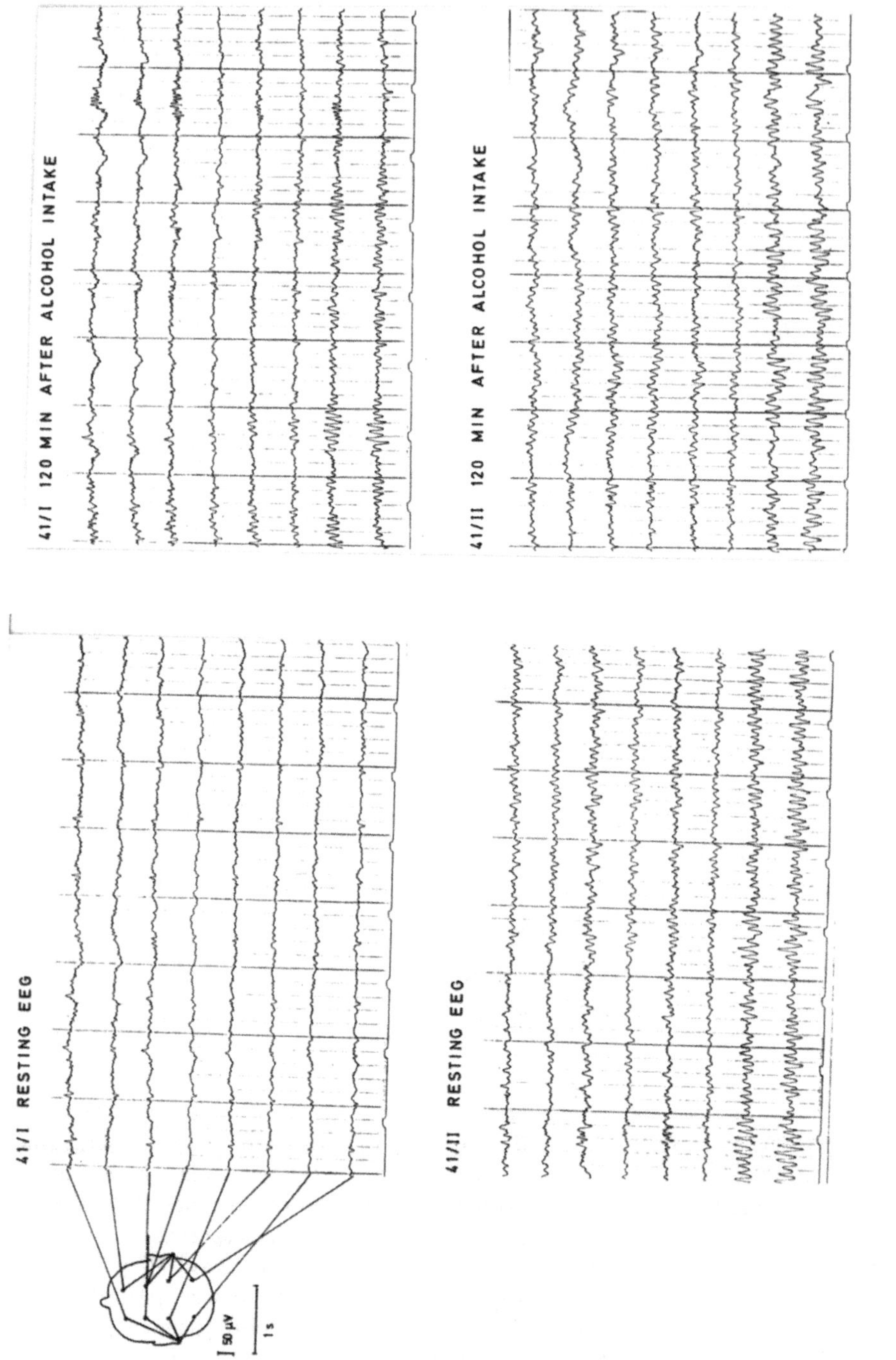

Fig. 7.4. DZ twin pair. The "low-voltage" EED of sibling 1 exhibits α waves after alcohol intake, while the α EEG of sibling 2 is only slightly impaired

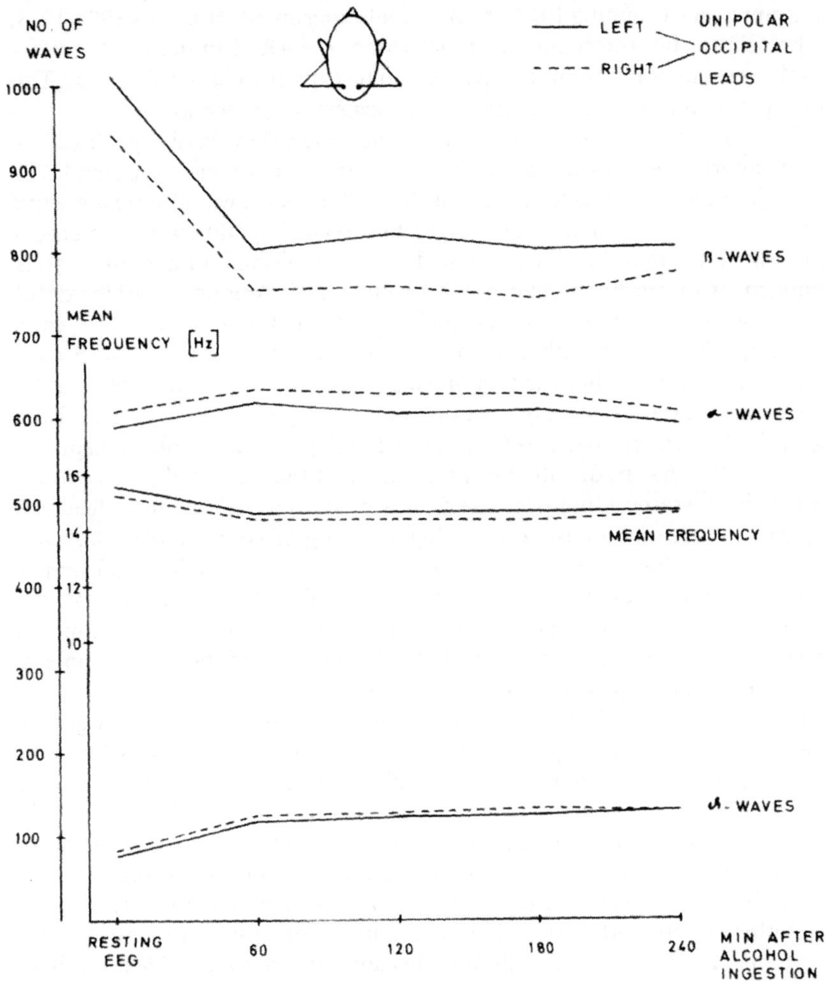

Fig. 7.5. Effect of 1.2 ml/kg ethanol on number of beta, alpha, and theta waves and on mean frequency. For the calculation of the alcohol effect only sibling 1 of each twin pair was used (Propping)

The Propping twin series was examined somewhat later by Christian et al. (1988), using a modified method of computerized EEG analysis. In this study, the β waves were examined. For the percentage of β waves (occipital leads) in 38 twin pairs, for which complete data were available, the intraclass correlation coefficients range between 0.85 and 0.91 in MZ twins before and after alcohol, while in DZ twins, it fell from 0.54 before alcohol to 0.05 2 h later. Heritability estimates based on these intraclasss correlations (h_3^2 according to Vogel and Motulsky 1996, Appendix 5) went up from 0.68 before alcohol to 1.73 (!)2 h later. Theoretically, heritability can go up only to 1.0 (if the entire variation is genetically caused). The authors remarked correctly that this absurd result may be caused by the linear statistical model used; they did not remark that the heritability estimate based on intraclass correlations may be subject to strong biases. In any case, this result also points to a strong effect of genetic variation on reaction of the EEG to alcohol.

It was known (see Propping 1977) from animal experiments (Caspers 1957, 1958) that alcohol diminishes the spontaneous activity of the ARAS in the rat. Therefore the alcohol effects in humans on α activity could be explained in the same way. This led to an explanation for a genetic effect on the causation of alcoholism.

It had been described repeatedly that alcoholics often show badly synchronized brain wave patterns, i.e., only few α and ϑ waves (for references see Propping 1977). Of course, this could be a long-term alcohol effect. However, it was also possible that persons having such an EEG are more susceptible to alcohol addiction than others. To obtain some hints that the twins, who had not been selected for drinking habits, were arranged also according to their usual alcohol intake. Among those who drank more than 60 g/day alcohol, 11 subjects had less, and 6 had more than 30% α waves in their resting EEGs. On the other hand, there were 8 with less and 22 with more than 30% α waves among those with a maximum daily alcohol intake of 10 g; the difference is significant statistically. This suggested the hypothesis that a genetically determined badly synchronized EEG causes a predisposition for alcoholism (see also Naitoh 1973). It has frequently been reported that the increased production of α waves (or the corresponding decrease in β waves), especially after biofeedback training, leads to pleasant sensations, giving a feeling of comfortable relaxation. Alpha-feedback has therefore been proposed for treatment of anxiety and tension (Brown 1975). Sometimes, these results have been doubted. Nevertheless, it is possible that alcohol-induced EEG synchronization may lead to similar feelings as bio-feedback experience. Therefore alcohol addiction could be an example of reward learning in predisposed humans (see below).

This hypothesis – or at least that part of it that alcoholics may have a genetic predisposition expressed by a poorly synchronized EEG with relatively little and irregular α activity – was tested by family studies (Propping et al. 1981). However, this could not be carried out by studying of other alcoholics in families of alcoholic probands, since this would not have permitted a distinction of EEG patterns caused by alcohol abuse from those indicating a genetic predisposition for alcoholism. The study had to be performed on nonalcoholic relatives of alcoholic probands.

The sample to be studied consisted of 115 inpatients of a psychiatric hospital (78 males, 37 females) who had been admitted because of alcoholism. Each alcoholic was matched with a healthy control subject of the same age and sex (mostly employees of an industrial company). The EEG recordings of alcoholics were grouped accordingly to synchronization by visual inspection. Then two extreme groups of patients were identified: Those with poor α wave activity (35 individuals) and those with particularly good α activity (12 individuals); 34 first-degree relatives of patients with poor α EEGs and 17 first-degree relatives of alcoholics with good α activity. Only relatives who did not show evidence for alcohol abuse and were drug free for at least 1 week were included in the study. Each relative was matched with an unrelated control individual of the same age and sex, the EEG recordings were analyzed using a program for amplitude-interval analysis. The results were the following:

- In the female alcoholics, α waves were reduced in comparison with the matched controls. β activity was increased and average frequencies were higher. A higher standard deviation of frequencies in frontal and precentral leads pointed to high irregularity.

- The male alcoholics did not show any consistent differences in comparison with their controls. In contrast to the females, the basic hypothesis of the study that an irregular EEG with weak α activity predisposes its carriers for alcohol abuse could not be confirmed in the male sample.
- The studies on the two groups of nonalcoholic relatives had the result that the first-degree relatives of the good α group also tend to have good and regular α activity. Relatives of the irregular α group of patients differed from the relatives of the good α group in the same direction; this difference was more pronounced in male than in female relatives.

In conclusion, the higher frequency of irregular EEGs in female alcoholics in comparison with their controls is caused by a higher genetic predisposition for alcohol abuse. In male alcoholics of this population group, however, this genetic predisposition has not been important for alcohol addiction. To find an explanation for this sex difference, the patients were subdivided into Jellinek's types alpha, beta, gamma and delta (Jellinek 1960). Among 37 female alcoholics, there were 31 alpha ("conflict drinkers") and 6 beta ("occasional drinkers") while among male patient, there were 26 alpha and 45 beta alcoholics at the beginning of their abuse. Shortly before admission to the hospital, 30 males showed signs of the gamma type ("addicts"), while 35 belonged to the delta group ("habitual drinkers"). Among 32 females, however, there were 31 cases of gamma and only one case of delta alcoholism. In a number of cases, clearcut classification into one of these groups proved to be impossible. However, the preponderance of the alpha/gamma types in female patients has been reported before (Feuerlein 1979). It can be concluded that psychological factors leading to alcoholism may be much more important in females than in males and a higher irritability might manifest itself sometimes by their EEG type; in males, environmental factor such as induction to excessive drinking by the social environment could be more important (it should be remarked that this study has been performed in the largest wine-growing area of Germany).

In another study by the same group (Propping et al. 1980), carriers of hereditary EEG variants (Chap. 4) were studied after the same standardized alcohol load that has also been used during the twin study and with the same design (see above). Altogether 59 individuals showing the following variants were examined: low-voltage EEG (N), diffuse β waves (BD), monomorphic α waves (R), and borderline α EEG. The carriers of these EEG variants were students from the student sample described above (and not alcoholics, Chap. 6). Blood alcohol concentrations did not differ significantly between these groups. Their EEG was again analyzed using the same program of amplitude-interval analysis that had been used in other studies of this group. This analysis revealed clearcut differences between EEG types: The most pronounced effect was produced in the borderline α EEG. Particularly in this type, the alcohol load shifted the frequency distribution toward lower frequencies; i.e., α activity became more pronounced and more regular. Again, as in the twin study described above, probands having a very regular resting EEG with monomorphic α waves only showed a weak reaction to the drug.

These results have induced some further studies on EEG in alcoholics and their close relatives. For example, young sons of alcoholics (19–20 years old), had, on the average, higher EEG frequencies than adequate controls. Moreover, they reacted to ethanol with a stronger reduction in mean EEG frequencies (Gabrielli et al. 1982; Pollock et al. 1983).

In a subsequent study, the same group (Pollock et al. 1995) examined middle-aged and elderly nonalcoholic men and women who had alcoholic relatives and compared them with sex- and age-matched persons without alcoholic relatives. Comparisons were performed at two levels: Psychological characteristics were assessed using a tridimensional personality questionnaire, while at the neurobiological level, the EEG was studied using quantitative criteria. While the personality test did not distinguish between the two groups, the EEG showed a clearcut difference: the relatives of alcoholics showed elevated β activities.

Other studies of sons of alcoholics were published by Ehlers et al. (1991, 1995). In their 1991 report, they compared computer analyzed EEG data from 24 sons of alcoholics with matched controls. The sons of patients had more energy in the fast-frequency α range in the resting EEG. Another study on α activity was published by Bauer and Hesselbrock; they also found significantly more α activity in individuals at risk than among controls. Other studies, however, failed to show any differences between sons of alcoholics and controls in the resting EEG (Cohen et al. 1991). They studied 15 males at risk, aged 19–24, and 15 matched controls. Their negative results are similar to those of Propping et al. (1981) in male alcoholics and their relatives; they again demonstrate that alcoholics are not a homogeneous group. Unfortunately, all these authors did not study children – sons and daughters – of female alcoholics. Ehlers et al. (1995) tried to apply approaches from chaos theory to understand EEG phenomena. It would go beyond the scope of this review to describe this approach in any detail; suffice it to say that a similar approach was used by Anokhin et al. (1996) to describe increasing EEG complexity with advancing age. Ehlers et al. calculated EEG "dimension" as described by Havstadt and Ehlers (1989). Data from 36 subjects were available: 17 high risk and 19 age-matched low risk men. A clearcut difference was revealed in this comparison; while low risk individuals, on the average, showed high dimension values, these values were much lower among the high risk persons. By comparison of the EEG records of two men, one with high and another one with low dimension values showed that there may be only small differences in usual aspects of their EEG, as well as in more traditional power spectra.

Another aspect of the resting EEG that has been studied is coherence. Coherence functions are useful measures for quantifying the relationship between EEG signals from different leads in the same individuals (Lopes da Silva 1993), for example, between the left-hand and right-hand sides. Michael et al. (1993) compared coherence scores in 27 probands suffering from alcohol dependence, 21 nonalcoholic first-degree relatives of alcoholics and 21 healthy subjects without a family history of alcoholism. The relatives of alcohol-dependent persons had significantly higher coherence scores in fronto- and centroparietal leads than the alcoholics and the probands without alcohol-dependent relatives. The authors suggested that a high coherence may be a trait marker for resilience in persons at risk for alcohol dependence. This finding probably accords well with the above observations above that individuals showing "good" α activity are less endangered to become alcohol dependent that those with a more irregular α pattern: Coherence is expected to be higher in the former group.

Results of studies on the resting EEG, alcoholism and risk for alcoholism can be summarized as follows:

- Alcohol intake, even in moderate doses, leads to more or less accentuated changes in the resting EEG. In most instances, α activity is enhanced and α amplitudes are increased. Especially in individuals normally showing an irregular α pattern, α activity becomes more regular. β activity tends to be reduced accordingly. In some persons, however, EEG changes after alcohol intake, are quite different: Typical low-voltage EEGs may not show any changes; and in other instances, β activity, especially in anterior leads, is increased.
- As shown by high similarities in MZ twins, individual variation in kind and extent of these EEG changes is due to genetic factors. These factors do not act at the level of ethanol metabolism but at the brain level.
- EEG records from alcoholics have often been compared with those of non-affected individuals. Many of them show significant differences, mainly reduced and more irregular α activity. Sometimes, increased β activity is reported; this impression may be created, in part, by higher power in the β range in central and occipital leads, i.e., in areas where, in the majority of individual EEG records, α waves prevail. However, not all series of alcoholics show these differences. In some series, no consistent differences between alcoholics and adequately matched controls could be demonstrated. In one study, male alcoholics did not show any difference from normal controls while female addicts did show a significant difference in the expected direction. This difference between male and female addicts was shown to be caused by prevalence of different types of alcoholism: While among males, cases prevailed in which addiction appeared to be caused mainly by external factors, conflict drinkers were much more common among female patients. This result supports the notion that alcoholism is not a homogeneous anomaly. It is highly heterogeneous; various types should be distinguished (see also Cloninger 1987).
- As shown by studies on close relatives of alcoholics, shifts of EEG parameters in the normal range have a genetic basis; they constitute a predisposition for becoming addicted to the drug. It is an attractive hypothesis suggested by experiences during α wave feedback that this predisposition involves positive feelings connected with a more regular and intense α activity. This aspect is discussed below in greater detail. However, regardless of whether this hypothesis can be maintained after additional studies, EEG shifts within the normal range are certainly not caused by too much alcohol drinking (of course, this does not exclude the possibility that excessive drinking may lead to organic brain damage and corresponding signs in the EEG).
- New methods of EEG evaluation such as quantification of coherence or dynamic analysis leading to measures of dimension or complexity may lead to new and more specific insights into the nature of predisposition to alcoholism.

7.2 Alcoholism and Evoked EEG potentials

Evoked (event-related) potentials (EPs) are being used increasingly for studying the functional state of the brain (Chap. 5). In recent years, varieties of the EP method have been used in an increasing number of studies in the hope of gaining deeper insight into the neurophysiological factors increasing predisposition for alcohol addiction (for an early review, see Porjesz and Begleiter 1991); in this paper many of the results on the resting EEG (see Sect. 7.1) are also reviewed. Some of the salient findings are the following: In one study, Begleiter et al. (1984) studied boys between the ages 7 and 13 with no prior experience with alcohol. Their fathers had been diagnosed as alcoholics. EPs were elicited by a relatively complex stimulus (recognition of a head with certain additional features). Amplitudes of the peak P3 were found to be significantly smaller in the group of children at risk as compared with matched controls. This finding has been replicated by a number of laboratories. O'Connor et al. (1986) studied a group of older persons at risk with the same result. Begleiter et al. (1987; see Begleiter et al. 1991) repeated the study in another series of sons of alcoholics to determine whether the effect was modality or task specific. This time, they used an auditory task. Twenty-three matched pairs of high- and low-risk males between 7 and 16 years of age were investigated. Again, reduced P3 amplitudes were observed, indicating that the P3 amplitude reductions are not modality- or task-specific. They seem to be present in auditory and visual experimental setups under speed and accuracy conditions. In another study, Whipple et al. (1988) examined EPs in prepubescent boys at high risk for alcoholism with a complex visual performance test where stimuli changed along the three dimensions shape, color, and identity of a numeral. They also found a reduction in the "late positive complex," which is identical or very similar to P3. Other studies, however, have failed to confirm this observation (Polich and Bloom 1988; Baribeau et al. 1987). This may in part be due to differences in details of the experimental setup as suggested in great detail by Begleiter et al. (1991). However, it is also possible that the difference is caused by the fact that amplitudes of the EPs depend on properties of the resting EEG. For example, they are especially high in the EEG variant with monomorphic α waves – an EEG type that appears to be underrepresented among alcoholics. On the other hand, EPs of persons having a low-voltage EEG are especially low, and those with β waves are in-between. In a sample of risk persons and alcoholics who show the EEG patterns described by various authors (irregular α waves; β waves etc.) a low P3 must be expected. This is not the case, however, if alcoholism in most probands belongs to a different type with special features of the resting EEG. Hill et al. (1988) reported increased cognitive efficiency as indicated by lower latency of P3 in nonaffected siblings of alcoholics. They suggest that this may offer protection against the development of alcoholism. For other studies with varying experimental setups and different – positive or negative – results, see again Begleiter et al. (1991). More recent studies on this problem were published by Lu and Chu (1991) from Taiwan; Lukas et al. (1991), Pfefferbaum et al. (1991), Hill and Steinhauer (1993 a,b), Berman et al. (1993) and Hesselbrock (1993). Pfefferbaum et al. confirmed that low P3 amplitude "reflects family history, but not alcohol consumption." In a study on 86 children (45 boys and 41 girls) at ages of 8–18 years, the high-risk again shows a P300 amplitude reduction; Hence a low P300 peak points to a genetic risk for alcoholism even at such a young age. There were no group differences in reaction time or EP latencies. A study by Hill and Steinhauer (1993) deserves special interest since it has been performed in women, while in most of the above studies above men were examined. Female alcoholics had significantly lower P300 amplitudes as compared with high-risk and low-risk controls. Together with a study of Propping et al. (1981) which showed a resting EEG with irregular α activity to be more common in alcohol-dependent females, the low P300 may constitute a specific vulnerability in women with irregular α activity and low P300. Here, again, the above association between resting EEG and EP amplitude (Vogel et al. 1986) comes to mind. It is a pity that many EP specialists pay so little attention to the resting EEG of their probands. A more specific experimental setup to test ability for reacting to stimulus specificity when stimuli of various types are offered was used by Berman et al. (1993a). According to their results, reduction in EPs in high-risk boys (and of alcohol addicts at ages 11–14) may express reduced sensitivity to information "about the frequency with which categories of events occur." It is not surprising that, among a sample of youth, high- and low-risk, alcohol misuse correlated not only with use of other substances but with delinquent behavior, as well. A similar association between reduced P300 amplitude and "antisocial personality disorder" in young men at risk for alcoholism was found by Hesselbrock et al. (1993).

In certain instances, alcohol may also have a short-time positive effect on the CNS. For example, Propping (1977 b) in their series of adult male twins (1977 a) described an MZ twin pair with concordant, autosomal-dominant essential tremor, the degree of which was reduced effectively by alcohol uptake. A similar reduction was observed in three brothers with dyssynergia cerebellaris myoclonica (Ramsay-Hunt; Lu and Chu 1991). In two of them, myoclonus improved considerably for about 6 h; in the third brother there was only a small reduction. Various EP components were also reduced, strongly in the first two brothers, but only slightly in the third. Latencies were not affected by the drug. Such observations may contribute to our understanding of neurophysiological changes caused by alcohol and to improved knowledge of genetic risk factors for alcohol addiction.

An interesting point of view was introduced into the discussion by a case report of Riikonen (1994). The DZ twin pair had been exposed to heavy alcohol consumption of the mother in the second part of pregnancy. One twin showed prenatal growth retardation delay in motor and cognitive development during the first year of life, brain atrophy as evidenced by the computer tomography, and, especially, slowing of background activity in the EEG. The other twin was normal at the end of the follow-up period (17 months). This observation raises the question whether EEG peculiarities in children of alcohol-dependent mothers, in addition to indicating genetic vulnerability, may also be caused in some instances by teratogenic effect during embyonic development.

We may conclude: in addition to certain aspects of the resting EEG, event-related potentials (EPs) may also indicate an increased susceptibility to alcohol dependence; peculiarities in individuals at risk (first-degree relatives of alcoholics) have been described, especially a reduction in amplitudes of late components (P300). Psychophysiological studies using various experimental setups were performed to elucidate the mechanisms involved. Studies on the relationships with performance in certain attention (and divided attention) tasks (see, for example, Lukas et al. 1991) may be rewarding. However, genetic variation in the resting EEG in relation to EPs should be considered in future studies. Moreover, there is another aspect of the problem that is difficult to study but may be rewarding in the long run: As noted above in the discussion of Propping's twin studies (Propping 1977a), the increase in amount and regularity of α waves in many individuals, especially those showing a somewhat irregular α activity in their resting EEG, is similar to that observed after α feedback, as described above. However, the increase in α activity has been described to be associated with a feeling of happy relaxation. Individuals may have an increased risk for becoming addicted to alcohol (and other drugs) when they obtain something from it, i.e., when they are gaining some sort of reward. In this way they learn to drink more and more, finally becoming addicts. Learning by reward not only correspondens to daily-life experience; it is one of the best confirmed results of learning theory. It is a reasonable hypothesis to assume that in individuals having a spontanously irregular α activity, this effect may be stronger than in those with α "strong" a activity whose EEG does not change very much under the influence of alcohol. This may make learning of alcohol misuse more enticing. Psychological studies have shown, for example, that hyperactive children are at an increased risk for alcoholism. The three dimensions of novelty seeking, harm avoidance and reward dependence assessed by a semistructured interview at ages 10–11 years were shown to be correlated with alcohol abuse in young adults. Alcoholism and depression were also reported to be associated frequently. According to Winokur, they may have a common cause; Winokur (1972) regards both conditions as belonging to a "depression spectrum disease." Studies, especially psychological studies on the resting EEG and on evoked potentials (EPs) in alcoholics and normal controls could be combined with those on genetic variants of the normal human EEG. Such combined studies may provide interesting results on genetic factors affecting personality, normal social functioning, and its disturbances. For example, it is a reasonable hypothesis that individuals showing the variant with monomorphic α waves (our R group) may have an especially low propensity to alcohol (and, possibly, to other drugs). Their stable and sthenic personality profiles (Sect. 6.6) as well as many of the above EEG results on alcoholics and their nonalcoholic relatives would fit into such a concept. As discussed above, however, alcoholism is not a uniform condition. The Jellinek types (Jellinek 1960) should be regarded. A more recent subdivision has been suggested by Cloninger (1987). He distinguished type 1 (low novelty seeking; high harm avoidance; high reward dependence) from type 2 (male-limited; high-novelty seeking; low harm avoidance; low reward dependence). Spontaneous alcohol seeking behavior or inability to obtain (type 2) and psychologic dependence or loss of control (type 1) should be associated with different personality traits.

Understanding the individually different ways in which a person may become alcohol dependent, and the various conditions that may help in this – disastrous – development at the neurophysiological and psychological levels, as well as their interaction, may help in prevention and therapy. This monograph cannot be the place for discussing in greater detail the entire problem of alcoholism, not even all its genetic problems. Propping (1992) gave a very useful review.

In this place, some brief remarks may be appropriate for another, very common kind of drug dependence: Smoking. Evidence has been provided by a number of twin studies that there is some genetic variation affecting the habit of smoking. Heritability estimates vary between these studies; they are generally moderate and, as a rule, not very high but still substantial (for references, see Boomsma et al. 1994). Therefore it was worthwhile to look for EEG differences between smokers and nonsmokers (Brown 1973). The sample examined by Brown consisted of 88 normal, healthy subjects (ages 21–65, 45% males). They were subdivided into four categories, from nonsmokers to very heavy smokers, and, in addition, two categories of former smokers. A program of amplitude-interval analysis was used. The following group differences were found:

- All active smokers, including the former smokers, showed significantly higher α frequencies than nonsmokers; as a rule, α frequencies also showed more intra-individual variation.
- One of the chief, usually distinguishing characteristics of heavy-smoker EEG was "an extraordinary amount of rhythmic β activity"; their β amplitudes were also much higher.
- There were no significant differences of ϑ activity, but the two groups of heavy and very heavy smokers tended toward a slightly higher ϑ activity.
- Desynchronized EEG activity in smokers appeared to be chiefly a mixture of fast activities, in nonsmokers a mixture of slower frequencies.
- A characteristic of the smoker' s EEG was stronger contamination by high-frequency muscular artifacts. As to personality characteristics, assessed by semi-quantitative scoring methods, the degree of the smoking habit was associated positively with aggression, anxiety, intelligence (for occupation), independence, physical activity and verbal activity, and negatively with contentment and sociability.

These findings suggest a higher level of general arousal as a more or less persistent state in smokers. They may use (and need) nicotine as a kind of "tranquilizer." Obviously, these EEG changes are clearly distinguished from those found in alcohol addicts. Unfortunately, it cannot be decided whether, and to what degree, these EEG traits are causes or effects of nicotine abuse; the similarity of the β pattern found with β waves elicited by other drugs such as barbiturates (Sect. 2.9) favors the second explanation but a comparison of differences in aspects of personality between different EEG variants (Chap. 6) may suggest a genetic component. Twin and family studies similar in design to those performed in alcoholism would be worthwhile.

7.3 The Low-Voltage EEG in Relation to Anxiety Disorders

So far, EEG variation and its genetic basis has been considered to normal psychological variation-intelligence, aspects of performance and personality (Chap. 6); and in relation to alcohol dependence and, very briefly, smoking. In most of the studies on alcohol effects and dependence the problem was considered carefully whether the EEG characteristics found were simply alcohol effects, or whether they indicated a genetic predisposition of brain function to alcohol addiction. The results pointed into the latter direction. As regards smoking, the situation is different: Here, genetic predisposition and nicotine effects are intimately intermingled. In most of the studies that are now to be discussed a major problem is this mixture of genetic variation with environmental effects in its broadest sense. One group of problems is posed by psychological conditions commonly called neuroses.

The problem whether and to what extent psychological difficulties commonly identified as "neuroses" may affect the EEG, leading astray scientists who think that certain EEG signs could constitute genetically determined "traits." This problem can be solved by examining the MZ twins discordant for neuroses. If their EEGs are as concordant as those of other MZ twins, it can safely be concluded that clinical signs of neurosis, at least those found in these twins, do not affect the EEG and could therefore be used as trait markers. As described in greater detail in Sect. 3.8, this problem was studied by Vogel et al. (1984), examining twins included in a long-term twin study on neuroses (see also Schepank 1974, 1996). In this study the degree of neurotic signs was quantified in a scoring system; differences between partners of a twin pair therefore could be quantified as well. On the average, these differences were smaller in MZ as compared with DZ twins but there were large differences in some of the MZ pairs. However, EEG records even in MZ pairs showing very discordant neurosis scores were quite as similar as in all other twin pairs. Hence it may be concluded with some caution that EEG characteristics in the "normal range" in individuals diagnosed as suffering from certain types of "neurosis" may be regarded as "trait markers."

Enoch et al. (1995), from the group of D. Goldman, studied individuals with low-voltage EEG (LV) and borderline low-voltage EEG (BLV) with regard to psychiatric diagnosis, especially anxiety disorder. Anxiety disorder, according to DSM III, comprises a number of disturbances in which anxiety is either the leading symptom, or in which anxiety arises when the patient tries to control symptoms (Propping 1989). In many of the patients diagnosed as suffering from anxiety neurosis (ICD 300.0) or phobia (ICD 300.2), the condition continues to be present over many years, the panic syndrome is an especially severe condition. In a comprehensive study on adult twins (Norwegian Twin Registry), Torgersen (1983) calculated a concordance rate of 34% in MZ as compared with 17% in DZ twins. However, MZ twins never showed precisely identical anxiety syndromes. Family studies of other authors showed an incidence of about 15% (three times the population incidence; see Propping 1989).

The result by Steinlein et al. (1992; see Sect. 4.3) that one of the genes leading to low-voltage EEG is located on chromosome 20q, together with the (weak) evidence reported by Knowles et al. (1995) that a gene for anxiety disorder may be located at 20q.13.2–13.3 had suggested to Enoch et al. (1995) the possibility that there is a relationship between the low-voltage EEG and anxiety-disorder. A sample of 124 subjects were studied, including 50 unrelated probands and 74 relatives (Table 7.1). The probands were paid volunteers recruited through newspaper advertisements which solely asked for volunteers with the relevant family structure. No mention was made of alcoholism or other psychiatric disease. However, since the name of the institute was mentioned (National Institute of Mental Health, Bethesda), it can be assumed that many of these volunteers may have had some complaints of psychiatric relevance. Candidates for the study were interviewed on the phone for medical history, alcohol, drugs and family history. Those having suffered from conditions that may have affected the EEG, for example, brain trauma or epilepsy, or whose family members refused to participate in this study were excluded. Of the remaining 50 index cases, 36 were male and 14 were female; the age range was 18–73 years (mean = 38.1 years). In addition, 74 family members were studied and their EEGs were included. All these individuals were examined medically and psychiatrically; psychiatric diagnoses were made blind as to the EEG. The EEG recording included, in addition to conventional clinical criteria, quantitative evaluation of information taken on tape (for the method, see Coppola 1979). The absolute power within the α band, averages of the two occipital recordings (O_1, O_2) was used as criterion. The 124 subjects studied included 19 low-voltage cases – 7 of them were regarded as

Table 7.1. EEG, anxiety states and other psychiatric diagnoses in 118 probands. Last column: Percentage of all cases with the psychiatric diagnosis (Enoch et al. 1995)

Psychiatric diagnosis	Low voltage (N + NG)	EEG Monomorphic alpha waves (R)	Normal alpha waves	% low voltage
No mental illness	2	1	21	8%
No alcoholism, anxiety disorder, drug abuse	2	2	40	5%
Alcoholism	9	2	26	24%[a]
Depression	3	2	19	12%
All anxiety disorders (phobia, general anxiety, panic)	14	5	29	29%[a]
Alcoholism and anxiety disorder	8	1	6	53%[a]
All subjects	17	8	93	14%

[a] χ^2 comparison of subjects with and without low-voltage EEG (N + NG) among all patients with the respective psychiatric diagnosis; significant difference ($p \leq 0.05$)

clearcut low-voltage (LVA) and 12 as borderline. The incidence 7/124 = 5.1% corresponds well with that given by Vogel and Fujiya (1969; 4.2%); the incidence of borderline cases is slightly higher possibly indicating some differences in classification. For assessment of these incidence figures, it should be considered that the majority of subjects were not ascertained independently but as relatives of probands. For 118 of the 124 subjects, a psychiatric diagnosis was available; Table 7.1 shows the distribution of these diagnoses. Obviously, there is a significant association of anxiety disorders with the low-voltage type as defined by these authors (group N + NG). Alcoholism is more common in this group as well, while there appears to be no relationship of the low-voltage types with depression.

Considering the heterogeneity of alcohol dependence, the data on alcoholism correspond fairly well with data on EEG and alcoholism discussed in Sect. 7.1. A relatively high α power of alcoholics in this sample as compared with subjects with various anxiety disorders could indicate that most alcoholics in this sample may belong not to the true low-voltage group (N, in our nomenclature) but to our borderline group NG. The combination of alcohol dependence with anxiety states in alcoholism seems not to have been considered expressly in earlier studies on EEG in alcohol dependence, as reviewed in Sect. 7.1. An association of low-voltage (N) and low-voltage borderline (NG) probands with anxiety states could hardly be anticipated from the results of our group in its attempts at characterizing persons showing these variants (Sect. 6.4). Here, however, the composition of the two samples investigated should be considered: soldiers belonging to an Air Force can hardly be expected to suffer from signs of an anxiety disorder. An appreciable prevalence of such disorders is not very likely in university students. Among our Air Force sample, N and NG probands even showed the lowest scores in "anxiety" (second stratum factor Q II of the 16-PF). In the student sample, they were also low. In both samples, they tended more toward "adjustment" than toward "anxiety." In addition to differences in composition of the samples used by Enoch et al. and by our group, it is also likely that the conceptualization of the second-stratum factor "anxiety"; as used by the psychologists who constructed the 16-PF differs from the psychiatric diagnosis of anxiety states as used by these authors. However, there appears to be one aspect in which the studies on the low-voltage and low-voltage borderline EEGs appear to coincide: They show a definite contrast to the "sthenic" and energetic attitude of subjects with very regular α activity (monomorphic α waves).

7.4 Psychopathy and Delinquiency

There have been many EEG studies on probands with dissocial behavior, "psychopathy" and delinquiency. Such studies have been performed to determine whether and to what extent such behavioral anomalies may have organic reasons. Such organic anomalies may be caused by exogenous factors such as brain trauma or intoxication during embryonic age, at the time of birth or later in life. However, they may also be inherited, being, for example, manifestations of a metabolic disease or a minor manifestation of a disposition for some type of epilepsy. Therefore it is doubtful whether the "state" of the EEG represents a "trait" indicating a genetic basis. These studies cannot be described here in greater detail; mentioning them in a table must suffice (Table 7.2).

Studies on MZ and DZ twins and comparisons of adopted children with their adoptive and biological parents have shown that genetic factors contribute significantly to the propensity of an individual for socially deviant behavior and delinquency (for references see Vogel and Motulsky 1996). Therefore some of the EEG anomalies found among delinquents of various kinds may have a genetic basis; a decision on this problems needs special analysis of individual cases and situations.

Tables 7.2 and 7.3 show a selection of results. Designs of the studies were very different, and the results are heterogeneous. However, they pose a relatively clearcut question to the geneticist. Hill (1944, 1952; Hill and Fenton 1969) described a posterior temporal slow phenomenon consisting of slow waves recorded from posterior and temporal leads of one or both hemispheres. The predominant frequency range was described as 3–5 c/s, but slower components also occur. These waves may be attenuated by the opening of the eyes and by photic stimulation. Their amplitude is often higher than that of the α rhythm and "their wave form often has a sharpened contour" (Fenton et al. 1974). This EEG type was described by Hill (1952) to occur in 2% of 146 healthy individuals as compared with 12% in 194 nonepileptic psychopaths. It was found to be associated with aggressiveness and antisocial conduct. Hill also described a decline in prevalence with advancing age. According to his opinion, such slow-wave activity indicated a delay in maturation of cerebral activity, since posterior slow waves are a predominant feature of the EEGs of healthy children. Jung (1941) pointing to similarities of the EEGs of such psychopaths and aspects of the children's EEG had also assumed a maturation defect. As evidenced from the selection of studies given in Tables 7.2 and 7.3, results on (mostly young) delinquents and individuals described as having a "psychopathic personality" are not uniform. Levy and Kennard (1953), for example, found a higher prevalence of this EEG anomaly in males scoring as "neurotic" in the MMPI but not in those showing high Pp (psychopathy) scores. Verdeaux et al. (1964) also found

Table 7.2. EEG and delinquency

Nature of the sample:	Studies performed:	Results and interpretation:	Reference:
Male inmates of a state penitentiary, age 18–55, I.Q. >70; 50 violent crime, 50 nonviolent crime	Psychological studies using the MMPI; clinical EEG studies	30% "abnormal" as compared to 5–10% in the normal population – 2 groups of offenders: 1) High Pp scores, normal EEG; 2) Normal or "neurotic" MMPI scores, high prevalence of 4–6 c/s EEG waves	Levy and Kennard 1953
120 male delinquents, 14–18 years old, + normal controls	EEG studies; clinical criteria, alpha frequency, occipital slow waves, etc.	3 groups: 1) Normal; 2) character anomalies; 3) delinquency. Deficiency: Lower alpha frequency (8 c/s); more occipital slow waves; stronger hyperventilation reaction; less maturity	Verdeaux et al. 1964
100 males, age 11–19, from an institution for delinquents; 50 males selected because of suspicion of organic damage; about 53% Blacks; nor normal controls	Clinical EEG and psychiatric assessment	23 abnormality in 100 unselected cases, mainly 14 and 6 c/s spikes – very few anomalies pointing to epilepsy or organic anomaly	Loomis 1965
30 young delinquents, mean age 15.1, and 24 normal controls (mean age 13.2)	Clinical EEG; Intelligence and Rorschach tests (only in the delinquent group)	10 delinquentes had spikes and theta waves, 11 only theta waves, 9 normal; of the younger controls, only 4 had theta waves. Theta group especially in violence disorders. Spike group: Violence and sex; normal group: Burglary etc.	Yoshii et al. 1961
229 delinquent males (age 14–19), comparison between EEG groups	Clinical EEG; I.Q. and Kraepeling performance test	90 with regular theta (mostly F, P); correlation with violence. 104 other EEG anomalies; no special correlations; 35 normal EEGs; mainly theft etc.	Yoshii et al. 1964

Table 7.2. (Continue)

Nature of the sample:	Studies performed:	Results and interpretation:	Reference:
43 juvenile delinquents, 23 normal controls	Clinical EEG; rating "dysrhythmic" (27) vs. "non-dysrhythmic" (23) 5 personality + performance tests	Significant personality differences between delinquents and normals but not between EEG types of delinquents	Beshai 1971
66 patients (majority males) with temporal-posterior slow waves, mean age about 30, and matched (delinquent) controls	Clinical EEG, psychiatric examination, including social history of families	No consistent differences between the two groups regarding intelligence; personality scores; and violence	Fenton et al. 1974
101 males (ages 14–¡6 at first test), at age 24 clinical status assessed	Clin. EEG and power spectra; testes for skin conductance; heart rate	Criminals-to-be had lower mean arousal (significantly more power in theta bands; tendency also for alpha and delta bands) – correlations between EEG and social parameters close to zero	Raine et al. 1990

Table 7.3. EEG and psychopathic personality

Nature of the sample:	Studies performed:	Results and interpretation:	Reference:
115 patients (Classification according to K. Schneider); among them 36 women; 50 normal controls	Clinical EEG; steandard reference leads	19 (53%) of women and 21 (27%) of men showed "dysrhythmia", often with slow, more often with fast waves (compared with 12% of normal controls)	Høncke et al. 1949
70 patients (Children, adolescents; adults) – no controls	Clinical EEG; neurological studies	41% had persistent theta rhythms; other slow waves were also present	Hodge 1945
192 cases, ages 12–30, 50 normal controls	Clinical EEG; psychological tests; especially tests showing aggression and low frustration tolerance	Increased theta activity in hostility and "acting-out" aggression. EEG in unstable persons "fluctuant and unstable"	Kennard et al. 1956
100 psychopaths (sociopaths)	Clinical EEG; Psychiatric diagnosis	High percentage (55%) of borderline and abnormal EEG; 4–7 c/s band (theta) twice as often as any other anomaly	Arthurs and Cahoon 1963
100 "Psychopathic personality" (age mostly 18–25)	Clinical EEG; Psychiatric diagnosis Craft scale	Among those younger than 25, 61% had an abnormal EEG; in the older group, EEGs were abnormal in 40%; 15% of patients had history of epileptic fits	Harper et al. 1973
Inmates of a security hosp. for abnormal offenders, mean age 33.9 (n = 80)	Clin. EEG and power spectra; psychol. tests mainly for hostility and aggression – orientation reaction + cold pressure response; adaptation to repeated auditory stimulation	No increased theta activity of the most aggressive subjects – slightly higher alpha frequency of high-aggressive group. Slightly lower theta response to auditory stimulation but higher cold-pressure (pain) response in high-aggressive group	Blackburn 1975
39 persons (36 female) with borderline personality disorders; age 20.3, compared with 20 unipolar depressed patients (13/20 females), mean age 52.4	Clin. EEG; three classes: Abnormal, possib.abnormal, normal. Psychiatric diagnosis – scores for many symptoms	46% abnormal in borderline group, 10% in depressive group; 41% posterior sharp waves in borderline vs. 5% in depressives. Age and medication effects? More complex partial seizure EEG in borderline group	Cowdry and Pickar

more occipital slow waves among their probands, and Yoshii et al. described an association of waves in the ϑ range especially with violence disorders. However, in their Japanese delinquents, these waves were found especially in frontoprecentral leads (Yoshii et al. 1964). It is not clear, whether this remarkable difference from results mainly found in Caucasians is due to the fact that these delinquents were Japanese or whether it had some technical reasons. According to our experiences, the range of variation in EEGs in normal individuals as well as frequencies of hereditary EEG variants did not differ from results found in Caucasians (Vogel and Fujiya 1969). Raine et al. (1990) examined a group of 101 school boys at the age of 15, and from three different schools with pupils from various social status and intelligence; EEG assessment included power spectra. Nine years later, when the probands had reached an age of 24, it was assessed by a search of data in the British Central Criminal Records office, in which all data on delinquency are collected. Future delinquents had shown at age 15 a significantly higher frequency of occipital slow waves in the ϑ range than those having no criminal record. There was also a nonsignificant tendency for more activity in the δ range and in the slower α range. Criminals had also shown at age 15 a slower heart rate, but no altered skin conduction. Considering these results together, the authors assumed "a lower level of central and autonomic arousal" in youths who were to come into conflict with law-enforcement authorities later in life. However, a "dissenting vote" was provided by the study of Fenton et al. (1974). These authors compared 66 delinquents with temporal posterior slow waves and the same number of matched controls – delinquents without this EEG type. There was no consistent difference between these groups regarding intelligence, personality scores and frequency of crimes involving violence.

Table 7.3 documents another group of studies in which the probands had been diagnosed as showing "psychopathic personality" or a similar diagnosis. In fact, some of them were also delinquents. Again, an increase in ϑ activity was found in some of them; other features described as abnormal or borderline were occipital sharp waves and sometimes, EEG signs pointing to a propensity for epileptic seizures. In another study, however, no increased ϑ activity was found in the group of most aggressive subjects when compared with less aggressive inmates of the same institution for delinquents.

It is not surprising that various groups of psychopaths and delinquents show a certain amount of heterogeneity; their age distribution, composition regarding kind and severity of crimes committed, and the methods of EEG recording and evaluation differ too greatly. For example, which EEG feature is hidden in Levy's and Kennard's (1952) "abnormal" records? Considering all these difficulties, it is remarkable, how often EEGs with increased occipital or occipital-temporal activities in the ϑ range have been described as being associated with delinquency or with certain types of delinquency; especially aggression, sometimes including sexual aggression and violence. Here, Hill recognized an important fact as early as 1944. The parallel with slow activity in EEGs of children is, indeed, striking. The concept of a "maturation" defect, while vague, may hit an important aspect. The studies of Raine et al. (1990) in which a slower mean heart rate at 15 was found in males having a criminal record at 24 points to a more general effect, possibly adequately described as lower central and autonomic arousal. Possibly, there is a connection with the finding reported in Sect. 4.7 on probands showing the hereditary EEG type with monomorphic α waves. As noted above, male subjects with this EEG type showed, on the average a higher level of DBH (dopamine-β-hydroxylase) in the blood; possibly a sign of high central and automatic arousal (Sect. 4.12). Moreover, the occipitotemporal ϑ waves reported in delinquents, while as a rule described slightly incompletely by the above authors, show similarities not only with many children's EEGs but also with the 4–5 c/s variant (Sect. 4.6). For example, the waves described in delinquents were sometimes described to be attenuated by opening of the eyes (Fenton 1974). On the other hand, a number of, sometimes major, neurotic signs and symptoms have been observed in probands showing the 4–5 c/s EEG variant; it may disappear some time during adult age (for details see Sect. 4.6); observations within families suggest a genetic basis. It is not likely that the observations of Hill and subsequent authors all relate to this EEG variant. With a prevalence of about 1‰ it is much too rare. However, it is very well possible, if not likely, that EEG types with occipital ϑ activity in adolescents and adults have a genetic basis; numerous twin studies indicate a strong genetic effect on all "normal" EEG activities, including ϑ waves (Chap. 3). Only in one MZ pair, age 11 years, we observed discordance of occipital slow activity (Fig. 3.6). Family studies starting with probands having become delinquent, and showing EEGs with occipital or occipitotemporal (and, probably, frontal) slow activity, especially in the ϑ range, would be worthwhile. They could help in elucidating genetic components contributing to a propensity for delinquency, especially to a propensity for aggression and violence. However, such studies would be difficult to perform.

Another EEG trait mentioned repeatedly in studies on delinquent behavior are the 14 and 16 c/s positive spikes, leading to the concept of "diencephalic epilepsy" (Gibbs; see Loomis 1965). This trait is now known to be part of the normal EEG in many young persons; as shown by twin studies, it has a clearcut genetic basis (Vogel 1965). Very critical studies are needed to clarify a possible relationship with dissocial and delinquent behavior.

In conclusion, genetic studies on the EEG may help in clarifying the kind of genetic predisposition involved in propensity for dissocial and criminal behavior.

7.5 Other Types of "Abnormal" and "Neurotic" Behavior: Psychosomatic Complaints

Almost from the beginning of EEG research, there were many studies on the EEG in conditions regarded as "neurotic," "psychosomatic," etc. An association with the low-voltage and low-voltage borderline EEG with anxiety states (Enoch et al. 1995) has been described in Sect. 7.2. Other studies involving anxiety states and panic disorders in relation to complex partial seizures have been performed by Handel et al. (1995), Strauss (1945), Abraham and Duffy (1991). Lower mean α and higher fast and slow activity in "anxiety-prone" normal individuals and differences in the photic driving response were shown by Ulett et al. as early as 1953. Flor-Henry et al. (1979) described signs of predominantly left frontal dysfunction as shown, for example, by reduced left-termporal variability, and an increase in the right-left parietal coefficients of variation, in patients suffering from an obsessive-compulsive syndrome. Some authors found EEG differences between individuals classified as predominantly "vagotonic," and those regarded as "sympathicotonic." Arndt et al. (1956) examining 69 healthy persons, described an association between a relatively slow basic α rhythm, a low heart minute volume and low oxygen consumption, as common signs of vagotony; sympathicotonic persons showed an opposite syndrome. Rubin and Bowman in 1942 compared a series of 100 patients with peptic ulcer with 100 "normal" persons and found a much higher prevalence of EEGs with "dominant α rhythm" in the ulcer patients, than in with the control group. A second group of ulcer patients showed "rare α waves." The majority of controls, however, were in-between these two extremes. A somewhat later study compared 49 patients with asthma with the same group of 100 healthy controls. Again, a much higher prevalence of "dominant α rhythm" was found among the patients (Rubin and Moses 1944). According to traditional views in medicine, both conditions, peptic ulcer and asthma, have a certain connection with vagotony. Crigel and Solomonovici (1968) examined 120 adults diagnosed as "neurosis" of various types, "neurasthenia" and anxiety or depression, or a combination of these two. In the latter group, both fast activity in the β range and spikes and spiky ϑ waves were observed predominantly in temporal leads. It is especially interesting that the authors also studied a limited number of children of 14 patients of this latter group (anxiety with or without depression). In nine cases, the children showed an "epileptoid activity," for example, febrile convulsions, epileptic or affective seizures, or psychomotor hyperexcitability: Hence a special genetic predisposition appears to be present in these cases. Family studies starting with certain diagnoses, or with certain, well-delimited EEG types, may be worthwhile. An excellent and very critical review of the older literature was given by Elllingson (1954, 1956). Now, more than 40 years later the problem should be taken up again in a systematic way and by a large-scale study.

7.6 The EEG in Behavioral Anomalies of Children and Youth

The development of the normal EEG in childhood and youth has been described briefly in Sect. 2.5 (see also Niedermeyer 1993). Numerous studies have been performed in children suffering from a variety of behavioral anomalies (see, for example, Christian 1968; Dumermuth 1972). Almost all authors agree that such children show in a high percentage of cases more or less distinct EEG anomalies; in most studies percentages vary between about 40 and 70%. Stronger dysrhythmias, ϑ rhythms mainly in occipital and parietal leads are common. These anomalies are sometimes similar to those observed in psychopaths or delinquents (Sect. 7.3). Various kinds of brain damage during infancy and early childhood are often discussed as possible causes. As discussed in Sect. 7.3, even early observers had identified similarities of certain aspects of EEG during childhood and EEG "anomalies" in adolescents and adults classified as psychopaths or sociopaths, especially various types of ϑ activity. This has led to the concept of maturation defect or retardation of brain maturation (Jung 1941; Hill 1944). Sometimes, EEG patterns were similar to those found among relatives among epileptic patients. The EEG during childhood shows an enormous range of interindividual variation in maturation speed as described in Sect. 2.5. Moreover, as documented extensively in Chap. 3, this variation at least in the "normal" range is determined largely by genetic differences.

Hence many of the behavior problems for which associations with EEG phenomena were shown may at least in part have a genetic basis. For some of these behavioral deviations, a genetic component had been shown before by twin studies (see Hallgren 1960 for enuresis; anorexia nervosa, Holland et al. 1984; Kendler et al. 1991).

A study of Boseus and Selldén (1979) deserves special interest. Unlike most other investigators, these authors did not select for their investigations a sample of patients with certain psychiatric diagnoses. They started with different EEG patterns and compared carriers of these patterns regarding clinical diagnoses. A total of 222 children, 112 girls and 110 boys, were taken from a series of 1500 children who had been selected using strict criteria of "normality" (Petersén and Eeg-Olofsen 1970/71). Of these children 165 were rated using the customary criteria as having a normal EEG; in 39 14 and 6 s positive spikes were found; in 29 of them (20 girls), paroxysmal activity was observed after activation. Thirteen children showed slight to moderate increase in slow-frequency activity and 15 children had paroxysmal activity, including a psychomotor variant pattern – "saw-tooth pattern" – in 7 children. The EEG symptoms "14 and 6 s positive spikes" in the normal EEG, paroxysmal activity on activation and, especially, slight or moderate increase in low-frequency activity and "paroxysmal EEG findings at rest" showed positive correlations with clinical "suspected lesion symptoms."

In children with slight-low frequency activity, there was also an association with sleep disturbance and, especially school problems. In the 126 children with normal EEG and without 14- and 6-s positive spikes, there were only negative correlations with prevalences of clinical signs. Differences of EEG patterns between various types of psychological abnormalities were observed, for example, by Müller and Shamsie (1968); severely inhibited persons had more β activity, an aggressive group showed more slow activity. Gross and Wilson (1964) described a syndrome of "subconvulsive cerebral dysrhythmia" with behavioral and learning difficulties in many children, for example, in one partner of an MZ twin pair, aged 9 years, 6 months. One twin was a "model" child with normal behavior and EEG, the other one had difficulties at school and an EEG with many left-temporal spikes. Antiepileptic treatment led to impressive recovery. In a study of 97 children with severe behavioral disorders (Stevens et al. 1968) distinctly abnormal EEGs were recorded in 47% of the children, compared with 9% and 19%, respectively, in two control groups of altogether 88 children, matched for age, sex and socioeconomic status. Mildly abnormal "borderline" EEGs were recorded from 29% of children in both the experimental and control groups. Only 3% of the children with behavioral disorders had a history of convulsive disorder. EEG and clinical status were assessed in a very detailed way; in addition to the expected correlations, for example, between EEG asymmetries and traumatic events around birth, there was a relationship between family history of "nervous and mental diseases" and disturbed parent-child relationships and frontal or frontotemporal amplitude anomalies. Withdrawal moodiness, antisocial or aggressive behavior were correlated positively with abnormal amplitude (paroxysmal activity) while hyperactivity was associated with slowing of EEG frequencies. Fortunately, improvement in EEG and behavior has been observed in a number of cases, sometimes even without therapy. In other instances, however, a syndrome consisting of hyperactivity and other behavioral anomalies may lead to deficiency or psychosis. The overwhelming majority of these children are boys; as shown above (Sect. 7.3), adolescent or adult psychopaths in which certain abnormal EEG signs such as different types of ϑ waves are a prominent clinical sign have often been observed. There are many other studies, some of them pointing to the above relationship of certain EEG signs with behavioral anomalies, especially those combined with hyperactivity; other authors stressed the frequency of normal EEGs among children with behavioral disturbances (for example, Zimányi 1972). Following the concept of Hill (1944, 1952) some authors stressed, and confirmed in their studies a maturation defect in children with behavioral anomalies (for example, Kidron and Weiss 1958), while others rather stress negative results (Turunen and Valleala 1967).

Autism in children is a relatively rare condition (see, for example, Propping 1989). Limited twin studies pointed to a participation of genetic factors (Folstein and Rutter 1977). An EEG study in 10 autistic children, 9 boys and 1 girl, average age 3 years, 10 months (Hutt et al. 1966) gave irregular low-voltage records ($<20\ \mu V$) without a dominant rhythm; only one case had a medium-voltage irregular record; another one had, in addition, paroxysmal, frontoprecentral δ waves. Etiologically, this syndrome is heterogeneous; combinations with severe hereditary diseases (see Propping 1989; and Chap. 8), especially with the FraX syndrome, have been observed but in other cases, exogenous brain damage is the most likely reason.

In conclusion, definite, and more often slight, anomalies of the EEG can be observed in many behavioral anomalies of children, while other children remain free from such anomalies. Some of these anomalies are caused by early exogenous brain damage before or during birth or during infancy and childhood. Others appear to indicate a genetic susceptibility, but this susceptibility has not been defined and identified properly. For some specific anomalies, such as enuresis or dyslexia, linkage studies suggest specific genes. For others, especially those explained in a very general way as "maturation retardation," little or no specific hints regarding the kind of the basic anomalies have become available. Here, a wide field of problems awaits the medical geneticist.

7.7 Affective Disorders

Affective disorders include manic-depressive or bipolar disease and unipolar depression. They are characterized mainly by cyclic anomalies of feeling tone – depression or mania. Studies using the customary biometric methods – twin and family studies – have established beyond any reasonable doubt a high genetic contribution (for details, see Vogel and Motulsky 1996; Propping 1989; Tsuang and Faraone 1990). For example, in a twin study on 55 MZ and 52 DZ pairs that was based on the famous Danish twin registry (Bertelsen et al. 1977), concordance in MZ twins for bipolar disease was 79% with narrow diagnostic classification and 97% with broad classification. For unipolar disease, the respective figures were 54% and 77%. In DZ pairs, the figures were 24% and 38% for bipolar, and 19% and 35% for unipolar disease. Prevalences in close relatives were also high. While the over-all family data indicate rather a multifactorial genetic model, some pedigrees suggest participation of main genes, or even a dominant mode of inheritance. So far, however, specific genes have not been identified convincingly; linkage studies were not successful. Some of them may have been "near misses."

Much of the literature on EEG studies in affective disorders has been reviewed by Vogel (1989). Such studies are hampered by the fact that most patients are under treatment or have been treated with psychotropic drugs. Perris (1980) reviewed some of the available studies, the results of which are conflicting. When increases or decreases in α activity or increases in slow activity were observed, it could not be determined in most instances whether they were traits, clinical signs of a disease state, or caused by drug therapy. Such distinction is possible using the research design of Knott et al. (1985) who compared the EEGs of 11 sib pairs, one of whom had suffered from bipolar disease but failed to show psychotic signs at the time of examination and the other one had never suffered from an affective disorder. On the average, the former patients showed "a significantly smaller percentage of time in alpha," and a higher amplitude of AEP peak 1. The data of Knott et al. paralleled the irregular and somewhat low α activity described in some alcoholics (Sect. 7.1). This, again, suggests the possibility noted above that overarousal and/or a certain weakness of the α-producing circuit between thalamus and cortex may lead to an increased vulnerability for mood swings, especially for certain types of depression. Another dimension may be added to these considerations by EEG studies in relation to suicide attempts. According to Struve (1986), paroxysmal EEGs are much more common among psychiatric patients who had attempted suicide than among other patients. Such EEG features regarded as "traits," i.e., as indicating a genetic predisposition must be distinguished from those occurring only during phases of depression or mania ("states"). Still, there may be a relationship between these two. Nyström et al. (1986), studying 25 outpatients with major depressive disorders (MDD, according to RDC) used quantitative computerized EEG diagnosis. Primary, MDD was related to an increase in temporal δ amplitude; recurrent unipolar MDD showed a relationship with a decrease in the normal α asymmetry in temporal and parieto-occipital leads. Retarded MDD was associated with increased amplitude of slow activity. There was a positive correlation of number of former depressive episodes, degree and amplitudes of β activity, and decrease in δ and total α asymmetry. Hence this study apparently shows that subdivision of major depressions into subgroups is biologically meaningful.

Other studies appear to agree more or less that EEG amplitudes and their variances are often reduced; that the combination of depressions and anxiety are related to high frequencies and that retardation may be related to low frequencies (see, for example, Monakhow and Perris 1980; Perris et al. 1980). There are few EEG studies on patients with mania. Results on two such patients were interesting (van Sweden 1986). The EEG of one patient showed poorly organized background activities with normal features, but also prominent, regular, and sustained sleep spindles within 190–200 s after closure of the eyes. The patient was not aware of his sleepiness. A second patient had a normal EEG, but prominent sleep spindles were recorded within 60–70 s after eye closure.

These observations are extreme signs of sleep abnormalities in patients suffering from affective disorders. Manic and depressive states are frequently accompanied by profound sleep disturbance; there are difficulties in falling asleep, frequent interruption and shortening of nocturnal sleep and awakening early in the morning. Other psychotically depressive patients suffer from hypersomnia during their depressive phases. In most studies, the decreased amount of REM sleep and a reduction in its percentage of total sleep was reported. In remission, the amount of REM sleep usually becomes normal, or even increases above the normal level. Few studies are available in hypomanic and manic patients; entire sleep time is usually shortened, and REM sleep is reduced markedly (for more references, see Kaneko and Hishikawa 1981). Mendlewicz et al. (1984) described a male MZ pair at the age of 14 years; both suffered from severe depression (RDC criteria), but one had somewhat more severe clinical signs than the other one. There were no REM latency disturbances, in contrast to such disturbances in a 16-year-old adolescent girl, in which such disturbances were found. The data confirm reports according to which there are no major sleep disturbances in depressive children (Puig-Antioh et al. 1982; Kupfer et al. 1976, 1978 1979; Young et al. 1982). How do these EEG results compare with those described in genetic variants of the normal EEG? There was a consistent association between the Ma (hypomania) score of the MMPI, and the EEG with monomorphic α waves (Chap. 6). Otherwise, no comparable results were found. And an energetic person with a high Ma score is quite different from a manic patient.

Depression of one or the other type is probably the most common clinical sign seen by the psychiatrist. It may have very different reasons, and in addition to exogenous factors, especially life events of various kinds, various biological causes are probably involved. It is well known that different groups of patients react in different ways to various psychotropic drugs. The effects of such drugs on the EEG may be helpful in classification of depressions into biological subtypes, as shown by Ulrich et al. (1982, 1984) for EEG effects of lithium therapy. A comprehensive review on reaction of the EEG to antidepressant drugs was provided by Itil (1983); according to this author, antidepressant properties of new drugs can be predicted from their effects on the EEG. Depression is common in old age; here, the EEG can help in distinguishing depression from dementia of Alzheimer and especially vascular types (Wagner et al. 1985).

7.8 Schizophrenia

The group of conditions named "schizophrenia" (for a precise and modern definition see the DSM-III-R) is not only fairly common; it shows impressive clinical signs some of which correspond to the popular notion of "madness." Therefore it came as a surprise, and for some of our pioneers as a disappointment, that no characteristic EEG changes were found in all or even the great majority of patients diagnosed as "schizophrenic." Davis et al. (1939, 1942) described the "choppy rhythm" as typical for schizophrenic patients. This is an EEG pattern with fairly low voltage and irregular and poorly developed a rhythm (see below). Hurst wrote as early as in 1952: "Choppy activity is low voltage, high frequency, irregular activity. The aspect of irregularity is to be stressed particularly, since too much emphasis is generally placed, except in epilepsy, on frequency and voltage as descriptive categories. There is reason to believe, however, that both choppy and epileptic records occur in schizophrenia, sharing the feature of disorganization." A certain tendency for spikes, and sometimes even atypical spike-wave complexes, especially in younger patients was described by Jasper et al. (1939). Meanwhile, very many studies have been published; often, the results are contradictory. Some problems must be considered:

- While the term "schizophrenia" was coined by Bleuler as early as 1911, replacing Kraepelin's "dementia praecox," diagnostic criteria remained relatively vague, and classification of patients was often ambiguous, until *Diagnostic and Statistical Manual of Mental Disorders,* 3rd edn, was accepted, making possible better conformity of diagnostic standards independently of local and national traditions.
- Twin, family and adoption studies performed over many decades had shown that genetic factors are involved in the causation of schizophrenia but were not the only causes; exogenous factors were suggested mainly by the many (up to about 50%) MZ twin pairs discordant for these diseases (Vogel and Motulsky 1996; Propping 1989; and many other sources). However, it was difficult to determine exactly which exogenous factors were most important.
- Clinical signs on which the schizophrenia diagnosis is commonly based were also found occasionally in patients suffering from a variety of anomalies and disases, from chromosomal aberrations such as the Klinefelter syndrome to some inherited metabolic diseases and Huntington disease (Propping 1983, 1989).
- Recent studies in which new methods for identification of genes were used to pinpoint individual genes contributing to the schizophrenia phenotype(s) are suggesting involvement of different genes in different populations (Moises et al. 1995).

One of the problems arising in genetic analysis and interpretation of any differences that may have been found between groups of patients diagnosed as schizophrenics, on the one hand, and adequately selected controls, on the other, is again the state-trait problem: Are these differences consequences of a disease process, or are they indications for a biological, and as a rule genetic, predisposition; a genetically determined "vulnerability"? From the point of view of the clinical electroencephalographer, Dongier et al. (1974) described this problem as follows: "One of the most difficult tasks is to differentiate the more permanent characteristics such as personality diagnosis, psychiatric nosology and their EEG correlates from fluctuating, unstable psychophysiological factors such as emotion, attention, alertness and their EEG correlates." And they added: "In this respect, one of the main deficiencies of the literature is the lack of longitudinal studies establishing the permanent characteristics, if any, of a group of patients." Despite the increase in our knowledge during recent decades, their second statement is still true, as well: "Both the physiology and the psychophysiology underlying most of the aspects under review are still poorly understood and their possible value in psychiatry must be defended on poorly empirical and statistical grounds." The problems have become still more complex since most schizophrenic patients are being treated some time during their lives with psychotropic drugs, mostly neuroleptics. Moreover, it is reasonable to assume that often, so-called "untreated" schizophrenics may have taken, on the average, more drugs of one or the other type than healthy controls. In the following, some of the available studies are classified as follows: First, some of the available conceptually related simple case-control studies are presented (Table 7.4). Most of the older studies have also been reviewed by Dongier et al. (1974). Studies using the EEG as vulnerability marker are then noted (Table 7.5). Finally, studies are discussed with more sophisticated designs by which the authors tried to elucidate neurobiological mechanisms.

Table 7.4. EEG and schizophrenia

Nature of the sample:	Studies performed:	Results and interpreation:	Reference:
111 schizophrenic patients; 53 male, 58 female; comparison between "nuclear" and "borderline" groups	Clinical resting EEG, activation by hyperventilation and metrazol injection	Differentiation between "nuclear" and "borderline" groups (Mitsuda); nucelar group: Slow activity and paroxysmal rare; peripheral group: abnormal records in 42.6% paroxysmal dysrhythmia in 29.6%. Confirmation of this difference by activation	Yamada 1960
42 schizophrenic patients without medication; 42 controls matched for age and sex	Clinical EEG; frequency analysis of right parieto-temporal region	Significantly higher amount of theta and alpha activity (but not beta) and more non-normal curves in patients. Abnormalities mostly diffuse. Maturation defect in Schizophrenia?	Volavka et al. 1966
124 psychiatric patients; comparison between schizophrenics and depressives	Clinical EEG; frequency analysis	Significantly higher amounts of delta activity and less fast activity in schizophrenic patients. Difference caused – at least in part – by higher average age of depressive group?	Funk et al. 1966
101 male chronic schizophrenics; 53 healthy volonteers; 51 male volonteers from the"State reformatory"	Clinical EEG; Drohocki amplitude integrator; recordings repeated after one week	Patients – especially catatonics – show less variability within a single examination or between examinations. No relation between examinations. No relation to percent-time alpha, age, or duration of disease. Higher general activation in patients	Goldstein et al. 1965
109 schizophrenic children with mentally sick first-degree relatives and without such relatives	Clinical EEG	59 (54%) had an excess of immature slow waves in posterior leads; such slow waves were more frequent in patients having relatives in mental institutions, as compared with 21% of patients without such relatives	Andermann 1960

Table 7.4. (Contiue)

Nature of the sample:	Studies performed:	Results and interpreation:	Reference:
88 schizophrenic patients; 28 chronic (mean age 48) and 60 acute cases (mean age 35.6) – 24 normal controls (mean age 34.2)	Clinical EEG, Drohocki amplitude integrator (Goldstein et al. 1965)	No significant differences of amplitudes but lower variability in chronic schizophrenics than acute cases and normals. Lower variability also in acute cases halluzinatory during EEG study. No relation between amplitude and variation	Marjerrison et al. 1968
25 chronic schizophrenics (mean age 48); 8 normal volonteers; all patients received phenothiazine	Clin. EEG and frequency analysis; CPT (continuous performance test) alpha reaction time test	Slow reaction time but higher level of fast activity in patients; attention dysfunction in patients, especially those having mentally ill relatives	Kornetzky and Orzak 1978
53 schizophrenic patients, compared with manic and depressive patients and normal controls	Clinical EEG, frequency analysis simple mental tasks; coherence analysis	Abnormal activation of the right hemisphere in schizophrenics (less in mania). Reduction of inter-hemispheric coherence	Flor-Henry and Koles 1984
50 first-episode schizophrenia patients, 55 relatives – 31 first-episode bipolar patients, 35 relatives; 113 non-psychotic patients and 42 relatives	Clin. EEG and frequency analysis; repetition of studies after 9 months	Generalized pattern of incrased delta and theta and decreased alpha activity in schizophrenic and bipolar patients – changes in the same direction also in female, unaffected relatives	Clementz et al. 1994
49 schizophrenic probands 106 first-degree relatives	Clinical EEG, frequency analysis; psychological tests	Discriminant functions including EEG and psychological parameters permitted discrimination between normal and high-risk individuals in 76–88% of cases	Trubnikow et al. 1995
Etiopathologically different paranoid-halluzinatory psychoses (40 patients and 22 alcohol psychoses)	Clin. EEG, frequency analysis; clin. classification of patients	Recution of delta power and increase of beta power in familial psychosis; slowing of dominant beta frequency and increase of fast-alpha power in sporadic psychosis; in cases with neuro-psychological deficits, there was a correlation between paranoid-halluzinatory symptoms and high-frequency beta waves	Neuwirth et al. 1995

Table 7.5. Studies with the EEG as "vulnerability marker for schizophrenia"

Nature of the sample:	Studies performed:	Results and interpretation:	Reference:
94 parents and siblings of schizophrenics; 43 normal controls	Clinical EEG; subdivision into "normal", "abnormal", and "doubtful"	6.5% of parents and 31% of sibs had abnormal EEG, as compared to 11.6% of controls; anomalies predominantly irregular or "choppiness"	Chamberlain and Russell 1952
100 parents of schizophrenics (acute and chronical)	Clinical EEG	Slight differences of EEG anomalies between parents of the two groups of schizophrenic patients	Kozushko et al. 1979
99 first-degree relatives of anxiety-neurotic and schizophrenic patients	Evoked potentials; augmenting-reducing; skin conductance; EMG	Slight differences between the two groups of relatives – higher slopes in schizophrenia relatives – interpretation: Weakening of CNS homeostasis, weaker cortical regulation of subcortical arousal mechanisms?	Claridge et al. 1985
50 first-degree relatives of schizophrenics;patients with major depression or bipolar disorder; 38 controls	Sleeping EEG (all-night; second night in the sleep laboratory)	Higher prevalence of depression-like sleep patterns (reduced slow-wave and increased REM sleep (But small sample size!)	Lauer et al. 1995

At first glance, the data reported in Table 7.4 seem to contain a number of inconsistencies. For example, some studies suggest an increase in slow waves (ϑ and even δ) among schizophrenic patients and sometimes even a decrease in fast waves while others stress the occurrence of fast frequencies. While irregularities in the EEG pattern are a commonly observed feature, low intraindividual variation has been reported in catatonics (Goldstein et al. 1965). Subdivisions within the schizophrenia diagnostic group are especially important: Yamada's (1960) result that slow activity and paroxysmal dysrhythmia were found more often in a "borderline" than in the "nuclear" group. Neuwirth found even a reduction in δ power together with an increase in β power in familial psychosis. Moreover, there was a correlation between paranoid-hallucinatory symptoms and high frequency β-activity. Studies on coherence of EEG patterns between various leads, for example, left- and right-sides, are especially revealing; the decrease in coherence helps in quantifying "irregularities" and "choppiness" described by older authors. This accords well with the general concept of coordination defects at the level of neurons in schizophrenia and various areas of the brain, and psychopathology. Here, something such as "excessive synaptic priming" (Keshawan et al. 1994) may be important at the neuronal level. Disturbances of coherence could play a role in producing functional asymmetries between the two hemispheres of the brain, especially its frontal areas (see, for example, Flor-Henry and Koles 1984; Uzarova et al. (1995). This problem has been discussed from a psychological point of view by Claridge and Broks (1984). The observation that almost half of MZ twin pairs, at least one of which is schizophrenic, are discordant for this disease (see Vogel and Motulsky 1996), as well as differences in details of neurocognitive deficits as well, and differences in the course of the disease even in concordant pairs point to the significance of additional and probably complex, epigenetic processes in neuronal development, despite the high concordance of EEG patterns with normal MZ twins. Here, observations such as that of Suddath et al. (1990) in which anatomical abnormalities of brains in MZ pairs discordant for schizophrenia, and of Condray et al. (1992) of a MZ pair concordant for schizophrenia but showing differences in neurocognitive tests may be important. A systematic EEG study of MZ twin pairs with schizophrenia, especially discordant ones, and especially inclusion of EEG coherence measures and other tests for hemispheric function and coordination, has been performed by Stassen et al. (1998).

These authors studied 27 pairs of MZ twins discordant for schizophrenia, 13 MZ pairs concordant for this disease, and 40 healthy pairs of control twins. Methods of quantitative EEG evaluation and statistical comparison used by this group are discussed in Chap. 3. The following problems were studied: (a) Within-pair similarities of brain waves patterns; (b) EEG characteristics that may allow discrimination between affected and unaffected individuals; (c) EEG indicators reflecting the severity of the illness; (d) possible relationships between brain wave patterns and subtle abnormalities of anatomy of the brain as revealed by magnetic resonance imaging; and (e) abnormal lateralization of brain wave patterns. The most important results were the following:

- MZ twins of the schizophrenia group showed much lower intrapair EEG similarities than the healthy control twins. However, these differences occurred both in MZ pairs concordant for and in those discordant for schizophrenia.

- In affected individuals, a generalized pattern of increased ϑ, and of decreased α activity was seen. These differences allowed the authors to reproducibly discriminate between affected and unaffected individuals by a multivariate discriminant function at an overall performance of 80%.
- The degree of EEG abnormality was closely related to the degree of severity of the disease
- MRI measures such as the vertricle-brain ratio did not permit distinguishing between healthy and affected cotwins as a group, but they did permit the affected cotwin to be identified within a pair.
- As to hemispheric asymmetries of brain wave patterns, multivariate discriminant analysis allowed distinguishing between affected and unaffected cotwin in about 60%–64% of cases. Hence the question whether abnormal lateralization of the brain plays a major role in schizophrenia (Crow 1987) can be answered by these results neither in a positive nor in a negative sense.
- In a small number only of MZ pairs discordant for schizophrenia, the affected twin did not take neuroleptics. This number is not sufficient to decide whether EEG anomalies in concordant or discordant MZ pairs could be caused, at least partially, by neuroleptic treatment.

The authors discuss the question whether their results rather suggest a state-dependent effect due to the schizophrenic illness, or reflect an irreversible, progressive change in the genetically determined EEG trait. They favor the second interpretation for a number of reasons: Slight anatomical changes as shown by MRI were present in almost every twin with schizophrenia; the reduced within-pair similarity of the EEG was independent of the actual state of illness; and it was of the same order of magnitude in pairs discordant and concordant for schizophrenia. The disease process as such may, for unknown epigenetic reasons, develop slightly differently even in genetically identical brains. Lower levels of α activity may reflect atrophy of the thalamus where the pacemaker cells for the α rhythm are located; higher level of ϑ activity may reflect hippocampal theta spiking, as defined by Shagass (1976).

This study shows how the twin method can be used to contribute significantly to the solution of important problems far beyond the classical genetics-environment alternative.

CHAPTER 8

8 The EEG in Hereditary Anomalies and Diseases

With the recent progress in identification and analysis of the molecular causes and mechanisms of diseases, a rapidly increasing number of genetically caused anomalies and diseases have been identified. In many of them, the normal function of the brain is impaired directly or indirectly, often leading, in addition to many other clinical signs, to deviation of the EEG. A comprehensive survey of syndromes caused by chromosomal aberrations can be found in Borgaonkar (1989) and Schinzel (1984). For hereditary diseases with mendelian modes of inheritance, the comprehensive catalogue by McKusick provides complete and reliable information (11th edn., 1995; and the following OMIM data base, which is being supplemented continuously and is accessible through the internet). For other monographs on groups of hereditary diseases see Vogel and Motulsky (1996, "Appendix 3"), and, from a more clinical viewpoint, Witkowski (1997). EEG anomalies in "degenerative disorders of the central nervous system" have been described by Naidu and Niedermeyer (1993). Most of the diseases mentioned in this chapter are either autosomal recessive or X-linked recessive or mitochondrial in origin. A great number of inherited diseases showing, in addition to various other clinical signs, some kind of epileptic seizures were compiled by Blandfort et al. (1987). The same paper also contains genetic risk figures for various clinical types of epilepsy. In addition to genetic counseling, it may help in diagnosing patients with seizures and, often, a variety of other clinical signs. This chapter is therefore confined to a small selection of conditions that offer special points of interest.

8.1 Syndromes Caused by Chromosomal Aberrations

The best known anomaly caused by a chromosomal aberration in humans is the Down syndrome. It is quite common (approx. 1–2 cases among 1000 newborns in populations without prenatal diagnosis) and is caused by trisomy 21. For the Down phenotype, the chromosome band 21q22 appears to be responsible (for a detailed description and references, see Vogel and Motulsky 1996). The most important clinical sign of this syndrome is mental retardation which is, in many instances, fairly severe. Therefore it is not surprising that the fine structures of brains from these patients have been examined repeatedly. For example, the average weight of the brain is about 24% lower than in normals (Coyle et al. 1986). In a series of 274 fetuses and children with trisomies 13, 18 and 21, macroscopic studies gave a corpus callosum defect also in some fetuses with trisomy 21. More important, neurons that had not reached their normal location during embryonic development (= heterotopy and micodysplasias) were quite common (Gulotta et al. 1981). However, such anomalies were also described in cytogenetically normal fetuses (Barth 1987). Micromorphological analyses in various types of mental deficiency, including the Down syndrome, have been claimed to share a common morphological substrate, an anomaly in dendrites of cortical neurons. Normally, these neurons show signs of intensive development during the last 3 months of fetal life. Numerous spines are formed that establish contacts with other neurons. In various types of mental deficiency, their numbers are diminished, and they often appear altered; some are unusually small and others are long and thin (Marin-Padilla 1975). In view of these clinical and morphological anomalies, results of the EEG studies must be interpreted.

The first EEG studies on the Down syndrome were published by Kreezer as early as 1939, who studied 50 individuals in the age range between 16 and 56. α index, α frequency and average α amplitude were measured in records from the right occipital electrodes. Within this group of patients, significant correlations were found between mental age-level and α index and amplitude but not α frequency. Unfortunately, patients were not compared with normal individuals. Gunnarson (1945) observed reduced α activity in children with Down syndrome. In a comprehensive study, Gibbs et al. (1965) examined 184 patients, the majority of whom were children between the first and the 14th year of life. Eighteen subjects had clinical seizures; in 17 of them, spike-wave patterns were seen. Of the 166 patients without clinical epilepsy, 20% showed spike-wave activity. Both results together indicate an increased susceptibility for epileptic fits in subjects with Down syndrome. Except for this finding, there appear to have been little EEG peculiarities in this series: In 72%, EEG frequencies were described as "normal"; in 11% slightly slow, and in 17% slightly fast. In 59% there was an average amplitude, in 29% a high amplitude, and in 11% a low amplitude. The fraction of cases showing 14- and 6-s positive spikes was lower than in other anomalies such as mental retardation of unknown origin (Gibbs et al. 1964). Some authors described impaired α development in older children (Clausen et al. 1977; Schlack and Schmidt-Schuh 1977).

For a more deep-rooting analysis, the studies of Schmid et al. (1985, 1992; Figs. 8.1–8.3) are of special interest, since these authors used more sophisticated methods of EEG analysis. In the first of these studies, 88 children with Down syndrome were examined every year in a longitudinal study from 6 months to 5 years and were compared with 277 normal children having been selected carefully by absence of any possible anomalies. Bipolar leads were used. Power spectra were registered and evaluated from frontocentral and parietal leads of the right hemisphere. The results were the following: In the frontocentral leads, the deviation of the relative power is rather low in younger children in subdelta, delta and theta bands. With increasing age, there is an increase in theta activity in Down children, reaching its maximum at the age of two. The most significant differences were found in the alpha and beta 1 bands: between the ages of 2–5 years, Down syndrome children show a clear decrease in alpha activity. Over the parieto-occpital areas, subdelta, relative delta and theta activities increase up to the ages 4–5; as in the frontocentral leads, differences between normal and Down syndrome children also increase with advancing age. The difference of beta 1 activity also increases but less constantly. The same

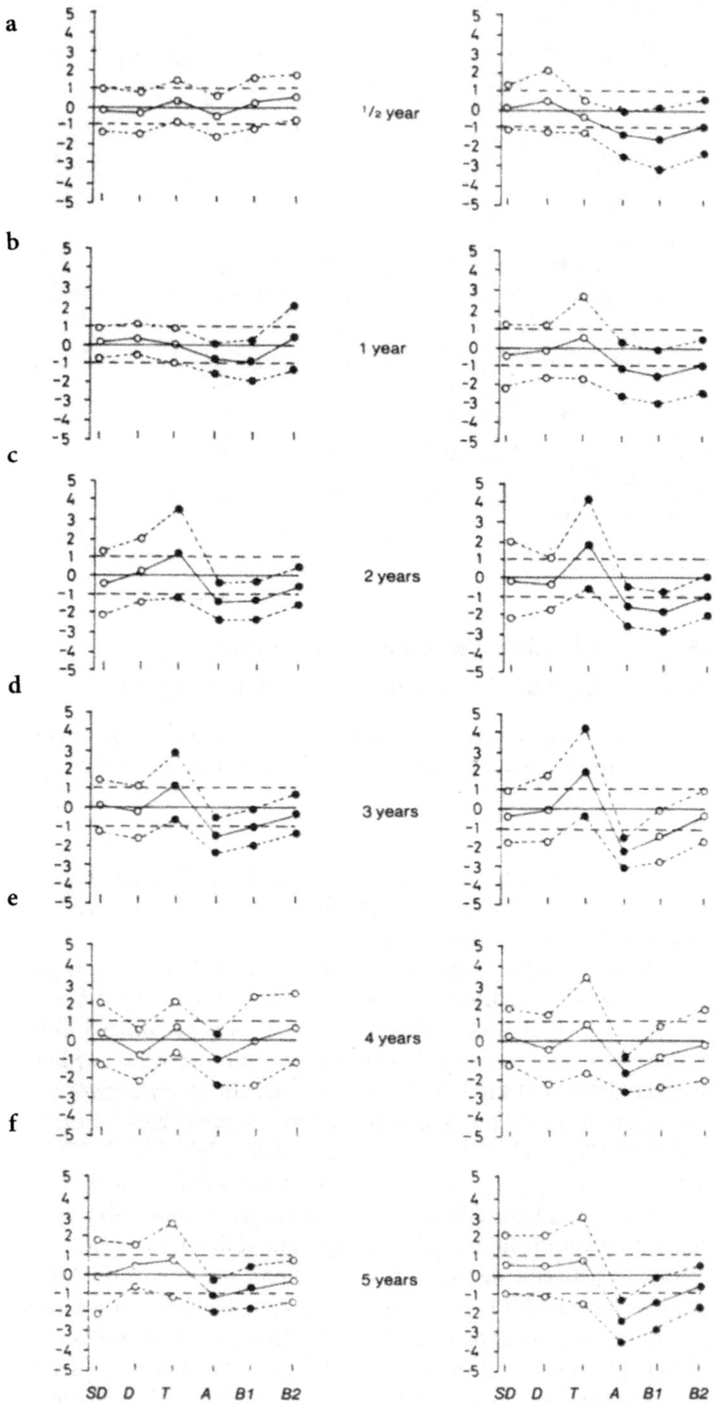

Fig. 8.1. Development of the z-transformed frequency band parameters for normal children and children with Down syndrome at the ages of 6 months–5 years over the frontocentral area. *Left*, F_4–C_4, the standard electrode placings of the 10–20 system (see Fig. 2.1). Frequency bands: *SD*, subdelta; *D*, delta; *T*, theta; *A*, alpha; *B1*, beta 1; *B2*, beta 2. *Straight lines*, means and standard deviations of the normal control population

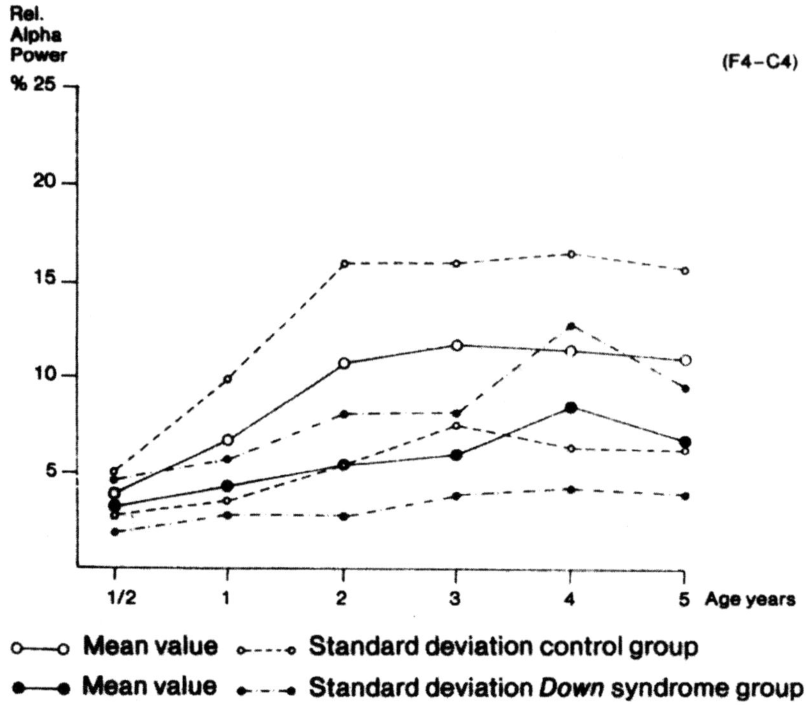

Fig. 8.2. Development of the relative alpha power over the frontocentral derivation. *Open circles,* control group; *closed circles,* Down syndrome group; *solid lines,* mean values; *broken lines,* standard deviation

tendency becomes visible when relative alpha power is considered: In children aged 4–5 years, it is much lower than in normal children, while slower activities, especially in the ϑ band, have a much higher power.

A few years later (Schmid et al. 1992) sample sizes had been enhanced including also older subjects (212 Down syndrome patients and 342 controls; aged from 6 months to 30 years). Analysis of frequency band coherences was performed. Here, the most distinct differences were found in the frontoprecentral interhemispheric coherence; the coherence deficits in the Down syndrome group became more prominent with increasing age from school age onward. On the other hand, intrahemispheric coherence in the "eyes closed" state was generally higher in the Down syndrome group. The authors suggest a correlation with the small number (and, partially abnormal shape) of dendritic spines in this syndrome, as noted above. It is a reasonable hypothesis that abnormally weak development of dendritic spikes lead to weaker communication between neurons in various parts of the brain. Other chromosomal syndromes for which EEG studies are available include those caused by numerical anomalies of the gonosomes. In 1959, the XXY karyotype was discovered for the Klinefelter syndrome, and the XO karyotype for the Turner syndrome (for details on these syndromes, see Vogel and Motulsky 1996). For both syndromes, in addition to somatic signs, certain psychological anomalies were described: Men with the Klinefelter syndrome often have an IQ slightly below average, and many of

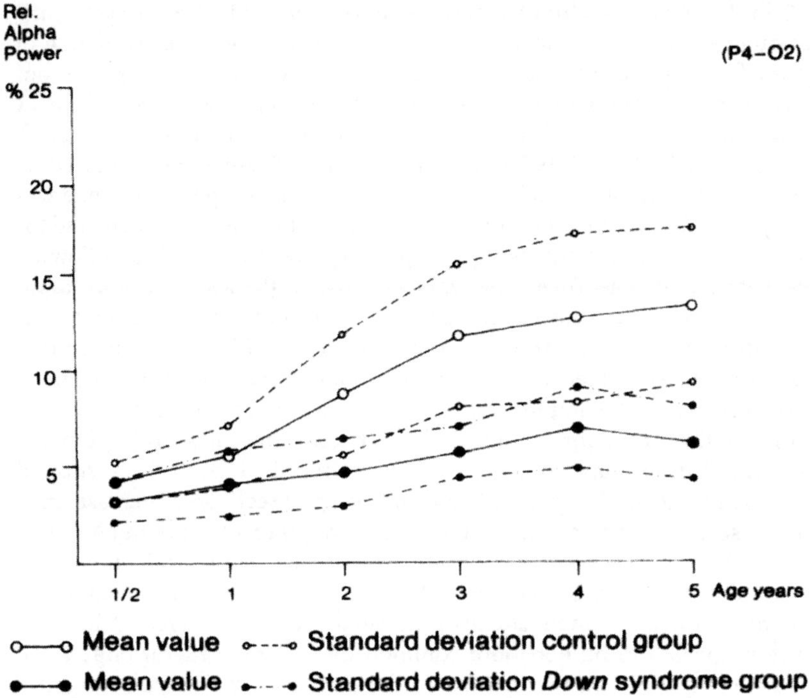

Fig. 8.3. Development of the relative alpha power over the parieto-occipital derivation. *Open circles,* control group; *closed circles,* Down syndrome group; *solid lines,* mean values; *broken lines,* standard deviation

them have certain difficulties in the personality field. Turner women show a fairly specific cognitive anomaly: They have difficulties in the perception of space and orientation.

There seems to be no systematic EEG study with modern methods such as coherences in the Klinefelter syndrome. This would be worthwhile not only because of the various problems of personality development but also because some reports indicate a higher prevalence of EEG anomalies (Hamlet and Frey 1964; Nielsen and Pedersen 1969; for more references from the older literature, see Ellingson 1972). α frequency could be below average, and it is possible (but not confirmed) that epileptic seizures may be somewhat more common in the general population. Elia et al. (1995) reported five patients with this syndrome who had seizures or epileptiform anomalies in the EEG (age range between 13 and 25 years). Four had the karyotype 47, XXY; one was a XY/XX mosaic. Two of these patients had epilepsy, one had only one isolated generalized tonic-clonic seizure, febrile convulsions were observed in one, and the last one showed focal epileptiform anomalies without seizures. Hence there was no typical pattern. A 30-year-old Klinefelter patient who had had epileptic seizures for 23 years, and was now suffering from pychotic signs such as auditory hallucinations and various delusions was observed by Miyamoto et al. (1992). A somewhat higher prevalence of symptoms normally leading to the diagnosis of “schizophrenia” has been observed (see Propping 1989).

The EEG in the Turner syndrome appears to have been studied more systematically. Poenaru et al. (1970) described a deficient modulation of the eye opening of the α rhythm, for example, little or no reaction to eye opening or closing in about half of their subjects. Anomalies characteristic for epilepsy were very rare. A thorough EEG study on many Turner cases had been performed by Tsuboi et al. (Tsuboi and Nielsen 1976, 1985 1988; Fig. 8.4, Table 8.1). These authors studied 62 Danish girls, 30 with karyotype 45,X and 32 with other karyotypes. Age range was from 6 to 47 years; 87% were 15 years old or older. Control women were matched for age. EEGs were analyzed visually and by computer (power spectra). The following differences were found: The Turner patients showed, on the average, more rapid frequencies in the β range; a lower amount of α waves but higher α amplitudes; higher amounts of ϑ waves; more δ waves, especially those with higher amplitudes. These findings in Turner subjects were more pronounced over the left hemisphere, and more typical, except the amplitudes of α waves, in Turner women with karyotype 45,X than in the others, for example, various kinds of mosaics. Both groups of women – some Turner patients and normal age-matched controls – showed basically the same mean changes with advancing age (Sect. 2.6): increase in β activity; decrease in amount and amplitudes of α waves; increase in ϑ and δ waves. Hemispheric differences found in the Turner patients were not specific; they were also present in the control group (Tsuboi et al. 1988). Paroxysmal activity was found only in one of 64 Turner women; slight paroxysmal activity was present in 13 of them. Hence it appears to be not more common than in the general population (Tsuboi and Nielsen 1985). In the opinion of these authors, their result suggest a certain functional brain disturbance, with an effect on the thalamocortical circuit. Coherence studies in these patients could be interesting.

An association with a "peculiar EEG pattern" was described for the 4p-syndrome (Wolf-Hirschhorm syndrome; Srgò et al. 1995; for clinical signs of this syndrome,

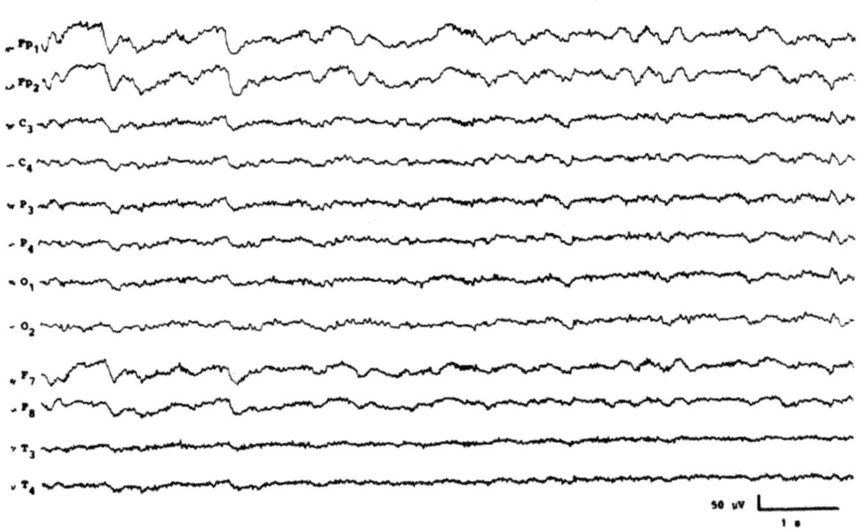

Fig. 8.4. EEG of a 17-year-old girl with Turner syndrome and 45,X karyotype. This EEG shows almost no α activity and a high amount of diffuse β activity. (From Tsuboi et al. 1988)

Table 8.1. A case-control study of the EEG background activity in 62 pairs of Turner subjects and controls. The number of pairs with a statistically significant difference at the 1% level was compared. The sign test was used to show significant differences between Turner subjects and controls. * $P < 0.05$; ** $P > 0.01$; *** $P < 0.001$. Hz, Frequency; µV, amplitude; T%, time % (From Tsuboi 1988)

Area	Alpha		Theta		Delta		Beta		
	µV	T%	Hz	µV	µV	T%	Hz	µV	T%
Fp_1		*a		*	*	*		**	
Fp_2		*a		*	*				
F_3									*
F_4									
C_3		**a						*	**
C_4									*
P_3		**a						*	**
P_4		*a							**
O_1		**a						*	***
O_2		*a					*		***
F_7	**			*	**			**	*
F_8					**				
T_3									
T_4	*		*	**		*a			*
T_5		*a							**
T_6			*						*

[a] Turner subjects < controls; alls other cases Turner subjects > controls

see Schinzel 1984). In four patients, the clinical picture showed generalized unipolar myoclonic seizures followed later by brief atypical absences. The EEG showed centroparietal or parietotemporal sharp waves. Spikes were superimposed creating unusual spike-wave complexes and complexes of spikes and waves, accompanied by frequent jerks. Since these anomalies are similar to those found in the Angelman syndrome (see below), in which the gene for the GABA-A receptor is lacking, the authors believe that this receptor may be involved in the 4p- syndrome, as well.

The XYY syndrome is much more common, and patients showing this karyotype were found to be more common among inmates of institutions for detention of persons because of criminal offenses than in the general population. On the other hand, most of these men never have conflict with the law. This problem has been discussed in greater detail by Vogel and Motulsky (1996). In an early study, various neurological anomalies were found in 10 of 12 XYY individuals (Daly 1969). Borgaonkar er al. (1968) described mild EEG anomalies; in this syndrome, coherence studies would be worthwhile.

The Angelman syndrome belongs to the syndromes that are caused by small deletions and are called "contiguous gene syndromes." It consists of a "happy puppet face," mental deficiency, paroxysmal laughing, lack of speech and epleptic seizures. It occurs, if the abnormal chromosome (mostly deletion of chromosome 15q11.2) is inherited from the mother (genomic imprinting; see Vogel and Motulsky 1996). Matsumoto et al. (1992), observing eight cases of this rare syndrome, described development of EEG and seizures as follows: The seizures start in early childhood; seizure type develops with advancing age. EEG changes from high-voltage slow bursts in infancy to diffuse spikes and waves in middle childhood; atypical absences; and diminution of seizures and seizure discharges after puberty. The authors think that untreatable epilepsies in childhood are often caused by the Angelman syndrome. The counterpart of the Angelman syndrome is the Prader-Willi-syndrome. It occurs if the same deletion comes from the father. Main clinical signs are hypotonia, small hands and feet, hypogonadism, obesity, small stature and mental retardation. Mild EEG anomalies are seen during respiratory anomalies in sleep (Kaplan et al. 1991). EEG anomalies in some other chromosomal syndromes were reported, for example, in ring 14 chromosome (with complex partial seizures; Itoh et al. 1992); in the 11 q- syndrome (Canabate et al. 1993); in the West syndrome (Mizukawa et al. 1992) and in the Miller-Dieker syndrome (deletion of 17q13.3; Bode and Bubl 1992). On the other hand, Rodichok and Miller (1992) found normal visually evoked potentials (VEPs) in a case of 18q- syndrome despite absence of the gene for myelin basic protein. Clinical manifestations in this patient were confined to mild intellectual deficiency, involuntary movements and ataxia, a surprising result.

8.2 Hereditary Diseases Caused by Gene Mutations

Many thousands of hereditary diseases are known (see McKusick 1995 and the OMIM data bank of this compilation). In many of them, epileptic seizures may occur in addition to a variety of other clinical signs (see Blandfort et al. 1987 for a survey that is, of course, incomplete). In hundreds of others, structure and/or function of the brain is involved; here, certain EEG anomalies may be present. As a rule, they are not "specific" in a sense that they suggest the presence of a specific hereditary disease, much less presence of a specific mutation. It would be hopeless to try to enumerate even some of these conditions; moreover, such an enumeration would be outdated in the moment it has been written down. A few examples which may be of interest even beyond diagnosis of a special, and as a rule very rare, disease are presented:

Rett Syndrome

In 1966 Rett described a peculiar syndrome with severe mental retardation; only girls are affected. Mainly due to a workshop held in 1985 in Baltimore, and to publication of its proceedings in the *American Journal of Medical Genetics* in 1986, this syndrome has received world-wide recognition. Hagberg et al. (1986) subdivided the clinical course into four stages: Immediately after birth, development of the children seems to be quite normal. Starting at about 6 months, statomotoric, psychosocial, and mental retardation become more and more obvious. Epileptic seizures are common. Autistic behavior and peculiar manieristic "washing" movements of hands are characteristic features. In the third stage, which was called "pseudostationary," the condition seems to be stabilizing, but clinical signs such as ataxia and epileptic fits are common, and mental retardation is obvious. Finally, in a fourth step, a multihandicap syndrome develops; the patients are wheel-chair bound and become cachetic. Up to 1986, among about 600 observations, this condition was observed once in two sisters and once in two half-sisters; all the other cases were sporadic. There appears to be no increase in consanguineous matings between parents; abortions in mothers appear not to be increased. Since affected females do not reproduce, all affected patients must be new mutants. Considering the incidence in the population, a mutation rate of about 3.3×10^{-5}/locus/generation was estimated (Comings 1986). However, unlike many (not all) new mutations, no increase in the "mutation rate" with the age of the father has been observed. The mutation rate estimate is valid only if the Rett syndrome is, indeed, genetically determined and not caused by an environmental factor. However, the genetic causation is suggested by observation of MZ twins pairs.

One such twin pair has been described by Tariverdian et al. (1987) and has been observed since that time. All the typical clinical signs are concordant. Both twins had relatively frequent epileptic fits of the grand mal type (derivation about 1 min); especially during febrile infections. At the time of their first examination, they had been under treatment with Mylepsinum. The resting EEG was taken frequently; it always showed a relatively regular and synchronized ϑ activity of high amplitude ($\geq$100 µV) but no specific signs of epilepsy (Fig. 8.5). Another MZ pair was observed by Bruck et al. (1991). The most remarkable feature of these twins was their discordance at the time of birth: From the time of birth, twin 1 was hypotonic, moving slowly, and sleeping most of the time. She had seizures several times daily. She showed a certain development but deteriorated later. Twin 2 appeared fairly normal although somewhat hypotonic at birth; at the end of her first year, delay of α quiring speech and gait became obvious. At age 3, she had frequent daily seizures. At age 4, the time of examination, the twins were distinguishable clinically. In both twins EEGs were recorded repeatedly. In twin 1, an EEG at age 2 showed "epileptiform abnormalities with frontal predominance and independent spikes in the Rolandic area and in the right temporal area. The background was excessively low." In twin 2

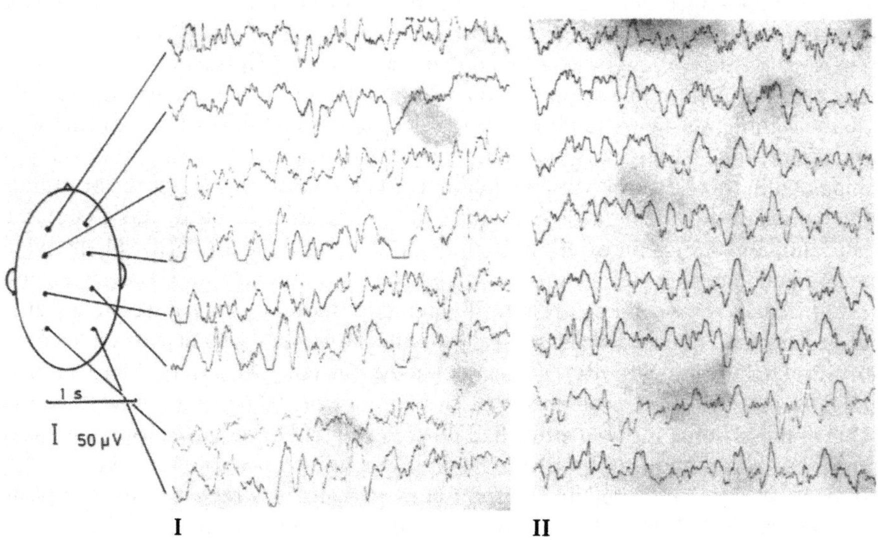

Fig. 8.5. EEG of 5-year-old twins with Rett syndrome. Both twins showed an almost rhythmic but irregular activity of about 4 c/s and high amplitude in all leads

"EEGs showed background abnormality slow for age at 2 years, 6 months and spikes in the right central temporal area one year later." Unfortunately, the EEGs were not shown in this report; therefore it cannot be decided exactly, how similar the EEGs of these twins were and whether clinical discordance at the beginning of their lives was also reflected in their EEGs.

Meanwhile, a few other twin pairs with Rett syndrome have been observed; 7 MZ pairs were recorded as being concordant (Zonghbi 1988).

FraX Syndrome

This syndrome is more common than the Rett syndrome. It is observed predominantly in males; females may also be affected but more rarely and, as a rule, in a much milder way. Two genes have been localized at the long arm of the X chromosome – Frax A and Frax B; mutants of Frax A are much more common. They belong to the trinucleotide expension mutants; the triplet expanded is CGG.52–200 repeats comprise a premutation, 200 to approx. 2000 comprise a full mutation. In this place, we cannot go into any further details (see, for example, Vogel and Motulsky 1996). Suffice it to say that: (a) male hemizygotes of such a mutant are very often severely mentally retarded; (b) female heterozygotes are often mentally quite normal – they may have a slightly subnormal intelligence, but some are also severely retarded; and (c) epileptic seizures are common especially in affected males.

Musumeci et al. (1985; see Musumeci et al. 1988) described a typical EEG pattern that was very similar to that described in Rolandic spike epilepsy: It is characterized by spikes of mean or high voltage that appear in the temporal regions bilaterally, often with diphasic shape, and sometimes with quasi-rhythmic course. They may be multifocal with two independent, occasionally alternating, foci in the two hemispheres. This pattern occurs predominantly during sleep, is reduced during REM sleep, but may be present rarely during wakefulness. A follow-up study on 18 affected males aged between 7 and 37 years (mean age 17.25 years) was performed by the same group. The background activity was normal in 4, and "slow" in 14 cases. The typical spike pattern described above was observed, at least once, in 8 cases; it was absent in two subjects younger than 8 years. These subjects showed sharp waves on the right temporal region both during sleep and wakefulness. On the other hand, the typical EEG pattern was present in only one man older than 16 years, and it disappeared in three cases during the follow-up. These findings suggest the presence of this pattern only during a certain phase of childhood and youth, and a characteristic anomaly of EEG maturation. A study on 29 cytogenetically verified hemizygous males and female heterozygotes was reported by Vieregge and Froster-Iskenius (1989). There were some neurological anomalies but no increased frequency either of seizures or EEG discharges typical for epilepsy. Some patients showed a slowing of EEG background activity. Of the 6 heterozygous female carriers, 3 had a normal EEG. In one case, 4 c/s was observed and another one showed a low-voltage EEG. One of these women, 26 years old, had posterior dysrhythmic discharges with sharp and slow waves. In this publication, a couple of studies have been reviewed in which frequency of epileptic seizures among FraX patients was reviewed for the period 1971–1989. Of 178 patients 43 were reported to have had seizures. Gorbachevskaia and Korsakowa (1997) studied the EEG background activity in 30 patients (age range 4–22 years). All cases show a reduction in occipital α rhythm, prevalence of ϑ rhythm in central-parietal and central-frontal regions and "epileptoid activity" in parietal and centroparietal regions. In heterozygous mothers, considerable EEG variation was found. Slow background activity was also observed in patients with and without seizures by Ribacoba-Montero et al. (1995) and in many FraX children (Lastochkina et al. 1990). The similarity of the EEG in youths with FraX syndrome and benign childhood epilepsy has been confirmed by other reports; however, there is no linkage with a dominant gene for this type of epilepsy (Rees et al. 1993). Latochkina et al. (1992) studied 21 heterozygous women whose intellectual level was described to correspond to the low norm. In 76% of these women, the α rhythm differed from the norm.

In conclusion, the following EEG features in the FraX syndrome appear to be confirmed:

- Epileptic seizures in adult patients and in children and youths are much more common than in the general population but the great majority of patients remain free from such seizures.
- The EEG pattern is similar to that observed in benign childhood epilepsy with centrotemporal spikes; such spikes are especially prominent during sleep (and are reduced in REM sleep).
- Background activity is often described as slow in the majority of cases. It is documented in some but not all reports that α activity is replaced, at least in part, by ϑ activity. While slow activity is noted in almost all reports, precise characterization is lacking in most of them.
- Female heterozygotes and their intellectual level are a common point of discussion in the literature on the FraX syndrome (for details, see Vogel and Motulsky 1996). EEG studies tend to corroborate results from clinical observations and from molecular studies: There is a wide range in variation, from completely normal to abnormal. However, slowing of background α activity, and occasional, dysrhythmic abnormalities are observed, and appear to be more common than in the general population.

The genetic anomalies and diseases described in this chapter have the advantage that they are being analyzed step by step down to their last causes. The way from the genes and chromosomes and their mutations is then be pursued, again step by step through neurobiological mechanisms up to the phenotype. This could make them useful tools for elucidation of mechanisms involved in normal variation and disease.

Huntington Disease

This is an autosomal dominant disease that usually manifests some time during middle age, often in the fifth decade of life. Therefore the problem had been discussed repeatedly whether a diagnosis of the preclinical life period is possible since children of manifest Huntington patients have a risk of 50% to be carriers of this dominant gene and to fall ill with this disease sooner or later. Meanwhile, this scientific problem has been solved since the gene has become known, and the specific mutation leading to this disease (a triplet amplification mutant) can be diagnosed directly by molecular studies (for details, see Vogel and Motulsky 1996). Before this direct diagnosis became possible, however, many research workers looked for subtle neurological signs that may be regarded as early indicators of the disease. Patterson et al. (1948) reported bilateral groups of slow waves in persons at risk; in a study of 25 children of Huntington patients, Harvald (1951) observed "low-voltage fast" EEGs in two individuals at risk who were diagnosed subsequently as choreatics. Some other borderline EEG patterns were also observed. In a study of 50 patients in various phases of the disease Vogel et al. (1961) observed a slightly higher frequency of low-voltage EEGs, often in combination with ϑ waves of relatively low amplitude. EEGs with α waves of low amplitudes in combination with ϑ waves were quite common, and there was a close relationship between severity of the clinical state and degree of EEG alteration. However, EEG patterns characteristic for epilepsies and impressive side differences are not characteristic for the EEG in chorea patients. Most patients in a preclinical phase of the disease have a normal EEG.

8.3 Hereditary EEG Variants Suggesting a Higher Suceptibility for Epilepsy

It is not the purpose of this monograph to describe the EEG phenomena found in the common types of epilepsies. However, some EEG variants are found in higher frequencies among close relatives of epileptics than in the population in general; apparently, they indicate an increased liability for epilepsy. Such EEG traits have been reviewed recently by Doose (1997). According to this author, the five most important EEG signs indicating such liability are: generalized irregular spikes and waves (SW) at rest and during hyperventialtion, the photo-paroxysmal reponse, 4–7 c/s rhythms, occipital 3–4 c/s rhythms and benign focal sharp waves. In healthy children at ages 1–16 years without known susceptibility to epilepsy, Gerken and Doose (1973) found prevalence of SW of 1.8%, the maximum prevalence (2.9%) occurring in 7- to 8-year-old children. Metrakos and Metrakos (1960, 1961) observed that 40% of 4.5- to 16.5-year-old sibs of epileptic probands showing generalized SW had this EEG pattern, while only 7% of their parents showed this trait. These authors concluded that this "centrencephalic trait" was caused by an autosomal dominant gene the penetrance of which was age-dependent. Later studies indicated that the matter is not quite as simple, as suggested by this hypothesis (Gerken and Doose 1973; Doose and Baier 1987). Metrakos and Metrakos did not, for example, differentiate between spontaneous and photically induced SW complexes; it is now obvious that they are different genetically (Doose and Gerken 1973). Spontaneous SW complexes, i.e., those not induced by photic stimulation, are much rarer and their age distribution is different: among 524 sibs of 272 SW-positive probands, the maximum percentage of positive findings was 13% as compared with 2.9% among controls. The distribution of prevalences per age was bimodal, with a primary peak of 13% between 3 and 6 years, and a secondary peak of 8% between 13 and 15 years. Similar prevalences were found in 302 sibs of children with absences, myoclonic and myoclonic-astatic seizures. There was no sex difference of prevalences among sibs. However, SW complexes were more frequent in sibs of female as compared with sibs of male probands (24% vs. 11%). A similar difference

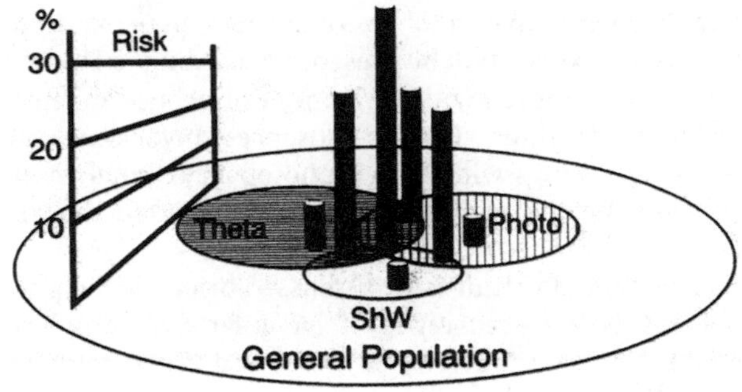

Fig. 8.6. Risk of seizure manifestation related to various susceptibility factors and their interactions. *Theta,* 4–7 c/s rhythm; *photo,* photoparoxysmal response; *shw,* sharp waves. (From Doose 1997)

between prevalences in relatives of female and male probands was also found in a series of relatives of patients with spontaneous myoclonias of myoclonic petit mal type (Tsuboi 1977).

Studies on children of parents showing spontaneous SW-patterns had especially interesting results: 24% of children of parents with primary generalized seizures and spontaneous SW complexes showed this pattern (Benninger et al. 1982; Scheffner 1982). The physiological basis of spontaneous and photically induced SWs appears to be different; the latter but not the former may be caused by a disturbance of dopamine metabolism as suggested by animal experiments (Quesney and Reader 1990). According to Doose (1997), another argument suggesting genetic heterogeneity of the SW complexes is their relationship to other genetically caused EEG patterns, especially its relationship to the 4–7 c/s rhythm of children. Some 63% of children with febrile convulsions and a 4–7 c/s rhythm developed spontaneous SW somewhat later, compared with only 23% of children with febrile convulsions but without 4–7 c/s rhythm (Doose et al. 1966; Baier and Doose 1987; Gundel and Doose 1986). Hence in many instances more than one genetic trait appears to cooperate in creating susceptibility to SW complexes which are a good sign of cortical hyperexcitability (Gloor 1979; (Figs. 8.6, 8.7)).

There seem to be no longitudinal studies on an unbiased series of children with SW complexes to determine their risk of getting epilepsy later in life; such series

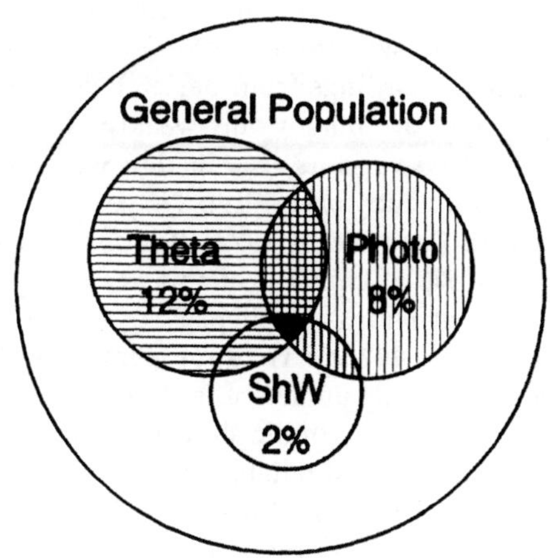

Fig. 8.7. Distribution of three genetic traits in the general population of children, with resulting overlap. *Theta,* 4–7 c/s rhythm; *photo,* photoparoxysmal response; *shw,* sharp waves. (From Doose 1997)

have been available from sibs of epileptic patients (in whom additional genetic risk factors are expected to be present). According to Doose and Baier (1987), the seizure risk of 272 children with SW complexes whose epileptic sibs suffer from idiopathic generalized minor seizures (absences; myoclonic-astatic seizures) was 33%. By contrast, siblings with only a photoparoyxysmal response or only 4–7 s rhythms became affected with seizures no more often than sibs showing a normal EEG (5%–7%).

The next EEG trait to be discussed briefly is the photoparoxysmal response. It is defined as the occurrence of irregular SW complexes after intermittent photic stimulation (for a review, see Doose and Waltz 1993). Many questions are still open; the PPR can show a wide range of expression using a wider definition of PPR (all types of responses, from spikes to full-fledged SW complexes). Doose et al. (1969, 1973) found an average prevalence of 7.6% in 662 healthy children between 1 and 16 years. There was a clear age dependency and girls were more often affected than boys. There are many reports on familial aggregation. Using the wide definition discussed above, PPR were observed in up to 40% of 390 sibs of photosensitive probands (Doose and Gerken 1973). The distribution was age-dependent with a peak between 5 and 15 years; sisters were positive more often than brothers. Prevalence of PPRs was equal in sibs of photosensitive probands with and without epilepsy (Waltz et al. 1992). However, probands with epilepsy and their sibs showed a high incidence of the photoconvulsive reponse. The mode of inheritance of PPRs is not quite clearcut; some observations suggest the contribution of a dominant gene (or dominant genes). In animal experiments, apomorphine, a dopamine receptor agonist, was shown to block PPR for a certain time; in humans suffering from photogenic seizures, such blockade was also observed (Quesney and Reader 1990).

The broad spectrum of clinical manifestations in children showing PPRs cannot be discussed here in greater detail; Doose (1997) estimated that only about 3% of children with a PPR manifest epilepsy up to the age of 20 (see also Scollo-Lavizzari 1971). Still, photosensitivity is often involved in the pathogenesis of various types of epilepsies (especially, obviously, in photogenic seizures). It is also related to other signs of cerebral irritability such as syncopal attacks, vasomotor headache and migraine.

Another EEG trait that is associated with a higher liability for epileptic seizures is the 4–7 c/s rhythm in children (Doose and Baier 1988; Fig. 8.8). These are runs of bilaterally synchronous monomorphic waves demonstrated most clearly by referential recordings from parietal electrodes. These rhythms are often spindle shaped; they are not, or only weakly, affected by opening of the eyes in distinction to the 4–5 c/s variants described in Sect. 4.6. The 4–7 c/s rhythm described here occurs predominantly in children 2–6 years old; usually it is more pronounced in boys than in girls (Doose et al. 1972). It is observed (more or less strongly expressed) in about 10%–15% of children of this age group. However, it is a constant feature in idiopathic generalized epilepsies of early childhood and febrile convulsions. In these instances, 4–7 c/s rhythms persisting during puberty or even adulthood are a prognostically unfavorable clinical sign. In epilepsies with complex partial seizures, for example, rhythmic slowing of EEG background activity, persistence into adulthood is the most reliable predictor of a complicated course with resistance to anticonvulsive therapy (for ref. see Doose 1997). Up to 30% of siblings of epileptic and nonepileptic children with this trait show this pattern compared to 2% of sibs of

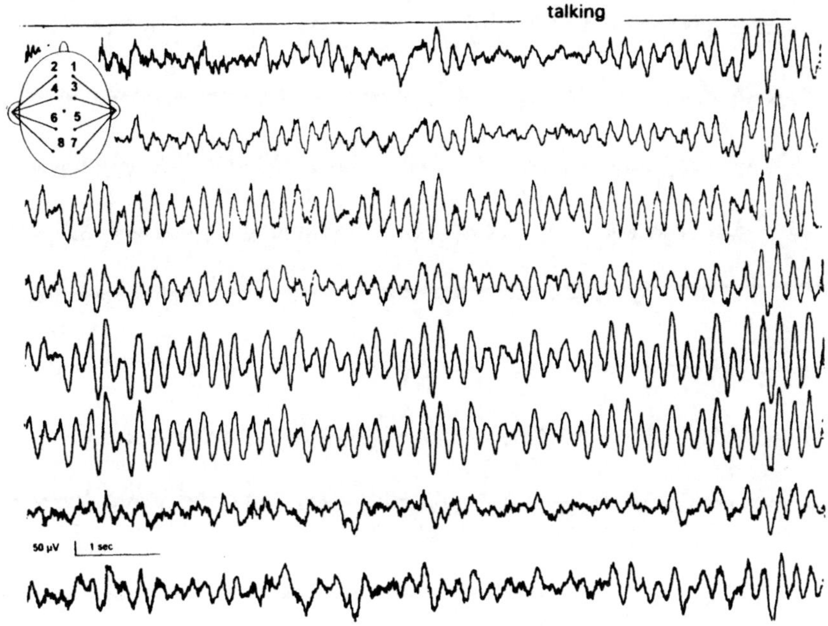

Fig. 8.8. EEG of a 2-year-old, fully awake boy with febrile convulsions; diffuse theta rhythms with parietal accentuation. (From Doose 1997)

children lacking this trait on repeated EEG examinations (Doose et al. 1972). These ϑ rhythms are transmitted genetically independently of other genetic EEG traits; their physiological basis appears to contribute one component within a multifactorial system contributing a genetic liability for epilepsy.

Occipital 3–4 c/s rhythms occurring in runs after eye closure, and consistently blocked by opening of the eyes are common findings in epilepsies and febrile convulsions in childhood (Cobb et al. 1961). They show aggregation in families but their mode of inheritance has not been clarified so far (Gerken and Doose 1972). In sibships of photosensitive children showing this occipital 3–4 c/s pattern, both a PPR and generalized SW complexes are less frequent than in sibs of photosensitive probands and no more frequent than in controls. Doose (1997) explained this as indication that the 3–4 c/s pattern may inhibit manifestation of a PPR and spontaneous SW complexes.

A different EEG trait showing an increased susceptibility for a certain type of epilepsy are focal sharp waves (Fig. 8.9). In sibships of probands showing this EEG pattern, it was found in 36%; an autosomal dominant mode of inheritance with age-dependent penetrance was proposed (Bray et al. 1964, 1965; Heijbel et al. 1975). Doose et al. (1997) found such sharp waves in 13% of sibships aged 4–10 years/only waking records); Degen and Degen (1990) observed sharp waves in only 5.8% of sibs of sharp-wave positive probands. They recorded EEGs during sleep; normally more pathological records are seen at sleep than in the wake state. MZ twins are almost completely concordant (Doose et al. 1997; Fig. 8.9). While earlier hypotheses on the mode of inheritance (Bray et al. 1964, 1965) may have been somewhat oversimplified, this EEG trait appears to be transmitted in families independently of other genetically determined EEG patterns. In healthy children, benign focal sharp

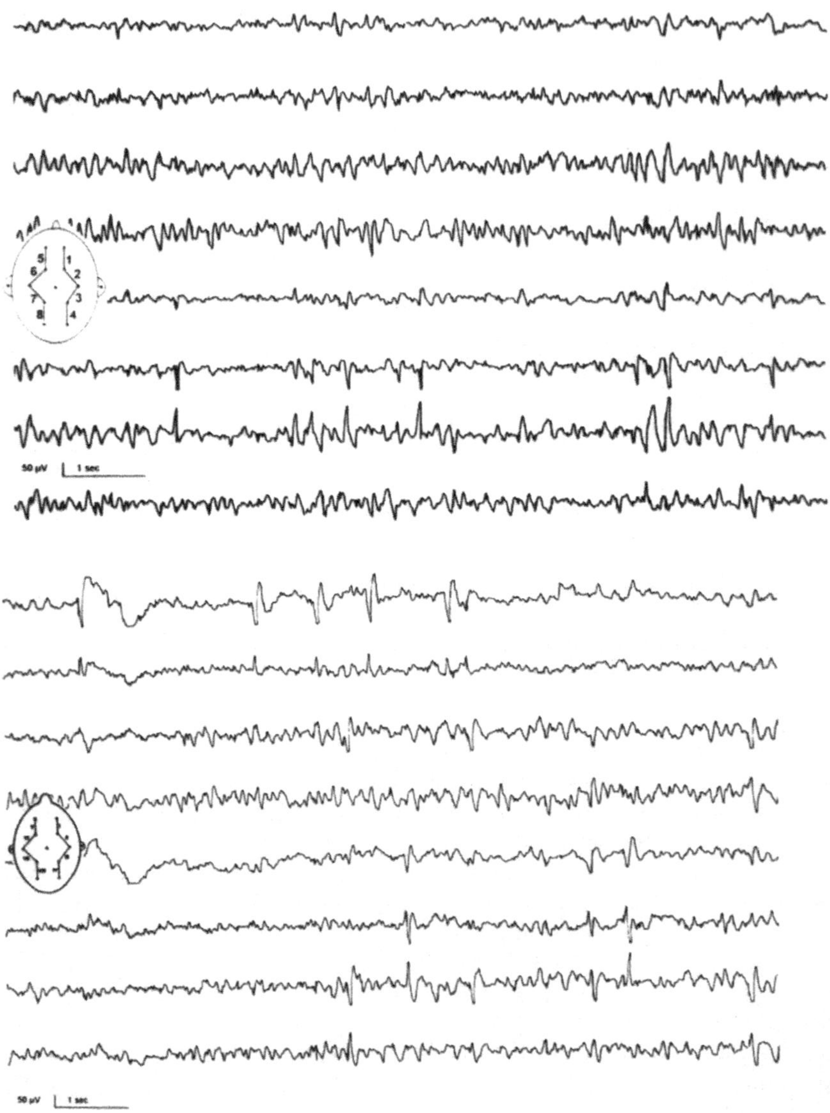

Fig. 8.9. Multifocal sharp waves in male MZ twins, 8 years old. Both suffer from learning problems, especially dyslexia. (From Doose 1997)

waves are to be seen in about 1%–2% only; only about 8% of carriers of this EEG trait may develop seizures. The detailed EEG pattern and clinical signs exhibit strong variability (for details see Doose et al. 1997; Fig. 8.10).

Obviously, different EEG patterns are markers of a genetically determined increased cerebral excitability for epilepsy. However, only a minority of individuals showing the EEG traits actually suffer from seizures. This raises the question: What circumstances may push the individual across the edge toward epilepsy? According

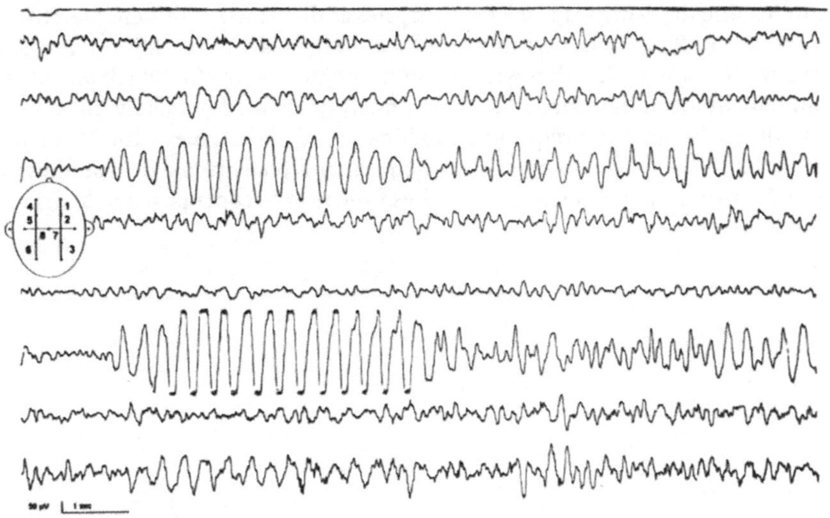

Fig. 8.10. Parieto-occipital delta rhythm after eye closure in a 4-year-old boy with febrile convulsions. (From Doose 1997)

to Doose (1997) who formulated especially clearly the opinion expressed by many observers "one very plausible explanation is that an interaction takes place between an inherited liabilty and exogenous lesional factors. In a large number of epilepsies, the EEG displays unequivocal signs of a constitutional seizure liability, such as PPR or SW ... The still widespread ... categorical differentiation between symptomatic and idiopathic epilepsies ... does not do justice to this pathogenic complexity.

A second plausible mechanism is an interaction between different genetic traits expressed by special EEG markers. If these liabilities are genetically independent of each other and widespread in the general population, as has been confirmed by comprehensive family studies" (for references see above and Doose 1997), "coincidences of these genetic factors must occur with a calculable statistical probability in some individuals ..." (Fig. 8.6, 8.7). "It is not surprising therefore but rather suspected that cases with such combinations of traits will aggregate in groups of epileptic children." This does not mean, however, that there must be a causal connection between these EEG traits; it is much more likely that a combination of anomalies of various neurobiological mechanisms, often in combination with exogenous factors, pushes the individuals beyond the edge toward epilepsy. This way of thinking is similar to the old concept of Krampfbereitschaft (Koch 1955); it is corroborated by the observation (see above) that twin studies have revealed a high but not complete concordance of MZ twins for epilepsy. For genetic counseling in families with epilepsies, empiric risk figures (Blandfort et al. 1987) could be refined by EEG studies in persons, especially children, at risk, and adequate consideration of the EEG traits described above.

These results also suggest new strategies for elucidation of genes and basic mechanisms involved in genetic epilepsies. As discussed in greater detail in Chap. 1, such mechanisms have been elucidated in two rare epilepsy types with simple autosomal dominant mode of inheritance. New family studies should be based on EEG traits leading to predispositions for epilepsies as described in this chapter: SW complexes; the PPR; 4–7 c/s rhythms and focal sharp waves. In addition, it would be worthwhile studying families with monomorpohic a waves for which an autosomal dominant mode of inheritance is not definitely confirmed but likely (Sect. 4.7). The task will not be simple; it requires a combination of EEG studies with DNA analyses, and, in addition, neurobiological, biochemical and pharmacological studies on the levels "in between." However, such studies have now become possible in principle.

Bibliography

Abraham HT, Duffy FH (1991): Computed EEG abnormalities in panic disorder with and without premorbid drug use. Biol. Psychiatr. 29, 687–690

Adams A (1959) Studies on the flat electroencephalogram in man. EEG Clin. Neurophysiol. 11, 34–41

Adams A (1968) Frequenzanalyse des flachen EEG. Dtsch. Z. Nervenheilk. 193, 57–72

Adrian ED, Matthews BH (1934) The Berger rhythm. Potential changes from the occipital lobes in man. Brain 57, 356–385

Amthauer R (1973) I-S-T 70. Intelligenz-Struktur-Test (4th ed.) Göttingen: Hogrefe

Andermann L (1968) The high incidence of mental disturbances in the family of schizophrenic children with excess of immature slow waves in the EEG. EEG Clin. Neurophysiol. 23, 494

Andersen P, Andersson SA (1968) Physiological basis of the alpha rhythm. New York: Appleton–Century–Crofts

Andersen P, Andersson SA (1974) Thalamic origin of cortical rhythmic activity. Handb. of Electroencephalography and Clin. Neurophysiology Vol. 2 Part C, pp. 2C-90-2c-118. Amsterdam: Elsevier

Anderson VE, Hauser WA, Perry JK, Sing CF (eds) (1982) Genetic basis of the epilepsies. New York: Raven Press

Anokhin AP (1986) On the genetic nature of individual peculiarities of the whole-brain EEG organization. The Soviet J. of Psychology 1986, 649–657

Anokhin AP (1987) On the genetic nature of individual peculiarities of the whole-brain EEG organization. The Psychological Journal 8, 146–153

Anokhin AP, Birbaumer N, Lutzenberger W (et al.) (1996) Age increases brain complexity. EEG Clin. Neurophysiol. 99, 63–68

Anokhin AP, Steinlein O, Fischer C (et al.) A genetic study of the human low-voltage electroencephalogram. Hum. Genet. 90, 99–112

Anokhin AP, Vogel F (1996) EEG alpha rhythm frequency and intelligence in normal adults. Intelligence 23, 1–14

Arndt T, Losse H, Hütwohl G (1956) Vegetative Tonuslage und Hirnstrombild. Die Medizinische, pp. 624–627

Arthurs RGS, Cahoon EB (1963–64) A clinical and electroencephalographic survey on psychopathic personality. Amer. J. Psychiatr. 120, 870–877

Baier WK, Doose H (1987) Interdependence of different genetic EEG patterns in siblings of epileptic patients. EEG Clin. Neurophysiol. 66, 483–488

Barideau JC, Ethier M, Braun CMJ (1987) Neurophysiological assessment of selective attention in males at risk for alcololism. In: Johmson R, jun. (et al., eds) Current trends in event-related potential res. (EEG Suppl. 40). New York: Elsevier; pp. 651–656

Barth PG (1987) Diseases of neuronal migration. Canad. J. Neurol. Sci. 14, 1–16

Bauer G (1993) EEG, drug effects and central nervous system poisoning. In: Niedermeyer E, Lopes da Silva F: Electroencephalography, 3rd ed. Baltimore: Williams & Wilkins; pp. 631–642

Bauer LO, Hesselbrock VM (1993) EEG, autonomic and subjective correlates of the risk for alcoholism. J.Stud.Alcohol 54, 577–589

Becker D (1972) Hirnstromanalysen affektiver Verläufe. Göttingen: Hogrefe

Begleiter H, Porjesz B, Bihari B (et al.) (1984) Event-retaled potentials in boys at risk for alcoholism. Science 225, 1493–1496

Benninger CK, Matthis P, Scheffner D (1982) EEG findings in children of epileptic parents. In: Anderson VE (et al.) (eds.) Genetic basis of the epilepsies. New York: Raven Press; pp. 95–99

Berger H (1929) Über das Elektrenkephalogramm des Menschen I. Arch Psychiatr. 87, 527–570

Berger H (1932) Über das Elektrenkephalogramm des Menschen. V. Arch Psychiatr. Nervenheilk. 98, 231–154

Berger H (1938) Das Elektrenkephalogramm des Menschen. Nova Acta Leopoldina 6, 173–309

Berman SM, Martinez RA, Noble EP (1993) Familial alcoholism and ERPs: differences in probability sensitivity? Alcohol – Alcohol. 28, 695–707

Berman SM, Whipple SC, Noble EP (1993) P3 in young boys as a predictor of adolescent substance use. Alcohol. 10, 69–76

Bertelsen A, Harvald B, Hauge M (1977) A Danish twin study of manic-depressive disorders. Brit.J.Psychiatr. 130, 330–351

Bievert C, Schröder BC, Kubisch (et al.) (1998) A potassium channel mutation in neonatal human epilepsy. Science 279, 403–406

Blackburn R (1975) Aggression and the EEG: a quantitative analysis. J. Abnorm. Psychol. 84, 358–365

Blandfort M, Tsuboi T, Vogel F (1987) Genetic counseling in the epilepsies.I.Genetic risks. Hum. Genet. 76, 303–331

Blinkhorn SF, Hendrickson DE (1982) Averaged evoked response and psychometric intelligence. Nature 295, 596–597

Bode H, Bubl R (1992) Lissenzephaliesyndrome. Schweiz. Rundschau Med. Praxis 81, 1529–1533

Boomsma DI, Koopmans JR, Van Doornen LJP, Orlebeke JF (1994) Genetic and social influences on starting to smoke: a study of Dutch adolescent twins and their parents. Addiction 89, 219–226

Borgaonkar S (1989) Chromosomal variation in man. A catalogue of chromosomal variants and anomalies (5th ed.) New York: A. Liss

Borgaonkar DS, Murdoch JL, McKusick VA, Borkow SP, Money JW (1968) The YY syndrome. Lancet 2, 461–462

Bosaeus E, Selldén U (1979) Psychiatric assessment of healthy children with various EEG patterns. Acta Psychiat. Scand. 59, 180–210

Bray PF, Wiser WC (1965) The relation of focal to diffuse epileptiform EEG discharges in genetic epilepsy. Arch. Neurol. 13, 223–237

Bray PF, Wiser WC (1964) Evidence for a genetic etiology of temporal-central abnormalities in focal epilepsy. New Engl. J. Med. 271, 926–933

Brickenkamp R (1962) Der Aufmerksamkeits-Belastungstest(d-2) Göttingen: Hogrefe

Brown BB (1973) Additional characteristic EEG differences between smokers and nonsmokers. In: Dunn WL (ed.) Smoking behavior: Motives and incentives. Washington: V. H. Winston & Sons; pp. 67–81

Brown BB (1975) New mind, new body: new directions of the mind. London: Hodder & Straighton

Bruck I, Philippart M, Giraldi G, Antoniuk S (1991) Difference in early development of presumed monozygotic twins with Rett syndrome Am. J. Med. Genet. 39, 415–417

Bouchard TJ, McGue M (1981) Familial studies of intelligence: a review. Science 212, 1055–1059

Buchsbaum MS (1974) Averaged evoked response and stimulus intensity in identical and fraternal twins. Physiol. Psychology 2, 365–370

Buchsbaum MS (1980) Genetic factors in EEG. Sleep and evoked potentials. In: Davidson RJ, Schwarz GE: Human consciousness and its transformations. New York: Plenum Press

Buchsbaum MS, Pfefferbaum A (1971) Individual differences in stimulus intensity response. Psychophysiology 8, 600–611

Bulayeva K, Pavlova T, Guseynov G (1993) Visual evoked potentials: Phenotypic and genotypic variability. Behavior Genetics 23, 443–447

Bunge M, Ardila R (1987) Philosophy of Psychology. Berlin etc.: Springer Verlag

Butler SR, Glass A (1974) Asymmetries in the EEG associated with cerebral dominance. EEG Clin. Neurophysiol. 36, 481–491

Callaway E (1973) Correlations between averaged evoked potentials and measures of intelligence. Arch. Gen. Psychiatr. 29, 553–558
Callaway E (1975) Brain electrical potentials and individual psychological differences. New York etc.: Grune & Stratton
Canabate-Reche F (et al.) (1993) The 11q- syndrome. Report of a new case. An. Esp. Pediatr. 38, 562–563
Caspers H (1958) Die Beeinflussung der kortikalen Krampferregbarkeit durch das aufsteigende Retikulärsystem des Hirnstammes.II.Narkosewirkungen. Z. Ges. Exp. Med. 129, 582
Caspers H, Abele G (1956) Hirnelektrische Untersuchungen zur Frage der quantitativen Beziehung zwischen Blutalkoholgehalt und Alkoholeffekt. Dtsch. Z. Gerichtl. Med. 45, 509
Cattell AB, Eber HW, Tatsuoka MM (1970) Handbook for the Sixteen Personality Factor Questionnaire (16 PF). Colorado Drive: Inst. f. Personality (etc.) Champaign
Chamberlain GHA, Russell JG (1952) The EEGs of relatives of schizophrenics. J. Ment. Sci. 98, 654–659
Charlier C, Singh NA, Ryan SG (et al.) (1998) A pore mutation in a novel KQT-like potassium channel gene in an idiopathic epilepsy family. Nature Genetics 18, 53–55
Christian JC, Li T-K, Norton JA (et al.) (1988) Alcohol effects on the percentage of beta waves in the electroencephalograms of twins. Genetic Epidemiology 5, 217–224
Christian W (1968) Klinische Elektroencephalographie. Stuttgart: Thieme Verlag
Christian W (1984) Das Elektroencephalogramm im höheren Lebensalter. Nervenarzt 55, 517–524
Cigánek L (1969) Variability of the human visual evoked potential: normative data. EEG Clin. Neurophysiol. 27, 35–42
Cigánek L (1975) Visual evoked responses. In: Rémond A (ed.) Handb. of Electroencephalography and Clin. Neurophysiol. Amsterdam: Elsevier, pp. 33–59
Claridge G, Broks P (1984) Schizotypy and hemisphere function I. Person. indiv. Diff. 5, 633–648
Claridge G, Robinson DL, Birchall P (1985) Psychophysiological evidence of 'psychoticism' in schizophrenic's relatives. Person. indiv. Diff. 6, 1–10
Clausen J, Sersen FA, Lidsky A (1977) Sleep patterns in mental retardation: Down's syndrome. EEG Clin. Neurophysiol. 43, 183–191
Clementz BA, Sponheim SR, Iacono WG, Beiser M (1994) Resting EEG in first-episode schizophrenic patients, bipolar psychosis patients, and their first-degree relatives. Psychophysiology 31, 486–494
Cloninger CR (1987) Neurogenetic adaptive mechanisms in alcoholism. Science 236, 410–416
Cobb WA, Gordon M, Matthews C, Niemann E (1961) Occipital delta rhythms in petit mal. EEG Clin. Neurophysiol. 13, 142
Cohen HL, Porjesz B, Begleiter H (1991) EEG characteristics in males at risk for alcoholism. Alcohol Clin. Exp. Res. 15, 858–861
Cohen J, Cohen P (1983) Applied multiple regression/correlation analysis for the behavioral sciences. Hillsdale, NJ: Erlbaum
Comings DE (1986) The genetics of Rett syndrome: the consequence of a disorder where every case is a new mutation. Am. J. Med. Genet. 24, 383–388
Conrad K (1936) Erbanlage und Epilepsie. III. Ein Beitrag zur Zwillingskasuistik: Die diskordanten Eineiigen. Z. Ges. Neurologie u. Psychiatrie 155, 509–542
Conrad K (1938) Epilepsie.Vererbung und Konstitution. Z. Ges. Neurologie u. Psychiatrie 161, 280–292
Coppola R (1979) Isolating low frequency activity in EEG spectrum analysis. EEG Clin. Neurophysiol. 46, 224–226
Cornil L, Gastaut H (1947) Étude EEG-phigue de la dominance sensorielle d'une hémisphère cérébrale. Presse Méd. 37, 421–422
Cotton NS (1979) The familial incidence of alcoholism. J. Stud. Alcohol. 40, 89–116
Cowdry R, Pickar D (1985/86) Symptoms and EEG findings in the borderlline syndrome. Intern. J. Psychiatry in Medicine 15, 201–211
Coyle JT, Oster-Granite ML, Gearhart JD (1986) The neurobiological consequences of Down syndrome. Brain Res. Bull. 16, 773–787

Crow TJ (1987) The scope for non-genetic factors in etiology: The retrovirus-transposon hypothesis. In: Helmchen H, Henn FA (eds.) Biological perspectives of Schizophrenia. New York: Wiley, pp. 85–105

Daly RF (1969) Neurological abnormalities in XYY males. Nature 221, 472–473

Davis H, Davis PA (1936) Action potentials of the brain. Arch. Neurol. 36, 1214–1224

Davis PA (1942) A comparative study of the EEGs of schizophrenic and manic-depressive patients. Amer. J. Psychiatr. 99, 210

Davis PA, Davis H (1939) Electroencephalograms of psychotic patients. Amer. J. Psychiatr. 95, 1007

Dawson GD (1954) A summation technique for the detection of small evoked potentials. EEG Clin. Neurophysiol. 6, 65–84

Degen R, Degen HE (1990) Some genetic aspects of rolandric epilepsy: Waking and sleep EEGs in siblings. Epilepsia 31, 795–801

Dencker SJ (1958) A follow-up study of 128 closed head injuries in twins using co-twins as controls. Acta Psychiat. Scand. 33, Suppl. 123:1–125

Dieker H (1967) Untersuchungen zur Genetik besonders regelmäßiger hoher Alpha-Wellen im EEG des Menschen. Hum. Genet. 4, 189–216

Dongier M (et al.) (1974) Mental diseases. In: Handb.Electroencephalography and Clin. Neurophysiolog. Vol.13, Clinical EEG III (Ed. H. Gastaut). Amsterdam: Elsevier, pp. 13B1–13B78

Doose H (1997) Genetic EEG traits in the pathogenesis of the epilepsies. J. Epilepsy 10, 97–110

Doose H, Baier WK (1987) Genetic factors in epilepsies with primary generalized minor seizures. Neuropediatrics 18 (Suppl.):1–64

Doose H, Baier WK (1988) Theta rhythms in the EEG: a genetic trait in childhood epilepsy. Brain Dev. 10, 347–354

Doose H, Baier WK (1989) Benign partial epilepsies and related conditions: multifactorial pathogenesis with hereditary impairment of brain maturation. Eur. J. Pediat. 149, 152–158

Doose H, Gerken H (1973) On the genetics of EEG anomalies in childhood. IV. Photoconvulsive reaction. Neuropädiatrie 4, 162–171

Doose H, Gerken H, Hien-Voelpel KF, Völzke E (1969) Genetics of photosensitive epilepsy. Neuropädiatrie 1, 56–73

Doose H, Gerken H, Koenig G, Völzke E (1978) Occipital 3-4/s rhythms in childhood EEG. Neuropädiatrie 10: 140–156

Doose H, Gerken H, Völzke E (1972) On the genetics of EEG anomalies in childhood. I. Abnormal theta rhythms. Neuropädiatrie 3, 386–401

Doose H, Neubauer B, Carlsson G (1996) Children with benign focal sharp waves in the EEG: developmental disorders and epilepsy. Neuropediatrics 27, 227–241

Doose H, Völzke E, Petersen CE, Herzberger E (1966) Fieberkrämpfe und Epilepsie:I. Ätiologie, klinisches Bild und Verlauf der sogenannten Infekt-oder Fieberkrämpfe. Arch. Psychiatr. Neurol. 208, 400–412

Doose H, Waltz S (1993) Photosensitivity: Genetics and clinical significance. Neuropediatrics 24, 249–255

Dumermuth G (1068) Variance spectra of electroencephalograms in twins. Kelleway P, Petersen I: Clinical electroencephalography of children.Stockholm: Almquist & Wiksell, pp. 119–154

Dumermuth G (1972) Elektroencephalographie im Kindesalter. Stuttgart: Thieme Verlag

Dustman RE, Beck EC (1963) Long-term stability of visually evoked potentials in man. Science 142, 1480–1481

Ehlers CL, Schuckit MA (1991) Evaluation of EEG alpha activity in sons of alcoholics. Neuropsychopharmacology 4, 199–206

Ellingson RJ (1954) The incidence of EEG abnormality among patients with mental disorders of apparently nonorganic origin: A critical review. Amer. J. Psychiat. 111, 263–275

Ellingson RJ (1956) Brain waves and problems of psychology. Psychol. Bull. 53, 1–34

Ellingson RJ (1966) Relationship betwen EEG and test intelligence: A commentary. Psychol. Bull. 65, 91–98

Ellingson RJ (1972) EEG in disorders associated with chromosome anomalies. Handb. Electroencephalography and Clin.Neurophysiol., Amsterdam: Elsevier,pp. 19–23

Engel R, Henderson NB (1973) Visual evoked responses and I.Q.scores at school age. Dev. Med. Child. Neurol. 15, 136–147

Enoch M-A,Rohrbough JW, Davis EZ (et al.) (1995) Relationship of genetically transmitted alpha EEG traits to anxiety disorder and alcoholism. Am. J. Med. Genet. (Neuropsychiatr. Genetics) 60, 400–408
Ertl B, Schafer EWP (1969) Brain response correlates of psychometric intelligence. Nature 22, 421–422
Evans DAP (1993) Genetic factors in drug therapy. Cambridge: Cambridge Univ. Press
Eysenck HJ (1967) The biological basis of personality. Springfield: Thomas
Eysenck HJ (1970) The structure of human personality. London: Methuen
Eysenck HJ (Ed.) (1982) A model for intelligence. Berlin etc.: Springer Verlag
Eysenck HJ & Eysenck SBG (1964) Eysenck Personality Inventory. London: Univ. of London Press
Falconer DS (1981) Introduction to quantitative genetics (2nd, ed.) Edinburgh: Oliver & Boyd
Fenton GW, Tennent TG, Fenwick PB, Rattray N (1974) The EEG in antisocial behavior: a study of posterior temporal slow activity in special hospital patients. Psychol. Med. 4, 181–186
Feuerlein W (1979) Alkoholismus – Mißbrauch und Abhängigkeit. Stuttgart: Thieme Verlag
Fink M, Itil T, Clyde D (1966) The classification of psychoses by quantitative EEG measures. Rec. Adv. Biol. Psychiatry 8, 305–312
Fischer C, Schweigert C, Spreckelsen, Vogel F (1996) Programs, data bases and expert systems for human geneticists – a survey. Hum. Genet. 97, 129–137
Fisher RA (1918) The correlation between relatives on the supposition of Mendelian inheritance. Trans. Roy. Soc. Edinburgh 52, 399–433
Flor-Henry P, Koles ZJ (1982) EEG characteristics of normal subjects: A comparison of men and women and of dextrals and sinistrals. Res. Comm. in Psychology, Psychiatry, and Behavior 7, 21–38
Flor-Henry P, Koles ZJ (1984) Statistical quantitative EEG studies of depression, mania, schizophrenia and normals. Biol. Psychology 19, 257–279
Förg B (1984) Über subjektive Beschwerden negativer Art bei Trägern genetisch bedingter Normvarianten des Elektroencephalogramms. Med. Dissertation Heidelberg
Folstein S, Rutter M (1977) Infantile autism: a genetic study on 21 twin pairs. J. Child. Psychol. Psychiatry 18, 297–321
Friedl W, Vogel F (1979) Geschlechtsunterschiede im normalen Ruhe-EEG bei jungen Erwachsenen. Z. EEG-EMG 10, 70–79
Friedländer WJ (1958) Electroencephalographic alpha-rate in adults as a function of age. Geriatrics 13, 29–31
Gabrielli WF, Mednick SA, Volavka J (et al.) (1982) Electroencephalograms in children of alcoholic fathers. Psychophysiology 19, 404–407
Gale A, Coles M, Blaydon J (1969) Extraversion-introversion and the EEG. Brit. J. Psychol. 60, 209–223
Galton F (1865) Hereditary talent and character. Macmillan's Magazine 12:157
Gerken H, Doose H (1972) On the genetics of EEG anomalies in childhood. II. Occipital 2–4/s rhythms. Neuropädiatrie 3, 437–454
Gerken H, Doose H (1973) On the genetics of EEG anomalies in childhood.III. Spikes and waves in the resting record and/or during hyperventilation. Neuropädiatrie 4, 88–97
Gesell A, Thompson H (1929) Learning and growth in identical infant twins: an experimental study by the method of co-twin control. Genet. Psychol. Monogr. 6, 5–124
Giannitrapani D (1969) EEG average frequency and intelligence. EEG Clin. Neurophysiol. 27, 480–486
Giannitrapani D (1985) The electrophysiology of intellectual functions. Basel etc.: Karger Verlag
Gibbs FA, Gibbs EL (1950; 1952) Atlas of electroencephalography, 2nd ed. Cambridge (Vol. 1, 1950; vol. 2, 1952).
Gibbs FA, Gibbs EL, Hirsch W (1965) Auffällige EEG-Befunde bei Mongoloiden. Elektromedizin 10, 73–75
Gibbs EL, Gibbs FA, Hirsch W (1964) Rarity of 14 and 6 per second positive spiking among mongoloids. Neurology 14, 581–583
Gloor P (1979) Generalized epilepsy with spike amd wave discharges: a reinterpretation of its electrographic and clinical manifestations. Epilepsia 20, 571–588

Götze W, Vogel F, Wolter M (1958) Findet man im Hirnstrombild von Zwillingen besonders häufig pathologische Veränderungen? Dtsch. Z. Nervenheilk. 177, 374–377
Goldberger AL (1996) Non-linear dynamics for clinicians: chaos theory, fractals, and complexity at the bedside. Lancet 347, 1312–1314
Goldstein L, Sugerman AA, Stolberg H (et al.) (1965) Electro-cerebral activity in schizophrenics and non-psychotic subjects: quantitative EEG amplitude analysis. EEG Clin. Neurophysiol. 19, 350–362
Golubeva EA (1980) Individual characteristics of human memory: A psychophysiological study. Moscow: Pedagogika
Gorbachevskaia NL, Denisova LV (1997) Zn-Nevral-Psikhiatr-Im-SS Korsakova 97, 33–37
Gottlober AB (1938) The inheritance of brain potential patterns. J. Exp. Psychol. 22, 193–200
Gross MD, Wilson WC (1964) Behavior disorders in children with cerebral dysrhythmias. Arch. Gen. Psychiatr. 11, 610–619
Gulotta F, Rehder H, Gropp A (1981) Descriptive neuropathology of chromosomal disorders in man. Hum. Genet. 57, 337–344
Gundel A, Doose H (1986) Genetic EEG patterns in febrile convulsions: a multivariate analysis. Neuropediatrics 17, 3–6
Gunnarson S (1945) Electroencephalography examinations of imbeciles. Acta Paediat. Scand. 32, 426–434
Hagberg BI, Wift-Engerström I (1986) Rett syndrome: a suggested staging system for describing impairment profile with increasing age towards adolescence. Am. J. Med. Genet. 24, 47–59
Haier RJ, Robinson DL, Braden WL, Williams D (1983) Electrical potentials of the cerebral cortex and psychometric intelligence. Person. Individ. Diff. 4, 591–599
Haken H (1996) Principles of brain functioning. Berlin etc.: Springer Verlag
Haken H, Haken-Krell M (1997) Gehirn und Verhalten. Stuttgart: Deutsche Verlagsanstalt
Hallgren B (1960) Nocturnal enuresis in twins. Acta Psychiat. Scand. 53, 73–90
Hambert G, Frey TS (1964) The electroencephalogram in the Klinefelter syndrome. Acta Psychiat. Scand. 40, 28–36
Handal NM, Masand P, Weilburg JB (1995) Panic disorder and complex partial seizures. A truly complex relationship. Psychosomatics 36, 498–502
Harper MA, Morris M, Bleyerveld J (1972) The significance of an abnormal EEG in psychopathic personalities. Aust. N. Z. J. Psychiatr. 6, 215–223
Harvald B (1951) On the possibility of predicting Huntington's chorea by electroencephalographic study. Amer. J. Psychiatr. 108, 295–297
Hathaway SR, McKinley JC: Minnesota Multiphasic Personality Inventory, Manual. Univ. of Minnesota, rev. 1967
Hathaway SR, McKinley JC, Spreen O (1963) MMPI Saarbrücken. Handbuch zur deutschen Ausgabe. Bern, Stuttgart, Wien: Huber
Havstadt JW, Ehlers CL (1989) Attractor dimension of nonstationary dynamical systems from small data sets. Phys. Rev. A 39, 845–853
Heijbel J, Blom S, Rasmuson M (1975) Benign epilepsy of childhood with centrotemporal EEG foci: a genetic study. Epilepsia 16, 285–293
Heintel H, Schalt E, Vogel F (1986) The 4-5 c/s rhythm changes in time. Europ. Arch. Psychiatr. Neurolog. Sci. 235, 299–300
Hendrickson AE (1982) The biological basis of intelligence, Part I: Theory. In: Eysenck HJ (ed.) A model for intelligence. Berlin etc.: Springer Verlag, pp. 151–196
Hendrickson DE (1982) The biological basis of intelligence. Part II: Measurement. In: Eysenck HJ (ed.) A model for intelligence. Berlin etc.: Springer Verlag
Herrmann T (1972) Lehrbuch der empirischen Persönlichkeitsforschung. Göttingen: Hogrefe
Herrnstein RJ, Murray C (1994) The bell curve. Intelligence and class structure in American life. New York etc.: The Free Press
Heuschert D (1963) EEG-Untersuchungen an eineiigen Zwillingen im höheren Lebensalter. Diss. Berlin 1963
Heuschert D (1963) EEG-Untersuchungen an eineiigen Zwillingen im höheren Lebensalter. Z. Menschl. Vererb.- u. Konst.-Lehre 37, 128–172

Hesselbrock V, Bauer L, O'Connor S, Gillen R (1993) Reduced P300 amplitude in relation to family history of alcoholism and antisocial personality disorder among young men at risk for alcoholism. Alcohol - Alcohol.-Suppl. 2, 95–100

Hill D (1944) Central dysrhythmia: its significance in aggressive behavior. Proc. Roy. Soc. Med. 37, 317–328

Hill D (1952) EEG in episodic psychotic and psychopathic behavior. EEG Clin Neurophysiol. 4, 419–442

Hill D, Fenton GW (1969) The temporal lobe: EEG and disorders of behavior. Curr. Probl. in Neuropsychiatr., pp. 49–54; Brit. J. Psychiatr. Special Publ. No. 4

Hill SY, Steinhauer SR, Zubin J (et al.) (1988) Event-related potentials as markers for alcoholism in high density families. Alcohol Clin. Exp. Res. 12, 545–554

Hill SY, Steinhauer SR (1993) Assessment of prebubertal and postpubertal boys and girls at risk for developing alcoholism with P300 from a visual discrimination task. J. Stud. Alcohol. 54, 350–358

Hill SY, Steinhauer SR (1993) Event-related potentials in women at risk for alcoholism. Alcohol. 10, 349–354

Höchel G (1942) Der Wellenindex, eine Methode zur zahlenmäßigen Auswertung des menschlichen Elektroencephalogramms. Z. ges. Neurol. Psychiatr. 174, 281–294

Høncke P, Strömgren E, Zahle V (1949) Elektrencephalographische Untersuchungen an Psychopathen. Arch. Psychiat. Z. Neurolog. 183, 55–63

Höpp HP (1983) Entwicklung eines Versuchsprogramms zur Untersuchung genetischer Hirnstromvarianten mit Hilfe von evozierten Potentialen. Med. Dissertation Heidelberg

Holland AJ, Hall A, Murray R (et al.) (1984) Anorexia nervosa: a study of 34 twin pairs and one set of triplets. Brit. J. Psychiatr. 145, 414–419

Holland AJ, Sicotte N, Treasure J (1988) Anorexia nervosa: evidence for a genetic basis. J. Psychosomatic Res. 32, 561–571

Horn W (1962) Performance Testing System. Göttingen: Hogrefe

Hurst LA (1952) Electroencephalographic support for a genetically oriented organic concept of schizophrenia. J. Nerv. Ment. Dis. 115, 95–120

Inoue E (1960) Observations on forty twin index cases with chronic epilepsy and their co-twins. J. Nerv. Ment, Dis. 130, 401–416

Jasper HH, Fitzpatrick CP, Solomon P (1939) Analogies and opposites in schizophrenia and epilepsy; electroencephalographic and clinical studies. Amer. J, Psychiat. 95, 835

Jensen AR (1973) Educability and group differences. London: Methuen

Jellinek EM (1960) Alcololism, a genius and some of its species. Canad. Med. Ass. J. 83, 1341–1346

Juel-Nielsen N (1965) Individual and environment. A psychiatric-psychological investigation of monozygotic twind reared apart. Acta Psychiat. Scand. (Suppl.) 183

Juel-Nielsen N, Harvald B (1958) The electroencephalogram in uniovular twins brought up apart. Acta Genet. Statist. Med. 8, 57–64

Jung R (1941) Das Elektroencephalogramm und seine klinische Anwendung.II. Das EEG des Gesunden, seine Variationen und Veränderungen und deren Bedeutung für das pathologische EEG. Nervenarzt 14, 57,104

Jung R (1953) Die Tätigkeit des Nervensystems. Neurophysiologische Untersuchungsmethoden. Hdb. Inn. Med. 4. Auflage Bd. V, 1; Berlin etc.: Springer Verlag

Jung R (1958) Neuropharmakologie: Zentrale Wirkungsmechanismen chemischer Substanzen und ihre neurophysiologischen Grundlagen. Klin.Wschr. 36, 1153–1165

Juolasmaa A, Toivakka E, Outakovski J (et al.) (1986) Relationship of quantitative EEG and cognitive test performance in patients with cardiac valvular disease. Scand. J. Psychol. 27, 30–38

Kagan J, Moss HA, Sigel IE (1963) Psychological significance of conceptualization. In: J. C. Wright and J. Kagan (eds.) Basic cognitive processes in children. Monographs of the Society for Research in Child Development, No. 86

Kagan J, Rosman BL, Day D, Albert J, Phillips W (1964) Information processing in the child: significance of analytical and reflective attitudes. Psychological Monographs, Whole Nr. 10

Kaneko Z, Hishikawa Y (1981) Paradoxical sleep in psychiatric disorders and narcolepsy. Internat. J. Neurol. 15, 40–55

Kaplan J, Fredrickson PA, Richardson JW (1991) Sleep and breathing in patients with the Prader-Willi syndrome. Mayo Clin. Proc. 66, 1124–1126

Kendler KS, McLean C, Neale M (et al.) (1991) The genetic epidemiology of bulimia nervosa. Amer. J. Psychiatr. 148, 1627–1637

Kennard MA, Rabinovich MS, Schwartzman AE, Fister WP (1956) Factor of aggression as related to the electroencephalogram. Dis. of the Nervous System 17, 3–7

Keshavan MS, Anderson S, Pettegrew JW (1994) Is schizophrenia due to excessive synaptic pruning in the prefrontal cortex? The Feinberg hypothesis revisited. J. Psychiatr. Res. 28, 239–265

Keuth U, Schmidt E, Tzieply G (1965) Katamnestische Untersuchungen einschließlich EEG zur perinatalen Schädigung von Zwillingen. Mschr. Kinderheilk. 113, 280–281

Kidron DP, Weiss AA (1958) Maturation defect. Elerctroencephalographic and psychological correlation. Psychiat. Neurol. Basel 135, 378–401

Kilian W (1986) On the genetics of Rett syndrome: analysis of family pedigree data. Am. J. Med. Genet. 24, 369–376

Klimesch W, Schimke H, Pfurtscheller G (1993) Alpha frequency, cognitive load and memory performance. Brain Topography 5, 241–251

v. Knorring L, Monakhow K, Perris C (1978) Augmenting-reducing: an adaptive switch mechanism to cope with incoming signals in healthy subjects and psychiatric patients. Neuropsychobiology 4, 150–179

Knott V, Waters B, Lapierre Y,(et al.) (1985) Neurophysiological correlates of sibling pairs discordant for bipolar affective disorders. Amer. J. Psychiatr. 142, 248–250

Koch G (1955) Krampfbereitschaft. Roma: Analecta Genetica

Kopun M, Propping P (1977) The kinetics of ethanol absorption and elimination in twins and supplemenrary repetition experiments in singleton subjects. Eur. J. Clin. Pharmakol. 11, 337–344

Kornetzky C, Orzack MH (1978) Physiological and behavioral correlates of attention dysfunction in schizophrenic patients. J. Psychiatr. Res. 14, 69–79

Kozhushko LF, Kozlova IA, Leibovich FA (1979) (EEG characteristics of the parents in relation to the form of the course of schizophrenia in the children) (Russian) Zh. Nevropatol. Psikhiatr. 79, 585–591

Kreezer G (1939) Intelligence level and occipital alpha rhythm in the Mongolian type of mental deficiency. Amer. J. Psychol. 52, 503–532

Krüger J, Schalt E, Vogel F (1981) Charakterisierung erblicher EEG-Varianten mit Hilfe der Amplituden-Intervall-Analyse. III. Das Klassifizierungsproblem: Zuordnung eines neu abgeleiteten EEG zu einem der bekannten EEG-Typen auf Grund der Parameterwerte der Amplituden-Intervall-Analyse. Z. EEG-EMG 12, 113–119

Krüger J, Schnobel R, Vogel F (1985) Die Oszillation, ein neues Maß für die Gesamt-Amplitude evozierter Potentiale. Z. EEG-EMG 16, 169–170

Kuhlo W (1967) Die 4-5/sec EEG-Grundrhythmusvariante im Schlaf und nach Contusio cerebri. Arch. Psychiat. Nervenkrankh. 210, 68–75

Kuhlo W, Heintel H, Vogel F (1969) The 4-5 c/sec rhythm. EEG Clin. Neurophysiol. 26, 613–619

Kupfer DJ (1976) REM latency – a psychobiological marker for primary depressive disease. Biol. Psychiatr. 11, 159

Kupfer DJ, Foster FG (1978) EEG sleep and depression. In: RL Williams, I Karacan (Eds) Sleep disorders – diagnostics and treatment. New York: J. Wiley & Sons, pp. 163–204

Lastochkina NA, Kuprianova LM,Marincheva GS (1990) (Clinico-electrophysiological examination of children with Martin-Bell syndrome) (Russian). Zh. Nevropatol. Psikhiatr., -Im S-S-Korsakova 90, 69–75

Lauer CJ, Schreiber W, Holsbeer F, Krieg JC (1995) In quest of identifying vulnerability markers for psychiatric disorders by all-night polysonography. Arch. Gen. Psychiatr. 52, 145–153

Lebedev AN (1990) Cyclical neural codes for human memory and some quantitative regularities in experimental psychology. In: H.-G. Geissler (ed.) Psychophysiological explorations of mental structures. Toronto: Hogrefe & Huber

Lennox WG (1951) The heredity of epilepsy as told by relatives and twins. J. Amer. Med. Ass. 146, 529–536

Lennox WG, Gibbs FA, Gibbs EL (1945) The brain wave pattern, a hereditary trait. Evidence from 74 "normal" pairs of twins. J. Hered. 36, 233–243

Lennox WG, Jolly D (1954) The heredity of epilepsy as told by relatives and twins. A. Res. Nerv. & Ment. Dis. Proc. 33, 325–345
Leppert M, Anderson VE, Quattlebaum T (et al.) (1989) Benign familial neonatal convulsions linked to genetic markers on chromosome 20. Nature 337, 647–648
Levy S, Kennard M (1953) A study of the electroencephalogram as related to personality structure in a group of inmates of a state penitentiary. Amer. J. Psychiatr. 109, 832–839
Lewis TB, Leach RJ, Ward K (et al.) (1997) Genetic heterogeneity in benign familialneonatal convulsions: identification of a new locus. Amer. J. Hum. Genet. 53, 670–675
Lindsley DB (1939) A longitudinal study of the alpha rhythm in normal children: frequency and amplitude standards. J. Genet. Psychol. 55, 197–203
Lipák J,Zsadányi O, Baszó J, Kleininger O (1970) EEG abnormalities in normal twins. Acta Med. Acad. Sci. Hungaricae, Tomus 27, 31–43
Lopes da Silva F (1993) Computer-assisted EEG diagnosis: Pattern recognotion and brain mapping. In: Electroencephalography (E. Niedermeyer and F. Lopes da Silva, eds.) (3rd ed.) Baltimore: Williams & Wilkins, pp. 1063–1086
Lopes da Silva F (1993) Event-related potentials: Methodology and quantification. In: Electroencephalography (E. Niedermeyer and F. Lopes da Silva, eds. (3rd ed.) Baltimore: Williams & Wilkins, pp. 877–886
Loomis, Harvey, Hobart (1936) Electrical potentials of the human brain. J. Exp. Psychol. 19, 249–279
Loomis SD (1965) EEG abnormalities as a correlate of behavior in adolescent male delinquents. Amer. J. Psychiatr. 121, 1003–1007
Lowitzsch K, Maurer J, Hopf CH (1983) Evozierte Potentiale in der klinischen Diagnostik. Stuttgart: Thieme Verlag
Lu CS, Chu NS (1991) Effects of alcohol on myoclonus and somatosensoric evoked potentials in dyssynergia cerebellaris myoclonica. J. Neurol. Neurosurg. Psychiatry 54, 905–908
Lukas SE, Mendelson JH, Kouri E (et al.) (1991)Alterations in the distribution of the auditory P300 evoked response potential: similarities between ethanol and divided attention task performance. NIDA Res. Monogr. 105, 605–606
Lutzenberger W, Elbert T, Rockstroh B, Birbaumer N (1985) Das EEG. Berlin etc.: Springer Verlag
Lykken D, Tellegen A, Thorkelson K (1974) Genetic determination of EEG frequency spectra. Biolog. Psychology 1, 245–259
Lykken D, Tellegen A, Iacono W (1982) EEG spectra in twins: Evidence for a neglected mechanism of genetic determination. Physiolog. Psycholog. 10, 60–65
Malafosse A, Leboyer M, Dulac O (et al.) (1992) Confirmation of linkage of benign familial neonatal convulsions to D20S19 and D20S20. Hum. Genet. 89, 54–58
Malykh S, Ravich-Shcherbo I (1986) Genotypical dependence of movement related brain potentials. In: V. Gallai (ed.) Maturation of the CNS and evoked potentials. Amsterdam, Elsevier, pp. 247–252
Marin-Padilla M (1975) Abnormal neuronal differentiation (functional maturation) in mental retardation. Birth Defects 11, 133–153
Marjerrison G, Krause AE, Keogh RP (1968) Variability of the EEG in schizophrenia: Quantitative analysis with a modulus voltage integrator
Matsumoto A, Kumagai T,Miura K, (et al.) (1992) Epilepsy in Angelman syndrome associated with chromosome 15 deletion. Epilepsia 33, 1083–1090
McKusick VA (1995) Mendelian inheritance in man (11th ed.) Baltimore: Johns Hopkins Univ. Press
Mendel JG (1865) Versuche über Pflanzenhybriden. Verhandl. Naturforsch. Verein Brünn
Mendlewicz J, Hoffmann G, Kerkhofs M, Linkowski P (1984) Electroencephalogram and neuroendocrine parameters in pubertal and adolescent depressed children. J. Affective Disorders 6, 265–272
Meshkova TA (1992) Laterality effects in twins. Acta Genet. Med. Gemellol. 41, 325–333
Metrakos JD, Metrakos K (1960) Genetics of convulsive disorders.I.Introduction, problems, methods, and base lines. Neurology (Minn.) 10, 228–240
Metrakos K, Metrakos JD (1961) Genetics of convulsive disorders.II. Genetic and electroencephalographic studies in centrencephalic epilepsy. Neurology (Minn.) 11, 474–483

Michael A, Mirza KA, Mukunden CR, Channabasavanna SM (1993) Interhemispheric electroencephalographic coherence as a biological marker in alcoholism. Acta Psychiat. Scand. 87, 213–217

Miyamoto A, Kitawaki K, Hoida H, Nagao K(1992) Klinefelter's syndrome and epileptic psychosis: a case report. Japan. J. Psychiatr. Neurol. 46, 61–65

Mizukawa M, Ohtsuka Y, Murashima I (et al.) (1992) West syndrome associated with chromosome abnormalities: clinicoelectrical study. Japan. J. Psychiatry and Neurology 46, 435–436

Moises HW, Yang L, Kristbjarnason H (et al.) (1995) An international two-stage genome-wide search for schizophrenia susceptibility genes. Nature (Genetics) 11, 321–324

Monakhov K, Perris C (1980) Neurophysiological correlates of depressive symptomatology. Neuropsychobiology 6, 268–279

Money J, Erhardt AA (1972) Man and woman, boy and girl. Baltimore, Johns Hopkins Univ. Press

Müller HF, Shamsie SJ (1968) Classification des troubles du compartement des adolescents et données électroencéphalographiques. Canad. Psychiat. Ass. 3, 363–370

Müller-Küppers M, Vogel F (1965) Über die Persönlichkeitsstruktur von Trägern einer seltenen erblichen EEG-Variante. Jahrb. Psychol. Psychotherap. Med. Anthropol. 12, 75–101

Musumeci SA (et al.) (1985) Studio elettroclinico di 3 casi con ritardo mentale X-linked. Un nuovo marker EEG? XXiV Congr. Nazionale della Società Italiana di Neurologia. Pisa (Abstr.)

Musumeci SA (et al.) (1988) Prevalence of a novel epileptogenic EEG pattern in the Martin Bell syndrome. Am. J. Med. Genet 30, 207–212

Musumeci SA (et al.) (1991) Epilepsy and Fragile X syndrom: a foloow-up study. Am. J. Med. Genet. 38, 511–513

Naidu S, Niedermeyer E (1993) Degenerative disorders of the Central Nervous System. In: Niedermeyer E, Lopes da Silva F: Electroencephalography. Baltimore etc.: Williams & Wilkins, pp. 351–371

Naitoh P (1973) The value of electroencephalography in alcoholism. Ann. NY Acad. Sci. 215, 303–320

Neundörfer B (1970) Über die 4-5/sec EEG-Grundrhythmusvariante. Nervenarzt 41, 321–326

Neuwirth J, Andresen B, Seifert R (et al.)(1995) Quantitatives EEG, Basisstörungen und Rauchen bei ätiopathogenetisch differenten Gruppen paranoid-halluzinatorischen Psychosen – eine explorative Studie. Fortschr. Neurolog. Psychiatr. 63, 78–89

Niedermeyer E, Lopes da Silva F (1993) Electroencephalography. Basic principles, clinical applications, and related fields (3rd ed.) Baltimore etc.: Williams & Wilkins

Niedermeyer E (1993) Metabolic central nervous system disorders. In: Niedermeyer E, Lopes da Silva F, Electroencephalography (3rd ed.) Baltimore etc.: Williams & Wilkins. pp. 405–418

Niedermeyer E (1993) Maturation of the EEG; development of waking and sleep patterns. In: Niedermeyer E, Lopes da Silva F, Electroencephalography (3rd ed.) Baltimore etc.: Williams & Wilkins, pp. 167–191

Nielsen J, Pedersen E (1969) Electro-encephalographic findings in patients with Klinefelter's syndrome. Acta Neurol. Scand. 45, 87–94

Nolte R, Schulte FJ, Michaelis R, Juergens U (1968) Power spectra analysis of the electroencephalogram of newborn twins in active and quiet sleep. Aus: Kelleway P, Petersén I: Clinical electroencephalography of children. Stockholm: Almquist & Wiksell, pp.89–96

Nyström C, Matousek M, Hällström T (1986) Relationship between EEG and clinical characteristics in major depressive disorder. Acta Psychiat. Scand. 73, 390–394

O'Connor S, Hesselbrock V, Tasman A (et al.) (1987) P3 amplitudes in two distinct tasks are decreased in young men with a history of paternal alcoholism. Alcohol 4, 323–330

Ott J(1983) Linkage analysis and family classification under heterogeneity. Ann. Hum. Genet. 47, 311–320

Ott J(1991) Analysis of human genetics linkage. Baltimore: Johns Hopkins Univ. Press

Patterson RM, Baghi BK, Test A (1948) The prediction of Huntington's chorea. Amer. J. Psychiat. 104, 786–797

Perris C (1980) Central measures of depression. In: van Praag H et al. (eds): Handbook of Biological Psychiatry. Part II: Brain mechanisms and abnormal behavior. New York: Marcel Dekker; pp. 183–223

Perris C, v. Knorring L (1982) Evoked potentials (EP) and the individual's reactivity and vulnerability in psychiatric studies. In: Bonné-Tamir B (ed.) Human Genetics, part A: The unfolding genome. New York: Alan Liss; pp. 443–454

Petersén I, Eeg-Olofsen O (1970/71) The development of the electroencephalogram in normal children from the age of 1 through 15 years. Nonparoxysmal activity. Netropädiatrie 2-3: 1–63

Petersén I, Eeg-Olofsen O (1971) The development of the electroencephalogram in normal children from the age of 1 through 15 years. Neuropädiatrie 2, 247–304

Petersén I, Selldén U, Eeg-Olofsen O (1975) The evolution of the EEG in normal children and adolescents from 1 to 21 years. Handb. Electroencephalography and clinical Neurophysiology, Vol. 6B Amsterdam: Elsevier, pp. 31–68

Pfefferbaum A, Ford JM, White PM, Mathalon D (1991) Event-related potentials in alcoholic men: p3 amplitude reflects family history but not alcohol consumption. Alcohol Clin. Exp. Res. 15, 839–850

Phillips HA, Scheffer IE, Berkovic SF (et al.) (1995) Localization of a gene for autosomal dominant nocturnal frontal lobe epilepsy to chromosome 20q13.2. Nature (Genetics) 10, 117–118

Pietz J (1984) Visuelle evozierte Potentiale bei geistiger Retardierung und I.Q. Diplomarbeit Univ. Heidelberg, Psycholog. Institut

Pilz AJ, Willer E, Povey S, Abbott CM (1992) The genes coding for phosphoenolpyruvate carboxykinase-1 (PCK1) and neuronal nicotinic acetylcholine receptor alpha 4 subunit (CHRNA4) map to human chromosome 20, extending the known region of homology with mouse chromosome 2. Ann. Hum. Genet. 56, 289–293

Plomin R, McClearn GE, Smith DL (et al.) (1994) DNA markers associated with high versus low I.Q.: the I.Q. quantitative trait loci(QTL) project. Behav. Genet. 24, 107–118

Poenaru S, Stanesco V, Poenaru L, Stoian D (1970) Étude EEG dans le syndrome de Turner. Acta Neurol. Belg. 70, 509–522

Polich J, Bloom FE (1988) Event-related potentials in individuals at high and low risk for developing alcoholism: Failure to replicate. Alcohol Clin. Exp. Res. 12, 368–373

Polich J, Burns T (1987) P300 from identical twins. Neuropsychologia 25, 299–304

Polich J, Howard L, Starr A (1983) P300 correlates with digit span. Psychophysiology 20, 665–669

Pollock VE, Volavka J, Goodwin DM (et al.)(1983) The EEG after alcohol administration in men at risk for alcoholism. Arch. Gen. Psychiat. 40, 857–861

Porjecz B, Begleiter H (1991) Neurophysiological factors in individuals at risk for alcoholism. Recent Development in Alcoholism 9, 53–67

Pritchard WS (1981) Psychophysiology of the P300. Psychol. Bull. 89, 506–540

Propping P (1977) Genetic control of ethanol action on the central nervous system. Hum. Genet. 35, 309–334

Propping P (1977) Psychophysiological test performance in normal twins and in a pair of identical twins with essential tremor that is suppressed by alcohol. Hum. Genet. 36, 321–325

Propping P (1978) Pharmakogenetics. Rev. Physiol. Biochem. Pharmacol. 83, 124–173

Propping P (1983) Genetic disorders presenting as"schizophrenia". Karl Bonhoeffer's early view of the psychoses in the light of medical genetics Hum. Genet. 65, 1–10

Propping P (1989) Psychiatrische Genetik. Berlin etc.: Springer Verlag

Propping P (1992) Alcoholism. In: King RA, Rotter JI, Motulsky AG (eds.)The genetic basis om common disease. New York: Oxford Univ. Press; pp. 837–865

Propping P, Friedl W, Nebel B, Feige A (1979) Plasma DBH, platelet MAO and proteins of red blood cell membranesin individuals with variants of the normal EEG. Neuropsychobiology 5, 309–316

Propping P, Friedl W, Pluto R (1980) Further evidence for correlation of EEG synchronization and plasma DBH activity in normal subjects. J. Neur. Transm. 49, 167–178

Propping P, Krüger J, Janah A (1980) Effect of alcohol on genetically determined variants of the normal electroencephalogram. Psychiat. Res. 2, 85–98

Propping P, Krüger J, Mark N (1981) Disposition to alcoholism. An EEG study in alcoholics and their relatives. Hum.Genet. 59, 51–59

Puig-Antich J, Goetz R, Hanlon C (et al.) (1982) Sleep architecture and REM sleep measures in prebubertal children with major depression. Arch.Gen.Psychiat. 39, 932–939

Quesney LF, Reader TA (1990) Role of dopamine in generalized photosensitive epilepsy: Electroencephalographic and biochemical aspects. In: Avoli M. et al.(eds): Generalized epilepsies: Neurobiological Approaches. Boston etc.: Birkhäuser; pp. 298–303

Raine A, Venables PH, Williams M (1990) Relationships between central and autonomic measures of arousal at age 15 years and criminality at age 24 years. Arch. Gen. Psychiatry 47, 1003–1007

Raney ET (1937) Bilateral brain potentials and lateral dominance in identical twins. Psychol. Bull. 34, 543 (1937)

Raney E (1939) Brain potentials and lateral dominance in identical twins. J. Exp. Psychol. 24, 21–39

Raven J (1960) Guide to the standard progressive matrices. London: H. K. Lewis & Co.

Reed TE, Jensen AR (1992) Conduction velocity in a brain nerve pathway of normal adults correlates with intellectual level. Intelligence 16, 259–272

Rees M (et al.) (1993) Benign childhood epilepsy with centrotemporal spikes and the focal sharp wave trait is not linked to the fragile X region. Neuropediatrics 24, 211–213

Regan D (1972) Evoked potentials in psychology, sensory physiology and clinical medicine. London: Chapman & Hall

Reilly EL (1993) EEG recording and operation of the apparatus. In: Niedermeyer E, Lopes da Silva F: Electroencephalography (3rd ed.) Baltimore etc.: Williams & Wilkins, pp. 104–124

Reinke G (1966) Zur genetischen Grundlage der sogenannten Grenzfälle des Niederspannungs-EEG und der diffusen beta-Wellen bei jungen Männern. Med. Dissertation Heidelberg

Rémond A (ed.) (1976 and other years) Handbook of Electroencephalography and clinical Neurophysiology. Amsterdam: Elsevier

Rett A (1966) Über ein eigenartiges hirnatrophisches Syndrom bei Hyperammonämien im Kindesalter. Wien. Med. Wschr. 116, 723–738

Rett A, Teupel R (1964) Neugeborenenkrämpfe im Rahmen einer epileptisch belasteten Familie. Wien. Klin. Wschr 76, 609–613

Ribacoba-Montero R (et al.) (1995) (Fragile X syndrome and epilepsy) (Spanish) Neurologia 10, 70–75

Riikonen RS (1994) Difference in susceptibility to teratogenic effects of alcohol in discordant twins exposed to alcohol during the second half of gestation. Pediatr.-Neurol. 11, 332–336

Rodichok L, Miller G (1992) A study of evoked potentials in the 18q- syndrome which includes the absence of the gene locus for myelin basic protein. Neuropediatrics 23, 218–220

Rohracher H (1950) Ein einfacher Index zur Auswertung der Alpha-Wellen des Elektroencephalogramms. Arch. Psychiat. Nervenkrankh. 184, 487–492

Rubin S, Bowman KM (1942) Electroencephalographic and personality correlates in peptic ulcer. Psychosomatic Med. 4, 309–319

Rubin S, Moses L (1944) Electroencephalographic studies in asthma with some personality correlates. Psychosomatic Med. 6, 31–39

Ruchalla E, Schalt E, Vogel F (1985) Relations between mental performance and reaction time: new aspects of an old problem. Intelligence 9, 189–205

Rust J (1957) Genetic effects in the cortical auditory evoked potential: A twin study. EEG Clin. Neurophysiol. 39, 321–327

Rust J (1975) Cortical evoked potential, personality and intelligence. J. Comp. Physiol. Psycholog. 78, 59–68

Scheffer ES, Bhatia KP, Lopes-Lendes I (et al.) (1994) Autosomal dominant nocturnal frontal lobe epilepsy misdiagnosed as sleep disorder. Lancet 343, 515–517

Scheffer ES, Bhatia KP, Lopes-Lendes I (et al.) (1995) Autosomal dominant nocturnal frontal lobe epilepsy: a distinct clinical disorder. Brain 118, 61–73

Scheffner D (1982) EEG in offspring (newborns, infants, and children of epileptic parents). In: Janz D (et al.) (eds): Epilepsy, pregnancy, and the child. New York: Raven Press, pp. 449–455

Schepank H (1974) Erb-und Umweltfaktoren bei Neurosen. Berlin etc.: Springer Verlag

Schepank H (1996) Zwillingsschicksale. Stuttgart: F. Enke

Schinzel A (1984) Catalogue of unbalanced chromosome aberrations in man. Berlin: De Gruyter

Schlack HG, Schmidt-Schuh H (1977) Neurophysiological changes in children with Down's syndrome. Neuropädiatrie 8, 374–386

Schlag J (1974) Retikular influences on thalamocortical activity. In: Handb. of Electroencephalography and clin. Neurophysiol. Vol. 2, Part C, 2C-119-2C-134. Amsterdam: Elsevier
Schmettau A (1969) Korrelationsstatistische Untersuchung über den Zusammenhang zwischen EEG- und Persönlichkeitsmerkmalen. Dissertation Univ. Köln
Schmettau A (1970) Zwei elektroencephalographische Merkmalsverbände und ihre psychologischen Korrelate. Z. EEG–EMG 1, 169–182
Schmid RG, Sadowski K, Weinmann HM (et al.) (1985) Z-transformed EEG power spectra of children with Down syndrome vs. a control group. Neuropediatrics 16, 218–224
Schmid RG, Tirsch WS, Rappelsberger P (et al.) (1992) Comparative coherence studies in healthy volunteers and Down's syndrome patients from childhood to adult age. EEG Cin. Neurophysiol. 83, 112–123
Scollo-Lavizzari G (1971) Prognostic significance of epileptiform discharges in the EEG of nonepileptic subjects during photic stimulation (Abstract). EEG Clin. Neurophysiol. 31, 174
Sgrò V, Riva E, Canevini MP (et al.) (1995) 4p- syndrome: A chromosomal disorder associated with a particular EEG pattern. Epilepsia 36, 1206–1214
Shagass C (1976) An electroencephalographic view of schizophrenia. Biol. Psychiatr. 11, 3–30
Shiang R, Thompson LM, Zhu YZ (et al.) (1994)Mutation in the trans-membrane domain of FGFR-3 causes the most common genetic form of dwarfism, achondroplasia. Cell 78, 335–342
Shirasaka Y, Ito M, Okino T (et al.) (1992) Ring 14 chromosome with complex partial seizures: a case report. Brain-Dev. 14, 257–260
Shucard DW, Horn JL (1972) Evoked cortical potentials and measurements of human abilities. J. Comp. Physiol. Psychol. 78, 59–68
Silverman AJ, Busse EW, Barnes RH (1955) Studies in the process of aging: Electroencephalographic findings in 400 elderly subjects. EEG Clin.Neurophysiol. 7, 67–74
Sisson BD, Ellingson RJ (1955) On the relationship between"normal" EEG patterns and personality variables. J. Nerv. Ment. Dis. 121, 353–358
Singh N, Charlier C, Stauffer D (et al.) (1998) A novel potassium channel gene, KCNQ2, is mutated in an inherited epilepsy of newborns. Nature (Genetics) 18, 25–29
Smith SM (1954) Discrimination between electro-encephalograph recordings of normal females and normal males. Ann. Eugen. 18, 344–350
Smith J, Pabst W, Schuh H (1973)n A computer analysis of the aperiodic amplitude-interval parameters of the electroencephalogram. EDV in Medizin und Biologie 1, 8–15
Sorbel J, Mozorati S, O'Connor S (et al.) (1996) Alcohol effects on the heritability of EEG spectral power. Alcohol Clin. Exp. Res. 20, 1523–1527
Speckmann EJ, Elger CE (1993) Introduction to the neurophysiological basis of the EEG and DC potentials. In: Electroencephaligraphy, E. Niedermeyer and F. Lopes da Silva, eds. (3rd ed.) Baltimore etc.: Williams & Wilkins; pp. 15–26
Stassen HH, Coppola R, Gottesman I (et al.) (1998) EEG differences in monozygotic twins discordant and concordant for schizophrenia. Psychophysiology (in the press)
Stassen HH, Katsanis J, Malone S (et al.) (1998) Familial brain wave patterns. The Minnesota twin family study. (In the press)
Steinlein OK, Anokhin A, Mao Y-P (et al.) (1992) Localization of a gene for the human low-voltage EEG on 20q and genetic heterogeneity. Genomics 12, 69–73
Steinlein OK, Magnusson A, Stoodt J (et al.) An insertion mutation of the CHRNA4 gene in a family with autosomal dominant nocturnal frontal lobe epilepsy. Hum. Mol. Genet. 6, 943–947
Steinlein OK, Mulley JK, Propping P (et al.) (1995) A missense mutation in the neuronal nicotinic acetylcholine receptor alpha 4 subunit is associated with autosomal dominant nocturnal frontal lobe epilepsy. Nature (Genetics) 11, 201–203
Steinlein OK, Schuster V, Fischer C, Häussler M (1995) Benign familian neonatal convulsions: Confirmation of genetic heterogeneity and further evidence for a second locus on chromosome 8q. Hum. Genet. 95, 411–415
Steinlein OK, Smigrodzki R, Lindstrom J (et al.) (1994) Refinement of the localization of the gene for neuronal acetylcholine receptor alpha 4 subunit (CHRNA) to human chromosome 20q13.2–13.3. Genomics 22, 493–495
Steinmetz H, Herzog A, Huang Y, Hacklander T (1994) Discordant brain surface anatomy in monozygotic twins. New England J. Med. 331, 952–953

Steriade M, McCarley RW (1990) Brainstem control of wakefulness and sleep. New York: Plenum Press

Stevens JR, Sachdev K, Milstein V (1968) Behavior disorders of childhood and the electroencephalogram. Arch. of Neurol. 18, 160–177

Strauß H (1945) Clinical and electroencephalographic studies: The electroencephalogram in psychoneurotics. J. Nerv. Mental Dis. 101, 19–27

Struve FA (1986) Clinical electroencephalography and the study of suicide behavior. Suicide Life Threat Behav. 16, 133–165

Suddath RL, Christison GW, Fuller Torrey E (et al.) (1990) Anatomical abnormalities in the brains of monozygotic twins discordant for schizophrenia. New Engl. J. Med. 322, 790–794

Sulg IA, Dencker SJ (1968) Electroencephalographic findings in MZ twin pairs, discordant for closed head injury. Acta Genet. Med. Gemellol. 17, 389–401

Surwillo WW (1964) The relation of decision time to brain wave frequency and to age. EEG Clin. Neurophysiol. 16, 510–514

Surwillo WW (1980) Cortical evoked potentials in monozygotic twins and unrelated subjects: comparisons of exogenous and endogenous components. Behavior Genetics 10, 201–209

Sutton S, Braren M, Zubin J, John ER (1965) Evoked potential correlates of stimulus uncertainty. Science 150, 1187–1188

Szepetowski P, Monaco AP (1998) Recent progress in the genetics of human epilepsies. (Unpubl. Manuscript)

Tariverdian G, Kantner G, Vogel F (1987) A monozygotic twin pair with Rett syndrome. Hum. Genet. 75, 88–90

Torgersen S (1983) Genetic factors in anxiety disorders. Arch. Gen. Psychiatry 40, 1085–1089

Tsuang MT, Faraone SV (1990) The genetics of mood disorders. Baltimore: Johns Hopkins Univ. Press

Tsuboi T (1977) Primary generalized epilepsy with sporadic myoclonias of myoclonic petit mal type. Topics in Human Genetics, Vol. 4, Stuttgart: Thieme Verlag

Tsuboi T, Christian W (1976) Epilepsy. A clinical, electroencephalographic and statistical study of 466 patients. Berlin etc.: Springer Verlag

Tsuboi T, Nielsen J (1976) Electroencephalographic examination of 50 women with Turner's syndrome. Acta Neurol. Scand. 54, 359–365

Tsuboi T, Nielsen J (1985) Electroencephalographic examination of 64 Danish Turner girls. Acta Neurol. Scand. 72, 590–601

Tsuboi T, Nielsen J, Nagayama I (1988) Turner's syndrome: a qualitative and quantitative analysis of EEG background activity. Hum. Genet. 78, 206–215

Trubnikov VI, Afimova MV, Uvarova LG, Orlava VA (1995) (Multivariate genetic analysis of the data from a complex study of the predisposition to schizophrenia) (Russian). Zh. Nevropatol. Psikhiatr. Im. S. S. Korsakova 95, 50–56

Turunen S, Valleala P (1967) Psychoinfantilism in school children and the EEG. Acta Paedopsychiatrica 34, 162–166

Ulett G, Gleser G, Winokur G, Lawler A (1953) The EEG reaction to photic stimulation as an index of anxiety-proneness. EEG Clin. Neurophysiol. 5, 23–32

Ulrich G, Renfordt E, Zeller G, Frick K (1984) Interrelation between changes in the EEG and psychopathology under pharmakotherapy for endogenous depression. A contribution to the predictor question. Pharmacopsychiatry 17, 178–183

Ulrich G, Scheuler W, Müller-Oerlinghausen B (1982) Zur visuell-morphologischen Analyse des hirnelektrischen Verhaltens bei Patienten mit manisch-depressiven und schizoaffektiven Psychosen unter Lithiumprophylaxe. Fortschr. Neurol. Psychiatr. 50, 24–36

Uzarova LG, Alfimova MV, Trubnikov VI (1995) (Interhemispheric asymmetry of the resting EEG and its relationship to psychological parameters of cognitive activity in families of schizophrenic patients) (Russian). Fiziol. Cheloveka 21, 39–49

Van Baal C (1997) A genetic perspective on the developing brain. Electrophysiological indices of neural functioning in five to seven year old twins. Dissertation Vrije Univ. te Amsterdam

Van Beijsterveldt CEM (1996) The genetics of electrophysiological indices of brain activity. An EEG study in adolescent twins. Dissertation Vrije Univ. te Amsterdam

Van Beijsterveldt CEM, Boomsma D (1994) Genetics of the human electroencephalogram (EEG) and event-related potentials(ERPs): a review. Hum. Genet.94, 319–330

Van Sweden B (1986) Disturbed vigilance in mania. Biol. Psychiatr. 21, 311–313
Van Sweden B, Wauquier A, Niedermeyer E (1993) Normal aging and transient cognitive disorder in the elderly. In: Niedermeyer E, Lopes da Silva F (eds.) Electroencephalography (3rd ed.) Baltimore: Williams & Wilkins; pp. 329–338
Verdeaux G, Verdeaux J, Selosse J, Chirol Y (1964) Les anomalies fonctionelles de l'EEG chez les adolescents normaux, caractériels ou delinquants. Rev. Neurologique 111, 359–362
Vernon PA, Weese S (1993) Predicting intelligence with multiple speed of information processing tests. Persinality and Individ. Differences 14, 413–419
v. Verschuer O (1954) Wirksame Faktoren im Leben des Menschen. Wiesbaden: Steiner Verlag
Vieregge P, Froster-Iskenius U (1989) Clinico-neurological investigations in the Fra(X) form of mental retardation. J. Neurol. 236, 85–92
Vogel F (1957) Elektroencephalographische Untersuchungen an gesunden Zwillingen. Acta Genet. Statist. Med. 7, 334–337
Vogel F (1958) Über die Erblichkeit des normalen Elektroencephalogramms. Stuttgart: Thieme Verlag
Vogel F (1962a) Ergänzende Untersuchungen zur Genetik des menschlichen Niederspannungs-EEG. Dtsch. Z. Nervenheilk.184, 101–111
Vogel F (1962b) Untersuchungen zur Genetik der beta-Wellen des Menschen. Dtsch. Z. Nervenheilk. 184, 134–173
Vogel F (1965) "14 and 6/sec positive spikes" im Schlaf-EEG von jugendlichen ein-und zweieiigen Zwillingen. Hum. Genet. 1, 390–391
Vogel F (1966a) Zur genetischen Grundlage fronto-präzentraler Betawellengruppen im EEG des Menschen. Hum. Genet. 2, 227–237
Vogel F (1966b) Zur genetischen Grundlage occipitaler langsamer Betawellen im EEG des Menschen. Hum. Genet. 2, 238–245
Vogel F (1970) The genetic basis of the normal human electroencephalogram (EEG). Hum. Genet. 10, 91–114
Vogel F (1984) Relevant deviations in heterozygotes of autosomal-recessive diseases. Clin. genet. 25, 381–415
Vogel F (1986) Grundlagen und Bedeutung genetisch bedingter Variabilität des normalen menschlichen EEG. Z. EEG-EMG 17, 173–188
Vogel F (1989) Resting EEG as a genetic marker. In: New directions in affective disorders (Eds. B. Lerer, S. Gershon) New York etc.: Springer Verlag; pp.221–224
Vogel F, Fujiya Y (1969) The incidence of some inherited EEG variants in normal Japanese and German males. Hum. Genet. 7, 28–42
Vogel F, Götze W (1959) Familienuntersuchungen zur Genetik des normalen Elektroencephalogramms. Dtsch. Z. Nervenheilk. 178, 112–136
Vogel F, Götze W (1962) Statistische Betrachtungen über die Betawellen im EEG des Menschen. Dtsch. Z. Nervenheilk. 184, 112–136
Vogel F, Götze W, Kubicki S (1961) Der Wert von Familienuntersuchungen für die Beurteilung des Niederspannungs-EEG nach geschlossenem Schädel-Hirn-Trauma. Dtsch. Z. Nervenheilk. 182, 337–354
Vogel F, Helmbold W (1959) Koppelungsdaten für zwei wahrscheinlich einfach mendelnde EEG-Merkmale des Menschen. Z. Menschl. Vererb. Konst. L. 37, 28–37
Vogel F, Krüger J, Höpp HP (et al.) (1986) Visually and auditory evoked EEG potentials in carriers of four hereditary EEG variants. Human Neurobiolog. 5, 49–58
Vogel F, Krüger J, Schalt E (et al.) (1980) EEG differences in neurotic as compared with normal twin pairs. Hum. Genet. 54, 327–334
Vogel F, Krüger J, Schalt E (1981) Charakterisierung erblicher EEG-Varianten mit Hilfe der Amplituden-Intervall-Analyse. I. Varianten der alpha-Tätigkeit; Niederspannungs-EEG, Grenzfälle des Niederspannungs-EEG; occipitale langsame Betawellen; EEG mit monotonen Alphawellen. Z. EEG-EMG 12, 33–44
Vogel F, Krüger J, Schalt E (et al.) (1987) No consistent relationship between oscillations and latencies of visually and auditory evoked EEG potentials and measures of mental performance. Human Neurobiol. 6, 173–182
Vogel F, Motulsky AG (1996) Human Genetics. Problems and approaches (3rd ed.) Berlin etc.: Springer Verlag

Vogel F, Schalt E, Krüger J (et al.)(1979) The electroencephalogram (EEG) as a research tool in human behavior genetics: Psychological examinations in healthy males with various inherited EEG variants.I.Rationale of the study; material;methods. Heritability of test parameters. Hum. Genet. 47, 1–45

Vogel F, Schalt E, Krüger J (1979) II. Results. Hum. Genet. 47, 47–80

Vogel F, Schalt E (1979) III. Interpretation of the results. Hum. Genet. 47, 81–111

Vogel F, Schalt E, Krüger J, Klarich G (1982) Relationship between behavioral maturation measured by the "Baum"test and EEG frequency. A pilot study on monozygotic and dizygotic twins. Hum. Genet. 62, 60–65

Vogel F, Wendt GG, Oepen H (1961) Das EEG und das Problem einer Frühdiagnose der Chorea Huntington. Dtsch. Z. Nervenheilk. 182, 355–361

Vogel W, Browerman DM, Klaiber E (1968) EEG and mental abilities. EEG Clin.Neurophysiol. 24, 166–175

Volavka J, Matousek M, Roubicek J (1966) EEG frequency analysis in schizophrenia. Acta Psychiat. Scand. 42, 237–245

Waggoner CW, Bagchi BK (1943) Simultaneous intra-twin and inter-twin electroencephalograms. Univ. Michigan Hosp. Bull. 9, 102–104

Wagner O, Oesterreich K, Hoyer S (1985) Validity of the ischemic score in degenerative and vascular dementia and depression in old age. Arch. Gerontol. Geriatr. 4, 333-345

Walter C (1982) Die Variabilität kognitiver Stile bei Trägern erblicher Varianten des normalen Elektroencephalogramms. Dissertation Heidelberg

Walter GW (1963) Das lebende Gehirn (The living brain) München, Zürich: Knaur

Wall TL, Gallen CC, Ehlers CL (1993) Effects of alcohol on the EEG in Asian men with genetic variations of ALDH2. Biol. Psychiatr. 34, 91–99

Waltz S, Christen HJ, Doose H (1992) The different patterns of photoparoxysmal response: a genetic study. EEG Clin. Neurophysiol. 83, 138–145

Wauquier A (1993) EEG and neuropharmakology. In: Niedermeyer E, Lopes da Silva F (eds.): Electroencephalography (3rd ed.) Baltimore: Williams & Wilkins; pp. 619–629

Weiß V (1992) Major genes of human intelligence. Personality and Individ. Differences 13, 1115–1134

Whipple SC, Parker ES, Nobel EP (1988) An atypical neurocognitive profile in alcoholic fathers and their sons. J. Stud. Alcohol 49, 240–244

Winter H, Herschel M, Propping P (et al.) (1978) A twin study on three enzymes (DBH, COMT, MAO) of catecholamine metabolism. Psychopharmakology 57, 63–69

Winokur G (1972) Depression spectrum disease: description and family study. Comp. Psychiatry 13, 3–8

Wolpert E, Neundörfer B, Dömpf D, Braun J (1979) Untersuchungen zur Psychopathologie bei Merkmalsträgern der 4-5/s. EEG-Grundrhythmusvariante. Arch. Psychiat. Nervenheilk. 226, 269–282

Yamada T(1960) Heterogeneity of schizophrenia as demonstrable in electroencephalography. Bull. Osaka Med. School, 107–146

Yoshii N, Shimokochi M, Tani K (1961) The electroencephalograms in juvenile delinquents. Fol. Psychiat. Neurol. Jap. 15, 85–91

Yoshii N, Ishiwara T, Tani K (1964) Juvenile delinquents and their abnormal EEGs.(2) Continuous theta waves. Fol. Psychiat. Neurol. Jap. 18, 161–167

Young JP, Lader MH, Fenton GW (1972) A twin study on the genetic influences on the electroencephalogram. J. Med. Genet. 9, 13–16

Zimányi I, Abaffy M, Sigmund A (1972) Über die Korrelation des psychischen Zustands und des EEG-Befundes: Einige Beziehungen der Verhaltensanomalien. Acta Paed. Acad. Sci. Hungaricae 13, 169–176

Zoghbi HY (1988) Genetic aspects of Rett syndrome. J. Child. Neurol. (Suppl.) 3, S 76–S 78

Zoghbi HY, Ledbetter DH, Schultz R (et al.) (1990) Translocation in Rett syndrome. Am. J. Med. Genet. 35, 148–151

Zung W, Wilson WP(1967) Sleep and dream patterns in twins: Markov analysis of a genetic trait. Rec. Adv. in Biolog. Psychiatry 9, 119–130

Young W, Knowles JB, MacLean AW (et al.) (1982) The sleep of childhood depressives – comparison with age-matched controls. Biol. Psychiatry 17, 1163–1168

Subject Index

GPSR Compliance

The European Union's (EU) General Product Safety Regulation (GPSR) is a set of rules that requires consumer products to be safe and our obligations to ensure this.

If you have any concerns about our products, you can contact us on ProductSafety@springernature.com

In case Publisher is established outside the EU, the EU authorized representative is:

Springer Nature Customer Service Center GmbH
Europaplatz 3
69115 Heidelberg, Germany

Batch number: 10704713

Printed by Printforce, the Netherlands